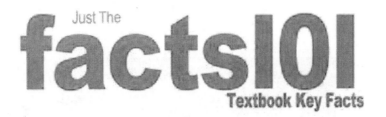

Just The
facts101
Textbook Key Facts

Textbook Outlines, Highlights, and Practice Quizzes

Pediatric Hospital Medicine

by Ronald M Perkin, 2nd Edition

All "Just the Facts101" Material Written or Prepared by Cram101 Publishing

Title Page

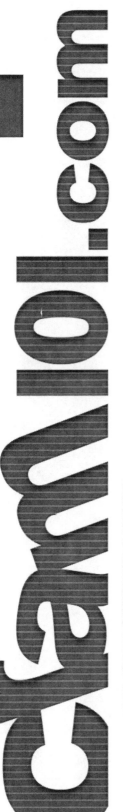
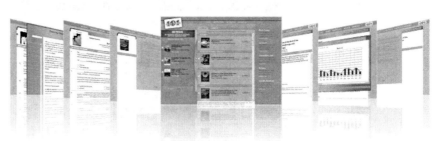

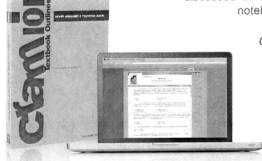

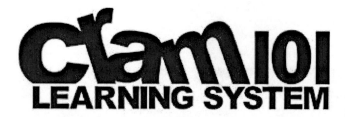

"Just the Facts101" is a Cram101 publication and tool designed to give you all the facts from your textbooks. Visit Cram101.com for the full practice test for each of your chapters for virtually any of your textbooks.

Cram101 has built custom study tools specific to your textbook. We provide all of the factual testable information and unlike traditional study guides, we will never send you back to your textbook for more information.

YOU WILL NEVER HAVE TO HIGHLIGHT A BOOK AGAIN!

Cram101 StudyGuides

All of the information in this StudyGuide is written specifically for your textbook. We include the key terms, places, people, and concepts... the information you can expect on your next exam!

Want to take a practice test?

Throughout each chapter of this StudyGuide you will find links to cram101.com where you can select specific chapters to take a complete test on, or you can subscribe and get practice tests for up to 12 of your textbooks, along with other exclusive cram101.com tools like problem solving labs and reference libraries.

Cram101.com

Only cram101.com gives you the outlines, highlights, and PRACTICE TESTS specific to your textbook. Cram101.com is an online application where you'll discover study tools designed to make the most of your limited study time.

By purchasing this book, you get 50% off the normal subscription free!. Just enter the promotional code **'DK73DW13357'** on the Cram101.com registration screen.

www.Cram101.com

Learning System

Pediatric Hospital Medicine
Ronald M Perkin, 2nd

CONTENTS

1. GENERAL ISSUES IN PEDIATRIC HOSPITAL MEDICINE 5
2. ETHICAL AND LEGAL ISSUES 17
3. COMMON PRESENTING SIGNS, SYMPTOMS, DIFFERENTIAL DIAGNOSIS 30
4. CARDIOVASCULAR 61
5. PULMONARY DISEASE 82
6. NEUROLOGIC 105
7. GASTROENTEROLOGY 127
8. HEMATOLOGY-ONCOLOGY 146
9. RENAL 163
10. VASCULITIS/ RHEUMATOLOGIC 178
11. INFECTIOUS DISEASES 195
12. ENDOCRINE 231
13. COMMON AND UNCOMMON PROBLEMS OF THE TERM NEWBORN 237
14. SURGICAL 291
15. HOSPITAL CARE OF CHILDREN WITH COMPLEX AND CHRONIC CONDITIONS 306
16. SEDATION AND PAIN MANAGEMENT 331
17. CHILD ABUSE AND NEGLECT 344
18. NUTRITION 352
19. Emergency MEDICINE 361
20. PSYCHIATRIC HOSPITALIZATION 379

Chapter 1. GENERAL ISSUES IN PEDIATRIC HOSPITAL MEDICINE

CHAPTER OUTLINE: KEY TERMS, PEOPLE, PLACES, CONCEPTS

Chronic disease

Health care

Home care

String searching algorithms

Primary care

Evidence-based medicine

Hospital medicine

Hospitalist

Medical error

Intensive care

Patient safety

Nurse practitioner

Joint Commission

High-mobility group

Communication

Medical education

Enteral formula

Life support

Pediatric

Chapter 1. GENERAL ISSUES IN PEDIATRIC HOSPITAL MEDICINE

CHAPTER OUTLINE: KEY TERMS, PEOPLE, PLACES, CONCEPTS

Advanced life support

Ductus arteriosus

Risk factor

Etiological myth

Physician assistant

Medical literature

Cochrane Library

Confidence interval

Relative risk

Relative risk reduction

Decision making

RBRVS

Resource-based relative value scale

Accounts receivable

Chronic disease	In medicine, a chronic disease is a disease that is long-lasting or recurrent. The term chronic describes the course of the disease, or its rate of onset and development. A chronic course is distinguished from a recurrent course; recurrent diseases relapse repeatedly, with periods of remission in between.
Health care	Health care is the diagnosis, treatment, and prevention of disease, illness, injury, and other physical and mental impairments in humans. Health care is delivered by practitioners in medicine, chiropractic, dentistry, nursing, pharmacy, allied health, and other care providers. It refers to the work done in providing primary care, secondary care and tertiary care, as well as in public health.
Home care	Home Care, (also referred to as domiciliary care or social care), is health care or supportive care provided in the patient's home by healthcare professionals (often referred to as home health care or formal care). Often, the term home care is used to distinguish non-medical care or custodial care, which is care that is provided by persons who are not nurses, doctors, or other licensed medical personnel, as opposed to home health care that is provided by licensed personnel. Professionals providing care Professionals providing home care include: Licensed practical nurses, Registered nurses, Home Care Aids, and Social workers.
String searching algorithms	String searching algorithms are an important class of string algorithms that try to find a place where one or several strings are found within a larger string or text. Let Σ be an alphabet (finite set). Formally, both the pattern and searched text are concatenations of elements of Σ.
Primary care	Primary care is the term for the health services by providers who act as the principal point of consultation for patients within a health care system. Such a professional can be a primary care physician, such as a general practitioner or family physician, or depending on the locality, health system organization, and patient's discretion, they may see a pharmacist, a physician assistant, a nurse practitioner, a nurse (such as in the United Kingdom), a clinical officer (such as in parts of Africa), or an Ayurvedic or other traditional medicine professional (such as in parts of Asia). Depending on the nature of the health condition, patients may then be referred for secondary or tertiary care.
Evidence-based medicine	Evidence-based medicine or evidence-based practice (EBP) aims to apply the best available evidence gained from the scientific method to clinical decision making. It seeks to assess the strength of the evidence of risks and benefits of treatments (including lack of treatment) and diagnostic tests.

Chapter 1. GENERAL ISSUES IN PEDIATRIC HOSPITAL MEDICINE

Hospital medicine	Hospital medicine in the United States is the discipline concerned with the medical care of acutely ill hospitalized patients. Physicians whose primary professional focus is hospital medicine are called hospitalists; this type of medical practice has extended beyond the US into Canada. The practical effect of the hospitalist is to act as transition coordinator and case manager, due to the tremendous growth in medical knowledge and resultant number of medical specialists.
Hospitalist	Hospital medicine in the United States is the discipline concerned with the general medical care of hospitalized patients. Physicians, physician assistants, and nurse practitioners whose primary professional focus is hospital medicine are called hospitalists; this type of medical practice has extended beyond the US into Canada. The practical effect of the hospitalist is to act as a case manager, due to the tremendous growth in medical knowledge and resultant number of medical specialists sometimes causing problems.
Medical error	A medical error is a preventable adverse effect of care, whether or not it is evident or harmful to the patient. This might include an inaccurate or incomplete diagnosis or treatment of a disease, injury, syndrome, behavior, infection, or other ailment. As a general acceptance, a medical error occurs when a health-care provider chose an inappropriate method of care or the health provider chose the right solution of care but executed it incorrectly.
Intensive care	intensive care medicine or critical care medicine is a branch of medicine concerned with the provision of life support or organ support systems in patients who are critically ill and who usually require intensive monitoring. Patients requiring intensive care may require support for hemodynamic instability (hypertension/hypotension), airway or respiratory compromise (such as ventilator support), acute renal failure, potentially lethal cardiac arrhythmias, or the cumulative effects of multiple organ system failure. They may also be admitted for intensive/invasive monitoring, such as the crucial hours after major surgery when deemed too unstable to transfer to a less intensively monitored unit.
Patient safety	Patient safety is a new healthcare discipline that emphasizes the reporting, analysis, and prevention of medical error that often leads to adverse healthcare events. The frequency and magnitude of avoidable adverse patient events was not well known until the 1990s, when multiple countries reported staggering numbers of patients harmed and killed by medical errors. Recognizing that healthcare errors impact 1 in every 10 patients around the world, the World Health Organization calls patient safety an endemic concern.

Nurse practitioner	A Nurse Practitioner is an Advanced Practice Nurse (APN) who has completed graduate-level education (either a Master's or a Doctoral degree). Additional APN roles include the Certified Registered Nurse Anesthetist (CRNA)s, CNMs, and CNSs. All Nurse Practitioners are Registered Nurses who have completed extensive additional education, training, and have a dramatically expanded scope of practice over the traditional RN role.
Joint Commission	The Joint Commission formerly the Joint Commission on Accreditation of Healthcare Organizations (JCAHO), is a United States-based not-for-profit organization that accredits over 19,000 health care organizations and programs in the United States. A majority of state governments have come to recognize Joint Commission accreditation as a condition of licensure and the receipt of Medicaid reimbursement. Surveys (inspections) typically follow a triennial cycle, with findings made available to the public in an accreditation quality report on the Quality Check Web site.
High-mobility group	High-Mobility Group is a group of chromosomal proteins that help with transcription, replication, recombination, and DNA repair. The proteins are subdivided into 3 superfamilies each containing a characteristic functional domain:•A - contains an AT-hook domain •A1•A2•B - contains a -box domain •B1•B2•B3•B4•N - contains a nucleosomal binding domain domain •N1•N2•N3•N4•Sex-Determining Region Y Protein•TCF Transcription Factors •Lymphoid enhancer-binding factor 1•T Cell Transcription Factor 1 Proteins containing any of these embedded in their sequence are known as motif proteins. -box proteins are found in a variety of eukaryotic organisms.
Communication	Communication is a process of transferring information from one entity to another. Communication processes are sign-mediated interactions between at least two agents which share a repertoire of signs and semiotic rules. Communication is commonly defined as 'the imparting or interchange of thoughts, opinions, or information by speech, writing, or signs'.
Medical education	Medical education is education related to the practice of being a medical practitioner, either the initial training to become a doctor (i.e., medical school and internship) or additional training thereafter (e.g., residency and fellowship). Medical education and training varies considerably across the world. Various teaching methodologies have been utilised in medical education, which is an active area of educational research.
Enteral formula	In medicine, an Enteral formula is a solution containing some or all of the nutrients that the body needs to function.

It can be introduced into the gastrointestinal tract either orally or through a feeding tube. For more information, please visit the page on Enteral nutrition.

Life support	Life support in medicine is a broad term that applies to any therapy used to sustain a patient's life while they are critically ill or injured, as part of intensive-care medicine. There are many therapies and techniques that may be used by clinicians to achieve the goal of sustaining life. Some examples include:•Feeding tube•Total parenteral nutrition•Mechanical ventilation•Heart/Lung bypass•Urinary catheterization•Dialysis•Cardiopulmonary resuscitation•Defibrillation•Artificial pacemaker These techniques are applied most commonly in the Emergency Department, Intensive Care Unit and, Operating Rooms.
Pediatric	Pediatrics is the branch of medicine that deals with the medical care of infants, children, and adolescents. The upper age limit of such patients ranges from age 12 to 21, depending on the country. A medical practitioner who specializes in this area is known as a pediatrician.
Advanced life support	Advanced Life Support is a set of life-saving protocols and skills that extend Basic Life Support to further support the circulation and provide an open airway and adequate ventilation (breathing). These include:•Tracheal intubation•Rapid sequence intubation•Cardiac monitoring•Cardiac defibrillation•Transcutaneous pacing•Intravenous cannulation (IV)•Intraosseous (IO) access and intraosseous infusion•Surgical cricothyrotomy•Needle cricothyrotomy•Needle decompression of tension pneumothorax•Advanced medication administration through parenteral and enteral routes (IV, IO, PO, PR, ET, SL, topical, and transdermal)•Advanced Cardiac Life Support (ACLS)•Pediatric Advanced Life Support or Pediatric Emergencies for Pre-Hospital Providers (PEPP)•Pre-Hospital Trauma Life Support (PHTLS), Basic Trauma Life Support (BTLS) or International Trauma Life Support (ITLS)2010 changes ALS is a treatment consensus for cardiopulmonary resuscitation in cardiac arrest and related medical problems, as agreed in Europe by the European Resuscitation Council, most recently in 2010. 2010 revisions include:•greater emphasis on continuous (uninterrupted) chest compression•less emphasis on airway and breathing•promotion of the intraosseous infusion of drugs and fluids if IV access not readily available•further demotion of the precordial thump•ongoing simplification•expanded role for post-arrest hypothermia and emphasis on post-arrest normo-glycaemiaALS algorithms

Ductus arteriosus	In the developing fetus, the ductus arteriosus also called the ductus Botalli, is a blood vessel connecting the pulmonary artery to the aortic arch. It allows most of the blood from the right ventricle to bypass the fetus's fluid-filled non-functioning lungs. Upon closure at birth, it becomes the ligamentum arteriosum.
Risk factor	In epidemiology, a risk factor is a variable associated with an increased risk of disease or infection. Sometimes, determinant is also used, being a variable associated with either increased or decreased risk. Risk factors or determinants are correlational and not necessarily causal, because correlation does not prove causation.
Etiological myth	Etiology is the study of causation, or origination. The word is most commonly used in medical and philosophical theories, where it is used to refer to the study of why things occur, or even the reasons behind the way that things act, and is used in philosophy, physics, psychology, government, medicine, theology and biology in reference to the causes of various phenomena. An etiological myth is a myth intended to explain a name or create a mythic history for a place or family.
Physician assistant	A Physician assistant is a healthcare professional licensed to practice medicine with supervision of a licensed physician. A Physician assistant is concerned with preventing, maintaining, and treating human illness and injury by providing a broad range of health care services that are traditionally performed by a physician. Physician assistants conduct physical exams, diagnose and treat illnesses, order and interpret tests, counsel on preventive health care, assist in surgery, and write prescriptions.
Medical literature	Medical literature refers to articles in journals and texts in books devoted to the field of medicine. Contemporary and historic views regarding diagnosis, prognosis and treatment of medical conditions have been documented for thousands of years. The Edwin Smith papyrus is the first known medical treatise.
Cochrane Library	The Cochrane Library is a collection of databases in medicine and other healthcare specialties provided by the Cochrane Collaboration and other organisations. At its core is the collection of Cochrane Reviews, a database of systematic reviews and meta-analyses which summarize and interpret the results of medical research. The Cochrane Library aims to make the results of well-conducted controlled trials readily available and is a key resource in evidence-based medicine.
Confidence interval	In statistics, a confidence interval is a kind of interval estimate of a population parameter and is used to indicate the reliability of an estimate. It is an observed interval (i.e.

it is calculated from the observations), in principle different from sample to sample, that frequently includes the parameter of interest, if the experiment is repeated. How frequently the observed interval contains the parameter is determined by the confidence level or confidence coefficient.

| Relative risk | In statistics and mathematical epidemiology, relative risk is the risk of an event relative to exposure. Relative risk is a ratio of the probability of the event occurring in the exposed group versus a non-exposed group. |

$$RR = \frac{p_{\text{exposed}}}{p_{\text{non-exposed}}}$$

Consider an example where the probability of developing lung cancer among smokers was 20% and among non-smokers 1%.

| Relative risk reduction | In epidemiology, the relative risk reduction is a measure calculated by dividing the absolute risk reduction by the control event rate. |

The relative risk reduction can be more useful than the absolute risk reduction in determining an appropriate treatment plan, because it accounts not only for the effectiveness of a proposed treatment, but also for the relative likelihood of an incident (positive or negative) occurring in the absence of treatment.

Like many other epidemiological measures, the same equations can be used to measure a benefit or a harm (although the signs may need to be adjusted, depending upon how the data was collected).

| Decision making | Decision making can be regarded as the mental processes (cognitive process) resulting in the selection of a course of action among several alternative scenarios. Every decision making process produces a final choice. The output can be an action or an opinion of choice. |

| RBRVS | Resource-Based Relative Value Scale (RBRVS) is a schema used to determine how much money medical providers should be paid. It is currently used by Medicare in the United States and by nearly all Health maintenance organizations (HMOs). |

RBRVS assigns procedures performed by a physician or other medical provider a relative value which is adjusted by geographic region (so a procedure performed in Manhattan is worth more than a procedure performed in El Paso).

| Resource-based relative value scale | Resource-based relative value scale is a schema used to determine how much money medical providers should be paid. It is partially used by Medicare in the United States and by nearly all Health maintenance organizations (HMOs). |

Accounts receivable	Accounts receivable is one of a series of accounting transactions dealing with the billing of a customer for goods and services he/she has ordered. In most business entities this is typically done by generating an invoice and mailing or electronically delivering it to the customer, who in turn must pay it within an established timeframe called 'creditor payment terms.' An example of a common payment term is Net 30, which means payment is due in the amount of the invoice 30 days from the date of invoice. Other common payment terms include Net 45 and Net 60 but could in reality be for any time period agreed upon by the vendor and the customer.

1. _____ is a group of chromosomal proteins that help with transcription, replication, recombination, and DNA repair.

   The proteins are subdivided into 3 superfamilies each containing a characteristic functional domain:•A - contains an AT-hook domain •A1•A2•B - contains a -box domain •B1•B2•B3•B4•N - contains a nucleosomal binding domain domain •N1•N2•N3•N4•Sex-Determining Region Y Protein•TCF Transcription Factors •Lymphoid enhancer-binding factor 1•T Cell Transcription Factor 1

   Proteins containing any of these embedded in their sequence are known as motif proteins. -box proteins are found in a variety of eukaryotic organisms.

   a. Hollywood
   b. Hormone response element
   c. Housekeeping gene
   d. High-mobility group

2. In epidemiology, a _____ is a variable associated with an increased risk of disease or infection. Sometimes, determinant is also used, being a variable associated with either increased or decreased risk.

   _____s or determinants are correlational and not necessarily causal, because correlation does not prove causation.

   a. Rule of three
   b. Sensitivity and specificity
   c. Risk factor
   d. Surrogate endpoint

3. . _____s is the branch of medicine that deals with the medical care of infants, children, and adolescents. The upper age limit of such patients ranges from age 12 to 21, depending on the country. A medical practitioner who specializes in this area is known as a pediatrician.

Chapter 1. GENERAL ISSUES IN PEDIATRIC HOSPITAL MEDICINE

a. Pediatric

b. Monitoring

c. Pediatric ependymoma

d. Receptor editing

4. In medicine, a _____ is a disease that is long-lasting or recurrent. The term chronic describes the course of the disease, or its rate of onset and development. A chronic course is distinguished from a recurrent course; recurrent diseases relapse repeatedly, with periods of remission in between.

a. symptom

b. Body temperature

c. Chronic disease

d. malignancy

5. _____ is the diagnosis, treatment, and prevention of disease, illness, injury, and other physical and mental impairments in humans. _____ is delivered by practitioners in medicine, chiropractic, dentistry, nursing, pharmacy, allied health, and other care providers. It refers to the work done in providing primary care, secondary care and tertiary care, as well as in public health.

a. Miguel de Cervantes Health Care Centre

b. Health care

c. Primary care physician

d. Primary care

1. d

2. c

3. a

4. c

5. b

You can take the complete Chapter Practice Test

for Chapter 1. GENERAL ISSUES IN PEDIATRIC HOSPITAL MEDICINE
on all key terms, persons, places, and concepts.

Online 99 Cents

http://www.epub219.49.13357.1.cram101.com/

Use www.Cram101.com for all your study needs

including Cram101's online interactive problem solving labs in

chemistry, statistics, mathematics, and more.

CHAPTER OUTLINE: KEY TERMS, PEOPLE, PLACES, CONCEPTS

Autonomy

Beneficence

Distributive justice

Informed consent

Nonmaleficence

Advance directive

Reasonable person

Periorbital cellulitis

Pulse oximetry

Regulation

Health care

Child abuse

Sexual abuse

Disclosure

Home care

Palliative care

Acute care

End-of-life care

Abdominal pain

Pain assessment

Conflict resolution

Intensive care

Life support

Mechanical ventilation

Organ donation

Medical examiner

Terminal sedation

Craniosacral therapy

Kangaroo care

Reflexology

Chest pain

Diabetic ketoacidosis

Alternative medicine

Epidemiology

Efficacy

CHAPTER HIGHLIGHTS & NOTES: KEY TERMS, PEOPLE, PLACES, CONCEPTS

Autonomy	Autonomy is a concept found in moral, political and bioethical philosophy. Within these contexts, it is the capacity of a rational individual to make an informed, un-coerced decision. In moral and political philosophy, autonomy is often used as the basis for determining moral responsibility for one's actions.
Beneficence	Beneficence is a concept in research ethics which states that researchers should have the welfare of the research participant as a goal of any clinical trial. The antonym of this term, maleficence, describes a practice which opposes the welfare of any research participant. The concept that medical professionals and researchers would always practice beneficence seems natural to most patients and research participants, but in fact, every health intervention or research intervention has potential to harm the recipient.
Distributive justice	Distributive justice concerns what some consider to be socially just with respect to the allocation of goods in a society. Thus, a community in which incidental inequalities in outcome do not arise would be considered a society guided by the principles of Distributive justice. Allocation of goods takes into thought the total amount of goods to be handed out, the process on how they in the civilization are going to dispense, and the pattern of division.
Informed consent	Informed consent is a phrase often used in law to indicate that the consent a person gives meets certain minimum standards. As a literal matter, in the absence of fraud, it is redundant. An informed consent can be said to have been given based upon a clear appreciation and understanding of the facts, implications, and future consequences of an action.
Nonmaleficence	Primum non nocere is a Latin phrase that means 'First, do no harm.' The phrase is sometimes recorded as primum nil nocere. Nonmaleficence, which derives from the maxim, is one of the principal precepts that all medical students are taught in medical school and is a fundamental principle for emergency medical services around the world. Another way to state it is that 'given an existing problem, it may be better to do nothing than to do something that risks causing more harm than good.' It reminds the physician and other health care providers that they must consider the possible harm that any intervention might do.
Advance directive	Advance health care directives, also known as living wills, Advance directives, are instructions given by individuals specifying what actions should be taken for their health in the event that they are no longer able to make decisions due to illness or incapacity. A living will is one form of Advance directive, leaving instructions for treatment. Another form authorizes a specific type of power of attorney or health care proxy, where someone is appointed by the individual to make decisions on their behalf when they are incapacitated.

Chapter 2. ETHICAL AND LEGAL ISSUES

Reasonable person	The reasonable person is a legal fiction of the common law that represents an objective standard against which any individual's understanding or conduct can be measured. It is used to determine contractual intent, or if a breach of the standard of care has occurred, provided a duty of care can be proven.

In contractual law: The intent of a party can be determined by examining the understanding of a reasonable person, after consideration is given to all relevant circumstances of the case including the negotiations, any practices which the parties have established between themselves, usages and any subsequent conduct of the parties. |
| Periorbital cellulitis | Periorbital cellulitis, which is behind the septum), is an inflammation and infection of the eyelid and portions of skin around the eye, anterior to the orbital septum. It may be caused by breaks in the skin around the eye, and subsequent spread to the eyelid; infection of the sinuses around the nose (sinusitis); or from spread of an infection elsewhere through the blood.

Periorbital cellulitis must be differentiated from orbital cellulitis, which is an emergency and requires intravenous (IV) antibiotics. |
| Pulse oximetry | Pulse oximetry is a non-invasive method allowing the monitoring of the oxygenation of a patient's hemoglobin.

A sensor is placed on a thin part of the patient's body, usually a fingertip or earlobe, or in the case of an infant, across a foot. Light of two different wavelengths is passed through the patient to a photodetector. |
Regulation	Regulation is 'controlling human or societal behavior by rules or restrictions.' Regulation can take many forms: legal restrictions promulgated by a government authority, self-regulation by an industry such as through a trade association, social regulation co-regulation and market regulation. One can consider regulation as actions of conduct imposing sanctions (such as a fine). This action of administrative law, or implementing regulatory law, may be contrasted with statutory or case law.
Health care	Health care is the diagnosis, treatment, and prevention of disease, illness, injury, and other physical and mental impairments in humans. Health care is delivered by practitioners in medicine, chiropractic, dentistry, nursing, pharmacy, allied health, and other care providers. It refers to the work done in providing primary care, secondary care and tertiary care, as well as in public health.
Child abuse	Child abuse is the physical, sexual or emotional mistreatment or neglect of a child or children.

In the United States, the Centers for Disease Control and Prevention (CDC) and the Department for Children And Families (DCF) define child maltreatment as any act or series of acts of commission or omission by a parent or other caregiver that results in harm, potential for harm, or threat of harm to a child. Child abuse can occur in a child's home, or in the organizations, schools or communities the child interacts with.

Sexual abuse

Sexual abuse is the forcing of undesired sexual behavior by one person upon another. When that force is immediate, of short duration, or infrequent, it is called sexual assault. The offender is referred to as a sexual abuser or (often pejoratively) molester. The term also covers any behavior by any adult towards a child to stimulate either the adult or child sexually. When the victim is younger than the age of consent, it is referred to as child sexual abuse.

Disclosure

Disclosure means the giving out of information, either voluntarily or to be in compliance with legal regulations or workplace rules.

· In computer security, full Disclosure means disclosing full information about vulnerabilities. · In computing, Disclosure widget · In journalism, full Disclosure refers to disclosing the interests of the writer which may bear on the subject being written about, for example, if the writer has worked with an interview subject in the past. · In psychology, Disclosure refers talking to others about one's feelings.

· In law:

· The law of England and Wales, Disclosure refers to a process that may form part of legal proceedings, whereby parties inform ('disclose') to other parties the existence of any relevant documents that are, or have been, in their control. This compares with the process known as discovery in the course of legal proceedings in the United States. · In U.S. civil procedure (litigation rules for civil cases), Disclosure is a stage prior to trial. In civil cases, each party must disclose to the opposing party the following: names of witnesses which it may use to support its side, copies of documents (or mere description of these documents) in its control which it may use to support its side, computation of damages claimed, and certain insurance information.

Home care

Home Care, (also referred to as domiciliary care or social care), is health care or supportive care provided in the patient's home by healthcare professionals (often referred to as home health care or formal care). Often, the term home care is used to distinguish non-medical care or custodial care, which is care that is provided by persons who are not nurses, doctors, or other licensed medical personnel, as opposed to home health care that is provided by licensed personnel. Professionals providing care

Chapter 2. ETHICAL AND LEGAL ISSUES

Palliative care	Palliative care is an area of healthcare that focuses on relieving and preventing the suffering of patients. Unlike hospice care, palliative medicine is appropriate for patients in all disease stages, including those undergoing treatment for curable illnesses and those living with chronic diseases, as well as patients who are nearing the end of life. Palliative medicine utilizes a multidisciplinary approach to patient care, relying on input from physicians, pharmacists, nurses, chaplains, social workers, psychologists, and other allied health professionals in formulating a plan of care to relieve suffering in all areas of a patient's life.
Acute care	Acute care is a branch of secondary health care where a patient receives active but short-term treatment for a severe injury or episode of illness, an urgent medical condition, or during recovery from surgery. In medical terms, care for acute health conditions is the opposite from chronic care, or longer term care.
	Acute care services are generally delivered by teams of health care professionals from a range of medical and surgical specialties.
End-of-life care	In medicine, end-of-life care refers to medical care not only of patients in the final hours or days of their lives, but more broadly, medical care of all those with a terminal illness or terminal condition that has become advanced, progressive and incurable.
	Regarding cancer care the United States National Cancer Institute writes:'
	When a patient's health care team determines that the cancer can no longer be controlled, medical testing and cancer treatment often stop. But the patient's care continues.'
Abdominal pain	Abdominal pain can be one of the symptoms associated with transient disorders or serious disease. Making a definitive diagnosis of the cause of abdominal pain can be difficult, because many diseases can result in this symptom. Abdominal pain is a common problem.
Pain assessment	Pain is often regarded as the fifth vital sign in regard to healthcare because it is accepted now in healthcare that pain, like other vital signs, is an objective sensation rather than subjective. As a result nurses are trained and expected to assess pain.
	Pain assessment and re-assessment after administration of analgesics or pain management is regulated in healthcare facilities by accreditation bodies, like the Joint Commission.
Conflict resolution	Conflict resolution is conceptualized as the methods and processes involved in facilitating the peaceful ending of social conflict. Often, committed group members attempt to resolve group conflicts by actively communicating information about their conflicting motives or ideologies to the rest of the group (e.g., intentions; reasons for holding certain beliefs), and by engaging in collective negotiation.

Intensive care	intensive care medicine or critical care medicine is a branch of medicine concerned with the provision of life support or organ support systems in patients who are critically ill and who usually require intensive monitoring. Patients requiring intensive care may require support for hemodynamic instability (hypertension/hypotension), airway or respiratory compromise (such as ventilator support), acute renal failure, potentially lethal cardiac arrhythmias, or the cumulative effects of multiple organ system failure. They may also be admitted for intensive/invasive monitoring, such as the crucial hours after major surgery when deemed too unstable to transfer to a less intensively monitored unit.
Life support	Life support in medicine is a broad term that applies to any therapy used to sustain a patient's life while they are critically ill or injured, as part of intensive-care medicine. There are many therapies and techniques that may be used by clinicians to achieve the goal of sustaining life. Some examples include:•Feeding tube•Total parenteral nutrition•Mechanical ventilation•Heart/Lung bypass•Urinary catheterization•Dialysis•Cardiopulmonary resuscitation•Defibrillation•Artificial pacemaker These techniques are applied most commonly in the Emergency Department, Intensive Care Unit and, Operating Rooms.
Mechanical ventilation	In medicine, mechanical ventilation is a method to mechanically assist or replace spontaneous breathing. This may involve a machine called a ventilator or the breathing may be assisted by a physician, respiratory therapist or other suitable person compressing a bag or set of bellows. Traditionally divided into negative-pressure ventilation, where air is essentially sucked into the lungs, or positive pressure ventilation, where air is pushed into the trachea.
Organ donation	Organ donation is the donation of biological tissue or an organ of the human body, from a living or dead person to a living recipient in need of a transplantation. Transplantable organs and tissues are removed in a surgical procedure following a determination, based on the donor's medical and social history, of which are suitable for transplantation. Such procedures are termed allotransplantations, to distinguish them from xenotransplantation, the transfer of animal organs into human bodies.
Medical examiner	A medical examiner is a medically qualified government officer whose duty is to investigate deaths and injuries that occur under unusual or suspicious circumstances, to perform post-mortem examinations, and in some jurisdictions to initiate inquests. In some jurisdictions with English origins or history, a coroner performs these and other duties.

Chapter 2. ETHICAL AND LEGAL ISSUES

Terminal sedation	In medicine, specifically in end-of-life care, terminal sedation is the palliative practice of relieving distress in a terminally ill person in the last hours or days of a dying patient's life, usually by means of a continuous intravenous or subcutaneous infusion of a sedative drug. This is a option of last resort for patients whose symptoms cannot be controlled by any other means. This should be differentiated from euthanasia as the goal of palliative sedation is to control symptoms through sedation but not shorten the patient's life, while in euthanasia the goal is to shorten life to relieve symptoms.
Craniosacral therapy	Craniosacral therapy is an alternative medicine therapy used by physiotherapists, osteopaths, massage therapists, naturopaths, and chiropractors. It was developed in 1899 by William Garner Sutherland. A craniosacral therapy session involves the therapist placing their hands on the patient, which allows them to 'tune into the craniosacral rhythm'.
Kangaroo care	Kangaroo care is a technique practiced on newborn, usually preterm, infants wherein the infant is held, skin-to-skin, with an adult. Kangaroo care for pre-term infants may be restricted to a few hours per day, but if they are medically stable that time may be extended. Some parents may keep their babies in-arms for many hours per day.
Reflexology	Reflexology, is an alternative medicine involving the physical act of applying pressure to the feet, hands, or ears with specific thumb, finger, and hand techniques without the use of oil or lotion. It is based on what reflexologists claim to be a system of zones and reflex areas that they say reflect an image of the body on the feet and hands, with the premise that such work effects a physical change to the body. A 2009 systematic review of randomised controlled trials concludes that 'The best evidence available to date does not demonstrate convincingly that reflexology is an effective treatment for any medical condition.' There is no consensus among reflexologists on how reflexology is supposed to work; a unifying theme is the idea that areas on the foot correspond to areas of the body, and that by manipulating these one can improve health through one's qi.
Chest pain	Chest pain may be a symptom of a number of serious conditions and is generally considered a medical emergency. Even though it may be determined that the pain is non-cardiac in origin, this is often a diagnosis of exclusion made after ruling out more serious causes of the pain. Causes of chest pain range from non-serious to serious to life threatening.
Diabetic ketoacidosis	Diabetic ketoacidosis is a potentially life-threatening complication in patients with diabetes mellitus. It happens predominantly in those with type 1 diabetes, but it can occur in those with type 2 diabetes under certain circumstances.

| Alternative medicine | Alternative medicine is any practice claiming to heal 'that does not fall within the realm of conventional medicine.' It may be based on historical or cultural traditions, rather than on scientific evidence.

Alternative medicine is frequently grouped with complementary medicine or integrative medicine, which, in general, refers to the same interventions when used in conjunction with mainstream techniques, under the umbrella term complementary and alternative medicine, or CAM. Critics maintain that the terms 'complementary' and 'alternative medicine' are deceptive euphemisms meant to give an impression of medical authority.

A 1998 systematic review of studies assessing its prevalence in 13 countries concluded that about 31% of cancer patients use some form of complementary and alternative medicine. |
| --- | --- |
| Epidemiology | Epidemiology is the study of the distribution and patterns of health-events, health-characteristics and their causes or influences in well-defined populations. It is the cornerstone method of public health research and practice, and helps inform policy decisions and evidence-based medicine by identifying risk factors for disease and targets for preventive medicine and public policies. Epidemiologists are involved in the design of studies, collection and statistical analysis of data, and interpretation and dissemination of results (including peer review and occasional systematic review). |
| Efficacy | Efficacy is the capacity to produce an effect. It has different specific meanings in different fields.

In a healthcare context, Efficacy indicates the capacity for beneficial change (or therapeutic effect) of a given intervention. |

Chapter 2. ETHICAL AND LEGAL ISSUES

1. _____ is a non-invasive method allowing the monitoring of the oxygenation of a patient's hemoglobin.

   A sensor is placed on a thin part of the patient's body, usually a fingertip or earlobe, or in the case of an infant, across a foot. Light of two different wavelengths is passed through the patient to a photodetector.

   a. Reflex bradycardia
   b. Registered Cardiovascular Invasive Specialist
   c. Regurgitant fraction
   d. Pulse oximetry

2. _____ may be a symptom of a number of serious conditions and is generally considered a medical emergency. Even though it may be determined that the pain is non-cardiac in origin, this is often a diagnosis of exclusion made after ruling out more serious causes of the pain.

   Causes of _____ range from non-serious to serious to life threatening.

   a. Coccydynia
   b. Chest pain
   c. Condylar resorption
   d. Congenital insensitivity to pain

3. _____ is a concept found in moral, political and bioethical philosophy. Within these contexts, it is the capacity of a rational individual to make an informed, un-coerced decision. In moral and political philosophy, _____ is often used as the basis for determining moral responsibility for one's actions.

   a. Earthscore
   b. Autonomy
   c. Eyeborg
   d. Inferential theory of learning

4. Beneficence is a concept in research ethics which states that researchers should have the welfare of the research participant as a goal of any clinical trial. The antonym of this term, maleficence, describes a practice which opposes the welfare of any research participant.

   The concept that medical professionals and researchers would always practice _____ seems natural to most patients and research participants, but in fact, every health intervention or research intervention has potential to harm the recipient.

   a. The Citadel
   b. Beneficence
   c. Justice
   d. Philoctetes

5. . _____ means the giving out of information, either voluntarily or to be in compliance with legal regulations or workplace rules.

· In computer security, full _____ means disclosing full information about vulnerabilities. · In computing, _____ widget · In journalism, full _____ refers to disclosing the interests of the writer which may bear on the subject being written about, for example, if the writer has worked with an interview subject in the past. · In psychology, _____ refers talking to others about one's feelings.

· In law:

· The law of England and Wales, _____ refers to a process that may form part of legal proceedings, whereby parties inform ('disclose') to other parties the existence of any relevant documents that are, or have been, in their control. This compares with the process known as discovery in the course of legal proceedings in the United States. · In U.S. civil procedure (litigation rules for civil cases), _____ is a stage prior to trial. In civil cases, each party must disclose to the opposing party the following: names of witnesses which it may use to support its side, copies of documents (or mere description of these documents) in its control which it may use to support its side, computation of damages claimed, and certain insurance information.

a. Premium
b. trabeculoplasty
c. Disclosure
d. Bone pain

1. d
2. b
3. b
4. b
5. c

You can take the complete Chapter Practice Test

for Chapter 2. ETHICAL AND LEGAL ISSUES
on all key terms, persons, places, and concepts.

Online 99 Cents

http://www.epub219.49.13357.2.cram101.com/

Use www.Cram101.com for all your study needs

including Cram101's online interactive problem solving labs in

chemistry, statistics, mathematics, and more.

Abdominal mass

Differential diagnosis

Computed tomography

Barium

Terminal sedation

Aplastic anemia

Cyanosis

Heart disease

Physical examination

Chest radiograph

Hyperoxia test

Pulse oximetry

Anorexia nervosa

Acetylcholinesterase inhibitor

Carbon monoxide

Methemoglobinemia

Arterial blood

Blood gas

Breath holding spells

CHAPTER OUTLINE: KEY TERMS, PEOPLE, PLACES, CONCEPTS

Methylene blue

Body fluid

Extracellular fluid

Intracellular fluid

Hyponatremia

Renal failure

Status epilepticus

Febrile seizure

Hypovolemia

Arginine vasopressin

Hypernatremia

Hypervolemia

Hyperkalemia

Hypokalemia

Symptom

Bartter syndrome

Gitelman syndrome

Chvostek sign

Hypocalcemia

Hypoparathyroidism

Serum

Bisphosphonate

Activation syndrome

Hypomagnesemia

Hypermagnesemia

Factor IX

Factor VII

Factor X

Factor XI

ACE inhibitor

Kawasaki disease

Fever of unknown origin

Heat stroke

Hypothermia

Beckwith-Wiedemann syndrome

Etiological myth

Glucose transporter

Hyperinsulinemic hypoglycemia

_____ | Hypoglycemia

_____ | Pathophysiology

_____ | Growth hormone

_____ | Reactive hypoglycemia

_____ | Inborn errors of metabolism

_____ | Lymphadenopathy

_____ | Bartonella henselae

_____ | Mycobacterium tuberculosis

_____ | Lymphangitis

_____ | Rheumatic fever

_____ | Organomegaly

_____ | Splenic vein

_____ | Abdominal pain

_____ | Diabetes insipidus

_____ | Chest pain

_____ | Ehlers-Danlos syndrome

_____ | Headache

_____ | Pain management

_____ | Prevalence

Nervous system

Brain tumor

Leukotriene antagonist

Triptan

Bronchopulmonary dysplasia

Arthralgia

Prevention

Prognosis

Purpura

Laryngomalacia

Stridor

Retropharyngeal abscess

Vocal cords

Croup

Septic arthritis

Subglottic stenosis

Tracheomalacia

Tuberculosis

Gastroesophageal reflux

CHAPTER OUTLINE: KEY TERMS, PEOPLE, PLACES, CONCEPTS

Proton pump

Vomiting

Cerebral palsy

Biliary dyskinesia

Binge eating

Binge eating disorder

Bulimia nervosa

Cyclic vomiting syndrome

Eating disorder

Sphincter of Oddi dysfunction

Beta-adrenergic agonist

Wheezing

Biliary atresia

Hepatitis

Hepatoblastoma

Hepatocellular carcinoma

Liver failure

Infectious hepatitis

Alagille syndrome

_____ | Autoimmune hepatitis

_____ | Crigler-Najjar syndrome

_____ | Cystic fibrosis

_____ | Hyperbilirubinemia

_____ | Cardiac output

_____ | Distributive shock

_____ | Septic shock

_____ | Stroke volume

_____ | Distributive

_____ | Anaphylactic shock

_____ | Cardiogenic shock

_____ | Neurogenic shock

Abdominal mass	An abdominal mass is any localized enlargement or swelling in the human abdomen. Depending on its location, the abdominal mass may be caused by an enlarged liver (hepatomegaly), enlarged spleen (splenomegaly), protruding kidney, a pancreatic mass, a retroperitoneal mass (a mass in the posterior of the peritoneum), an abdominal aortic aneurysm, or various tumours, such as those caused by abdominal carcinomatosis and omental metastasis. The treatments depend on the cause, and may range from watchful waiting to radical surgery.
Differential diagnosis	A differential diagnosis is a systematic diagnostic method used to identify the presence of an entity where multiple alternatives are possible (and the process may be termed differential diagnostic procedure), and may also refer to any of the included candidate alternatives (which may also be termed candidate condition). This method is essentially a process of elimination, or at least, rendering of the probabilities of candidate conditions to negligible levels. In this sense, probabilities are, in fact, imaginative parameters in the mind or hardware of the diagnostician or system, while in reality the target (such as a patient) either has a condition or not with an actual probability of either 0 or 100%.
Computed tomography	Computed tomography is a medical imaging method employing tomography created by computer processing. Digital geometry processing is used to generate a three-dimensional image of the inside of an object from a large series of two-dimensional X-ray images taken around a single axis of rotation. Computed tomography produces a volume of data which can be manipulated, through a process known as 'windowing', in order to demonstrate various bodily structures based on their ability to block the X-ray/Röntgen beam.
Barium	Barium is a chemical element with the symbol Ba and atomic number 56. It is the fifth element in Group 2, a soft silvery metallic alkaline earth metal. Barium is never found in nature as a free element, due to its high chemical reactivity. Its oxide is historically known as baryta, but this oxide (in a similar way to calcium oxide, or quicklime) must be artificially produced since it reacts avidly with water and carbon dioxide, and is not found as a mineral.
Terminal sedation	In medicine, specifically in end-of-life care, terminal sedation is the palliative practice of relieving distress in a terminally ill person in the last hours or days of a dying patient's life, usually by means of a continuous intravenous or subcutaneous infusion of a sedative drug. This is a option of last resort for patients whose symptoms cannot be controlled by any other means.

Chapter 3. COMMON PRESENTING SIGNS, SYMPTOMS, DIFFERENTIAL DIAGNOSIS

Aplastic anemia	Aplastic anemia is a condition where bone marrow does not produce sufficient new cells to replenish blood cells. The condition, as the name indicates, involves both aplasia and anemia. Typically, anemia refers to low red blood cell counts, but aplastic anemia patients have lower counts of all three blood cell types: red blood cells, white blood cells, and platelets, termed pancytopenia.
Cyanosis	Cyanosis is the appearance of a blue or purple coloration of the skin or mucous membranes due to the tissues near the skin surface being low on oxygen. The onset of cyanosis is 2.5 g/dL of deoxyhemoglobin. The bluish color is more readily apparent in those with high hemoglobin counts than it is with those with anemia.
Heart disease	Heart disease is an umbrella term for a variety of diseases affecting the heart. As of 2007, it is the leading cause of death in the United States, England, Canada and Wales, accounting for 25.4% of the total deaths in the United States. Coronary heart disease refers to the failure of the coronary circulation to supply adequate circulation to cardiac muscle and surrounding tissue. Coronary heart disease is most commonly equated with Coronary artery disease although coronary heart disease can be due to other causes, such as coronary vasospasm.
Physical examination	A physical examination, medical examination, or clinical examination (more popularly known as a check-up or medical) is the process by which a doctor investigates the body of a patient for signs of disease. It generally follows the taking of the medical history -- an account of the symptoms as experienced by the patient. Together with the medical history, the physical examination aids in determining the correct diagnosis and devising the treatment plan.
Chest radiograph	In medicine, a chest radiograph, commonly called a chest X-ray (CXR), is a projection radiograph of the chest used to diagnose conditions affecting the chest, its contents, and nearby structures. Chest radiographs are among the most common films taken, being diagnostic of many conditions. Like all methods of radiography, chest radiography employs ionizing radiation in the form of X-rays to generate images of the chest.
Hyperoxia test	A hyperoxia test is a test that is performed--usually on an infant-- to determine whether the patient's cyanosis is due to lung disease or a problem with blood circulation. It is performed by measuring the arterial blood gases of the patient while he breathes room air, then re-measuring the blood gases after the patient has breathed 100% oxygen for 10 minutes.

Pulse oximetry	Pulse oximetry is a non-invasive method allowing the monitoring of the oxygenation of a patient's hemoglobin.
	A sensor is placed on a thin part of the patient's body, usually a fingertip or earlobe, or in the case of an infant, across a foot. Light of two different wavelengths is passed through the patient to a photodetector.
Anorexia nervosa	The differential diagnoses of anorexia nervosa (AN) include various medical and psychological conditions which may be misdiagnosed as (AN), in some cases these conditions may be comorbid with anorexia nervosa (AN). The misdiagnosis of AN is not uncommon. In one instance a case of achalasia was misdiagnosed as AN and the patient spent two months confined to a psychiatric hospital.
Acetylcholinesterase inhibitor	An acetylcholinesterase inhibitor or anti-cholinesterase is a chemical that inhibits the cholinesterase enzyme from breaking down acetylcholine, increasing both the level and duration of action of the neurotransmitter acetylcholine.
	Uses
	Acetylcholinesterase inhibitors:•Occur naturally as venoms and poisons•Are used as weapons in the form of nerve agents•Are used medicinally: •To treat myasthenia gravis. In myasthenia gravis, they are used to increase neuromuscular transmission.•To treat Glaucoma•To treat Alzheimer's disease•To treat Lewy Body Dementia•As an antidote to anticholinergic poisoning
Carbon monoxide	Carbon monoxide also called carbonous oxide, is a colorless, odorless, and tasteless gas that is slightly lighter than air. It can be toxic to humans and animals when encountered in higher concentrations, although it is also produced in normal animal metabolism in low quantities, and is thought to have some normal biological functions. In the atmosphere however, it is short lived and spatially variable, since it combines with oxygen to form carbon dioxide and ozone.
Methemoglobinemia	Methemoglobinemia is a disorder characterized by the presence of a higher than normal level of methemoglobin (metHb) in the blood. Methemoglobin is an oxidized form of hemoglobin that has a decreased affinity for oxygen, resulting in an increased affinity of oxygen to other heme sites and overall reduced ability to release oxygen to tissues. The oxygen-hemoglobin dissociation curve is therefore shifted to the left.
Arterial blood	Arterial blood is the oxygenated blood in the circulatory system found in the lungs, the left chambers of the heart, and in the arteries. It is bright red in color, while venous blood is dark red in color (but looks purple through the opaque skin). It is the contralateral term to venous blood.

Chapter 3. COMMON PRESENTING SIGNS, SYMPTOMS, DIFFERENTIAL DIAGNOSIS

Blood gas	Blood gas is a term used to describe a laboratory test of blood where the purpose is primarily to measure ventilation and oxygenation. The source is generally noted by an added word to the beginning; arterial blood gases come from arteries, venous blood gases come from veins and capillary blood gases come from capillaries. •pH -- The acidity or basicity of the blood.•PaCO2 -- The partial pressure of carbon dioxide in the blood.•PaO2 -- The partial pressure of oxygen in the blood.•HCO3 -- The level of bicarbonate in the blood.•BE -- The base-excess of bicarbonate in the blood.Purposes for testing •Acidosis•Diabetic ketoacidosis•Lactic acidosis•Metabolic acidosis•Respiratory acidosis•Respiratory alkalosisAbnormal results Abnormal results may be due to lung, kidney, or metabolic diseases.
Breath holding spells	Breath holding spells are the occurrence of episodic apnea in children, possibly associated with loss of consciousness, and changes in postural tone. Breath holding spells occur in approximately 5% of the population with equal distribution between males and females. They are most common in children between 6 and 18 months and usually not present after 5 years of age.
Methylene blue	Methylene blue is a heterocyclic aromatic chemical compound with the molecular formula $C_{16}H_{18}N_3SCl$. It has many uses in a range of different fields, such as biology and chemistry. At room temperature it appears as a solid, odorless, dark green powder, that yields a blue solution when dissolved in water.
Body fluid	Body fluid, bodily fluids, or biofluids are liquids originating from inside the bodies of living people. They include fluids that are excreted or secreted from the body as well as body water that normally is not. The dominating content of body fluids is body water.
Extracellular fluid	Extracellular fluid or extracellular fluid volume (ECFV) usually denotes all body fluid outside of cells. The remainder is called intracellular fluid. In some animals, including mammals, the extracellular fluid can be divided into two major subcompartments, interstitial fluid and blood plasma.
Intracellular fluid	The cytosol or intracellular fluid is the liquid found inside cells. In eukaryotes this liquid is separated by cell membranes from the contents of the organelles suspended in the cytosol, such as the mitochondrial matrix inside the mitochondrion. The entire contents of a eukaryotic cell, minus the contents of the cell nucleus, are referred to as the cytoplasm.
Hyponatremia	Hyponatremia is lower than normal.

	Sodium is the dominant extracellular cation and cannot freely cross the cell membrane. Its homeostasis is vital to the normal physiologic function of cells.
Renal failure	Renal failure or kidney failure (formerly called renal insufficiency) describes a medical condition in which the kidneys fail to adequately filter toxins and waste products from the blood. The two forms are acute (acute kidney injury) and chronic (chronic kidney disease); a number of other diseases or health problems may cause either form of renal failure to occur. Renal failure is described as a decrease in glomerular filtration rate.
Status epilepticus	Status epilepticus is a life-threatening condition in which the brain is in a state of persistent seizure. Definitions vary, but traditionally it is defined as one continuous unremitting seizure lasting longer than 30 minutes, or recurrent seizures without regaining consciousness between seizures for greater than 30 minutes. Treatment is, however, generally started after the seizure has lasted 5 minutes.
Febrile seizure	A febrile seizure, is a convulsion associated with a significant rise in body temperature. They most commonly occur in children between the ages of 6 months to 6 years and are twice as common in boys as in girls. The direct cause of a febrile seizure is not known; however, it is normally precipitated by a recent upper respiratory infection or gastroenteritis.
Hypovolemia	In physiology and medicine, hypovolemia is a state of decreased blood volume; more specifically, decrease in volume of blood plasma. It is thus the intravascular component of volume contraction , but, as it also is the most essential one, hypovolemia and volume contraction are sometimes used synonymously. Hypovolemia is characterized by salt (sodium) depletion and thus differs from dehydration, which is defined as excessive loss of body water.
Arginine vasopressin	Arginine vasopressin, also known as vasopressin, argipressin or antidiuretic hormone (ADH), is a hormone found in most mammals, including humans. Vasopressin is a peptide hormone. It is derived from a preprohormone precursor that is synthesized in the hypothalamus and stored in vesicles at the posterior pituitary. Most of it is stored in the posterior pituitary to be released into the blood stream; however, some of it is also released directly into the brain.
Hypernatremia	Hypernatremia is defined by an elevated sodium level in the blood. Hypernatremia is generally not caused by an excess of sodium, but rather by a relative deficit of free water in the body. For this reason, hypernatremia is often synonymous with the less precise term, dehydration.

Chapter 3. COMMON PRESENTING SIGNS, SYMPTOMS, DIFFERENTIAL DIAGNOSIS

Hypervolemia	Hypervolemia, is the medical condition where there is too much fluid in the blood. The opposite condition is hypovolemia, which is too little fluid volume in the blood. Causes Excessive sodium or fluid intake:•IV therapy•Transfusion reaction by blood transfusions.•High intake of sodium Sodium or water retention:•Heart failure•Liver cirrhosis•Nephrotic syndrome•Corticosteroid therapy•Hyperaldosteronism•Low protein intake Fluid shift into the intravascular space:•Fluid remobilization after burn treatment•Administration of hypertonic fluids, e.g. mannitol or hypertonic saline solution•Administration of plasma proteins, such as albuminSymptoms The excess fluid, primarily salt and water, builds up in various locations in the body and leads to an increase in weight, swelling in the legs and arms (peripheral edema), and/or fluid in the abdomen (ascites).
Hyperkalemia	Hyperkalemia refers to the condition in which the concentration of the electrolyte potassium (K^+) in the blood is elevated. Extreme hyperkalemia is a medical emergency due to the risk of potentially fatal abnormal heart rhythms (arrhythmia). Normal serum potassium levels are between 3.5 and 5.0 mEq/L; at least 95% of the body's potassium is found inside cells, with the remainder in the blood.
Hypokalemia	Hypokalemia, also hypopotassemia or hypopotassaemia (ICD-9), refers to the condition in which the concentration of potassium (K^+) in the blood is low. The prefix hypo- means 'under' (contrast with hyper-, meaning 'over'); kal- refers to kalium, the Neo-Latin for potassium, and -emia means 'condition of the blood.' Normal serum potassium is 3.5 to 5.5 mEq/L; however, in persons with this condition, plasma potassium is 0.5 mEq/L lower. Normal plasma potassium levels are between 3.5 to 5.0 mEq/L; at least 95% of the body's potassium is found inside cells, with the remainder in the blood.
Symptom	A symptom is a departure from normal function or feeling which is noticed by a patient, indicating the presence of disease or abnormality. A symptom is subjective, observed by the patient, and not measured. A symptom may not be a malady, for example symptoms of pregnancy.
Bartter syndrome	Bartter syndrome is a rare inherited defect in the thick ascending limb of the loop of Henle.

	It is characterized by low potassium levels (hypokalemia), increased blood pH (alkalosis), and normal to low blood pressure. There are two types of Bartter syndrome: neonatal and classic.
Gitelman syndrome	Gitelman syndrome is an autosomal recessive kidney disorder characterized by hypokalemic metabolic alkalosis with hypocalciuria, and hypomagnesemia and caused by loss of function mutations of the thiazide-sensitive sodium-chloride symporter (also known as NCC, NCCT, or TSC) located in the distal convoluted tubule. Gitelman syndrome was formerly considered a subset of Bartter syndrome until the distinct genetic and molecular bases of these disorders were identified. Bartter syndrome is also an autosomal recessive hypokalemic metabolic alkalosis, but it derives from a mutation to the NKCC2 found in the thick ascending limb of the loop of Henle.
Chvostek sign	The Chvostek sign is one of the signs of tetany seen in hypocalcemia. It refers to an abnormal reaction to the stimulation of the facial nerve. When the facial nerve is tapped at the angle of the jaw (i.e. masseter muscle), the facial muscles on the same side of the face will contract momentarily (typically a twitch of the nose or lips) because of hypocalcemia (i.e. from hypoparathyroidism, pseudohypoparathyroidism, hypovitaminosis D) with resultant hyperexcitability of nerves.
Hypocalcemia	In medicine, Hypocalcemia is the presence of low serum calcium levels in the blood, usually taken as less than 2.1 mmol/L or 9 mg/dl or an ionized calcium level mm of less than 1.1 mmol/L (4.5 mg/dL). It is a type of electrolyte disturbance. In the blood, about half of all calcium is bound to proteins such as serum albumin, but it is the unbound, or ionized, calcium that the body regulates.
Hypoparathyroidism	Hypoparathyroidism is decreased function of the parathyroid glands with under production of parathyroid hormone. This can lead to low levels of calcium in the blood, often causing cramping and twitching of muscles or tetany (involuntary muscle contraction), and several other symptoms. The condition can be inherited, but it is also encountered after thyroid or parathyroid gland surgery, and it can be caused by immune system-related damage as well as a number of rarer causes.
Serum	In blood, the serum is the component that is neither a blood cell (serum does not contain white or red blood cells) nor a clotting factor; it is the blood plasma with the fibrinogens removed. Serum includes all proteins not used in blood clotting (coagulation) and all the electrolytes, antibodies, antigens, hormones, and any exogenous substances (e.g., drugs and microorganisms). The study of serum is serology, and may also include proteomics.

Bisphosphonate	Bisphosphonates (also called diphosphonates) are a class of drugs that prevent the loss of bone mass, used to treat osteoporosis and similar diseases. They are called bisphosphonates because they have two phosphonate (PO_3) groups and are similar in structure to pyrophosphate. Evidence shows that they reduce the risk of osteoporotic fracture in those who have had previous fractures.
Activation syndrome	Activation syndrome is a form of sometimes suicidal or homicidal stimulation or agitation that can occur in response to some psychoactive drugs. A study of paroxetine found that 21 out of 93 (23 percent) of youth taking Paxil reported manic-like symptoms which included hostility, emotional lability and nervousness. Pfizer has denied that sertraline can cause such effects.
Hypomagnesemia	Hypomagnesemia is an electrolyte disturbance in which there is an abnormally low level of magnesium in the blood. Normal magnesium levels in humans fall between 1.5 - 2.5 mg/dL. Usually a serum level less than 0.7 mmol/L is used as reference for hypomagnesemia. The prefix hypo- means low (contrast with hyper-, meaning high).
Hypermagnesemia	Hypermagnesemia is an electrolyte disturbance in which there is an abnormally elevated level of magnesium in the blood. Usually this results in excess of magnesium in the body. Hypermagnesemia occurs rarely because the kidney is very effective in excreting excess magnesium.
Factor IX	Factor IX (EC 3.4.21.22) is one of the serine proteases of the coagulation system; it belongs to peptidase family S1. Deficiency of this protein causes hemophilia B. It was discovered in 1952 after a young boy named Stephen Christmas was found to be lacking this exact factor, leading to hemophilia.. Factor IX is produced as a zymogen, an inactive precursor. It is processed to remove the signal peptide, glycosylated and then cleaved by factor XIa (of the contact pathway) or factor VIIa (of the tissue factor pathway) to produce a two-chain form where the chains are linked by a disulfide bridge.
Factor VII	Factor VII is one of the proteins that causes blood to clot in the coagulation cascade. It is an enzyme (EC 3.4.21.21) of the serine protease class. A recombinant form of human factor VIIa (NovoSeven, eptacog alfa [activated]) has U.S. Food and Drug Administration approval for uncontrolled bleeding in hemophilia patients.
Factor X	Factor X, also known by the eponym Stuart-Prower factor or as prothrombinase, is an enzyme (EC 3.4.21.6) of the coagulation cascade. It is a serine endopeptidase (protease group S1).

Factor XI	Factor XI is the zymogen form of factor XIa, one of the enzymes of the coagulation cascade. Like many other coagulation factors, it is a serine protease. In humans, Factor XI is encoded by the F11 gene.
ACE inhibitor	ACE inhibitors are a group of drugs used primarily for the treatment of hypertension (high blood pressure) and congestive heart failure. Originally synthesized from compounds found in pit viper venom, they inhibit angiotensin-converting enzyme (ACE), a component of the blood pressure-regulating renin-angiotensin system.
Kawasaki disease	Kawasaki disease also known as Kawasaki syndrome, lymph node syndrome and mucocutaneous lymph node syndrome, is an autoimmune disease in which the medium-sized blood vessels throughout the body become inflamed. It is largely seen in children under five years of age. It affects many organ systems, mainly those including the blood vessels, skin, mucous membranes and lymph nodes; however its rare but most serious effect is on the heart where it can cause fatal coronary artery aneurysms in untreated children.
Fever of unknown origin	Fever of unknown origin pyrexia of unknown origin (PUO) or febris e causa ignota (febris E.C.I). refers to a condition in which the patient has an elevated temperature but despite investigations by a physician no explanation has been found. If the cause is found it usually is a diagnosis of exclusion, that is, by eliminating all possibilities until only one explanation remains, and taking this as the correct one.
Heat stroke	Heat stroke is defined as a temperature of greater than 40.6 °C (105.1 °F) due to environmental heat exposure with lack of thermoregulation. This is distinct from a fever, where there is a physiological increase in the temperature set point of the body. Treatment involves rapid mechanical cooling. A number of heat illnesses exist including: · Heat stroke as defined by a temperature of greater than >40.6 °C (105.1 °F) due to environmental heat exposure with lack of thermoregulation. · Heat exhaustion · Heat syncope · Heat edema · Heat cramps · Heat tetany Heat stroke presents with a hyperthermia of greater than >40.6 °C (105.1 °F) in combination with confusion and a lack of sweating.
Hypothermia	Hypothermia is a condition in which core temperature drops below the required temperature for normal metabolism and body functions which is defined as 35.0 °C (95.0 °F).

	Body temperature is usually maintained near a constant level of 36.5-37.5 °C (98-100 °F) through biologic homeostasis or thermoregulation. If exposed to cold and the internal mechanisms are unable to replenish the heat that is being lost, a drop in core temperature occurs.
Beckwith-Wiedemann syndrome	Beckwith-Wiedemann syndrome is an overgrowth disorder present at birth characterized by an increased risk of childhood cancer and certain features. Five common features used to define BWS are: macroglossia (large tongue), macrosomia (birth weight and length >90th percentile), midline abdominal wall defects (omphalocele, umbilical hernia, diastasis recti), ear creases or ear pits, and neonatal hypoglycemia (low blood sugar after birth). Most children with BWS do not have all of these five features.
Etiological myth	Etiology is the study of causation, or origination. The word is most commonly used in medical and philosophical theories, where it is used to refer to the study of why things occur, or even the reasons behind the way that things act, and is used in philosophy, physics, psychology, government, medicine, theology and biology in reference to the causes of various phenomena. An etiological myth is a myth intended to explain a name or create a mythic history for a place or family.
Glucose transporter	Glucose transporters (GLUT or SLC2A family) are a family of membrane proteins found in most mammalian cells. Structure Glucose transporters are integral membrane proteins that contain 12 membrane-spanning helices with both the amino and carboxyl termini exposed on the cytoplasmic side of the plasma membrane. Glucose transporter proteins transport glucose and related hexoses according to a model of alternate conformation, which predicts that the transporter exposes a single substrate binding site toward either the outside or the inside of the cell.
Hyperinsulinemic hypoglycemia	Hyperinsulinemic hypoglycemia describes the condition and effects of low blood glucose caused by excessive insulin. Hypoglycemia due to excess insulin is the most common type of serious hypoglycemia. It can be due to endogenous or injected insulin.
Hypoglycemia	Hypoglycemia, hypoglycæmia or low blood sugar (not to be confused with hyperglycemia) is an abnormally diminished content of glucose in the blood. The term literally means 'low sugar blood' . It can produce a variety of symptoms and effects but the principal problems arise from an inadequate supply of glucose to the brain, resulting in impairment of function (neuroglycopenia).

Pathophysiology	Pathophysiology sample values
	Pathophysiology is the study of the changes of normal mechanical, physical, and biochemical functions, either caused by a disease, or resulting from an abnormal syndrome. More formally, it is the branch of medicine which deals with any disturbances of body functions, caused by disease or prodromal symptoms.
	An alternative definition is 'the study of the biological and physical manifestations of disease as they correlate with the underlying abnormalities and physiological disturbances.'
	The study of pathology and the study of pathophysiology often involves substantial overlap in diseases and processes, but pathology emphasizes direct observations, while pathophysiology emphasizes quantifiable measurements.
Growth hormone	Growth hormone is a peptide hormone that stimulates growth, cell reproduction and regeneration in humans and other animals. Growth hormone is a 191-amino acid, single-chain polypeptide that is synthesized, stored, and secreted by the somatotroph cells within the lateral wings of the anterior pituitary gland. Somatotropin (STH) refers to the growth hormone 1 produced naturally in animals, whereas the term somatropin refers to growth hormone produced by recombinant DNA technology, and is abbreviated 'HGH' in humans.
Reactive hypoglycemia	Reactive hypoglycemia, is a medical term describing recurrent episodes of symptomatic hypoglycemia occurring within 4 hours after a high carbohydrate meal in people who do not have diabetes. It is thought to represent a consequence of excessive insulin release triggered by the carbohydrate meal but continuing past the digestion and disposal of the glucose derived from the meal.
	The prevalence of this condition is difficult to ascertain and controversial, because a number of stricter or looser definitions have been used, and because many healthy, asymptomatic people can have glucose tolerance test patterns said to be characteristic of reactive hypoglycemia.
Inborn errors of metabolism	Inborn errors of metabolism comprise a large class of genetic diseases involving disorders of metabolism. The majority are due to defects of single genes that code for enzymes that facilitate conversion of various substances (substrates) into others (products). In most of the disorders, problems arise due to accumulation of substances which are toxic or interfere with normal function, or to the effects of reduced ability to synthesize essential compounds.
Lymphadenopathy	Lymphadenopathy is a term meaning 'disease of the lymph nodes.' It is, however, almost synonymously used with 'swollen/enlarged lymph nodes'. It could be due to infection, auto-immune disease, or malignancy.

Chapter 3. COMMON PRESENTING SIGNS, SYMPTOMS, DIFFERENTIAL DIAGNOSIS

Bartonella henselae	Bartonella henselae is a proteobacterium that can cause bacteremia, endocarditis, bacillary angiomatosis, and peliosis hepatis. It is also the causative agent of cat-scratch disease (Bartonellosis) which, as the name suggests, occurs after a cat bite or scratch. The disease is characterized by lymphadenopathy (swelling of the lymph nodes) and fever.
Mycobacterium tuberculosis	Mycobacterium tuberculosis is a pathogenic bacterial species in the genus Mycobacterium and the causative agent of most cases of tuberculosis (TB). First discovered in 1882 by Robert Koch, M. tuberculosis has an unusual, waxy coating on its cell surface (primarily mycolic acid), which makes the cells impervious to Gram staining, so acid-fast detection techniques are used, instead. The physiology of M. tuberculosis is highly aerobic and requires high levels of oxygen.
Lymphangitis	Lymphangitis is an inflammation of the lymphatic channels that occurs as a result of infection at a site distal to the channel. The most common cause of lymphangitis in humans is Streptococcus pyogenes (Group A strep). Lymphangitis is also sometimes called 'blood poisoning'.
Rheumatic fever	Rheumatic fever is an inflammatory disease that occurs following a Streptococcus pyogenes infection, such as streptococcal pharyngitis or scarlet fever. Believed to be caused by antibody cross-reactivity that can involve the heart, joints, skin, and brain, the illness typically develops two to three weeks after a streptococcal infection. Acute rheumatic fever commonly appears in children between the ages of 6 and 15, with only 20% of first-time attacks occurring in adults.
Organomegaly	Organomegaly is the abnormal enlargement of organs. For example, clitoromegaly is the enlargement of the clitoris, hepatomegaly is enlargement of the liver, cardiomegaly is enlargement of the heart, and splenomegaly is enlargement of the spleen.
Splenic vein	In anatomy, the splenic vein is the blood vessel that drains blood from the spleen. It joins with the superior mesenteric vein, to form the hepatic portal vein and follows a course superior to the pancreas, alongside of the similarly named artery, the splenic artery. Unlike the splenic artery, the splenic vein is intraperitoneal as it courses along the superior border of the body of the pancreas, whereas the splenic artery is retroperitoneal.
Abdominal pain	Abdominal pain can be one of the symptoms associated with transient disorders or serious disease. Making a definitive diagnosis of the cause of abdominal pain can be difficult, because many diseases can result in this symptom. Abdominal pain is a common problem.
Diabetes insipidus	Diabetes insipidus is a condition characterized by excessive thirst and excretion of large amounts of severely diluted urine, with reduction of fluid intake having no effect on the concentration of the urine. There are several different types of DI, each with a different cause.

Chest pain	Chest pain may be a symptom of a number of serious conditions and is generally considered a medical emergency. Even though it may be determined that the pain is non-cardiac in origin, this is often a diagnosis of exclusion made after ruling out more serious causes of the pain.
	Causes of chest pain range from non-serious to serious to life threatening.
Ehlers-Danlos syndrome	Ehlers-Danlos syndrome is a group of inherited connective tissue disorders, caused by a defect in the synthesis of collagen. The collagen in connective tissue helps tissues to resist deformation. In the skin, muscles, ligaments, blood vessels, and visceral organs collagen plays a very significant role and with reduced elasticity, secondary to abnormal collagen, pathology results.
Headache	A headache is pain anywhere in the region of the head or neck. It can be a symptom of a number of different conditions of the head and neck. The brain tissue itself is not sensitive to pain because it lacks pain receptors.
Pain management	Pain management is a branch of medicine employing an interdisciplinary approach for easing the suffering and improving the quality of life of those living with pain. The typical pain management team includes medical practitioners, clinical psychologists, physiotherapists, occupational therapists, and nurse practitioners. Pain sometimes resolves promptly once the underlying trauma or pathology has healed, and is treated by one practitioner, with drugs such as analgesics and (occasionally) anxiolytics.
Prevalence	In epidemiology, the prevalence of a health-related state (typically disease, but also other things like smoking or seatbelt use) in a statistical population is defined as the total number of cases of the risk factor in the population at a given time, or the total number of cases in the population, divided by the number of individuals in the population. It is used as an estimate of how common a disease is within a population over a certain period of time. It helps physicians or other health professionals understand the probability of certain diagnoses and is routinely used by epidemiologists, health care providers, government agencies and insurers.
Nervous system	The nervous system is an organ system containing a network of specialized cells called neurons that coordinate the actions of an animal and transmit signals between different parts of its body. In most animals the nervous system consists of two parts, central and peripheral. The central nervous system of vertebrates (such as humans) contains the brain, spinal cord, and retina.
Brain tumor	A brain tumor is an intracranial solid neoplasm, a tumor (defined as an abnormal growth of cells) within the brain or the central spinal canal.
	Brain tumors include all tumors inside the cranium or in the central spinal canal.

Chapter 3. COMMON PRESENTING SIGNS, SYMPTOMS, DIFFERENTIAL DIAGNOSIS

Leukotriene antagonist	A leukotriene antagonist is a drug that inhibits leukotrienes, which are fatty compounds produced by the immune system that cause inflammation in asthma and bronchitis, and constrict airways. Leukotriene inhibitors (or modifiers), such as montelukast, zafirlukast and zileuton, are used to treat those diseases. They are less effective than corticosteroids and thus less preferred in the treatment of asthma.
Triptan	Triptans are a family of tryptamine-based drugs used as abortive medication in the treatment of migraines and cluster headaches. They were first introduced in the 1990s. While effective at treating individual headaches, they do not provide preventative treatment and are not considered a cure.
Bronchopulmonary dysplasia	Bronchopulmonary dysplasia is a chronic lung disorder that is most common among children who were born prematurely, with low birthweights and who received prolonged mechanical ventilation to treat respiratory distress syndrome. The classic diagnosis of BPD may be assigned at 28 days of life if the following criteria are met (Bureau of Maternal and Child Health, 1989): (1) Positive pressure ventilation during the first 2 weeks of life for a minimum of 3 days.(2) Clinical signs of abnormal respiratory function.(3) Requirements for supplemental oxygen for longer than 28 days of age to maintain PaO2 above 50 mm Hg.(4) Chest radiograph with diffuse abnormal findings characteristic of BPD.
Arthralgia	Arthralgia literally means joint pain; it is a symptom of injury, infection, illnesses (in particular arthritis) or an allergic reaction to medication. According to MeSH, the term 'arthralgia' should only be used when the condition is non-inflammatory, and the term 'arthritis' should be used when the condition is inflammatory. Diagnosis and causes Diagnosis involves interviewing the patient and performing physical exams.
Prevention	Prevention refers to: · Preventive medicine · Hazard Prevention, the process of risk study and elimination and mitigation in emergency management · Risk Prevention · Risk management · Preventive maintenance · Crime Prevention · Prevention, an album by Scottish band De Rosa · Prevention a magazine about health in the United States · Prevent (company), a textile company from Slovenia
Prognosis	Prognosis is a medical term to describe the likely outcome of an illness.

When applied to large populations, prognostic estimates can be very accurate: for example the statement '45% of patients with severe septic shock will die within 28 days' can be made with some confidence, because previous research found that this proportion of patients died. However, it is much harder to translate this into a prognosis for an individual patient: additional information is needed to determine whether a patient belongs to the 45% who will succumb, or to the 55% who survive.

Purpura	Purpura is the appearance of red or purple discolorations on the skin that do not blanch on applying pressure. They are caused by bleeding underneath the skin. Purpura measure 0.3-1 cm (3-10 mm), whereas petechiae measure less than 3 mm, and ecchymoses greater than 1 cm.
Laryngomalacia	Laryngomalacia is an unusual condition, in which the soft, immature cartilage of the upper larynx collapses inward during inhalation, causing airway obstruction. It can also be seen in older patients, especially those with neuromuscular conditions resulting in weakness of the muscles of the throat. However, the infantile form is much more common.
Stridor	Stridor is a high pitched wheezing sound resulting from turbulent air flow in the upper airway. Stridor is a physical sign which is produced by narrow or obstructed airway path. It can be inspiratory, expiratory or biphasic.
Retropharyngeal abscess	Most commonly seen in infants and young children, retropharyngeal abscess is an abscess located in the tissues in the back of the throat behind the posterior pharyngeal wall (the retropharyngeal space). Because RPA's typically occur in deep tissue, they are difficult to diagnose by physical examination alone. RPA is a relatively uncommon illness, and therefore may not receive early diagnosis in children presenting with stiff neck, malaise, difficulty swallowing, or other symptoms listed below.
Vocal cords	The vocal folds, also known commonly as Vocal cords, are composed of twin infoldings of mucous membrane stretched horizontally across the larynx. They vibrate, modulating the flow of air being expelled from the lungs during phonation. Open during inhalation, closed when holding one's breath, and vibrating for speech or singing , the folds are controlled via the vagus nerve.
Croup	Croup is a respiratory condition that is usually triggered by an acute viral infection of the upper airway. The infection leads to swelling inside the throat, which interferes with normal breathing and produces the classical symptoms of a 'barking' cough, stridor, and hoarseness. It may produce mild, moderate, or severe symptoms, which often worsen at night.
Septic arthritis	Septic arthritis is the purulent invasion of a joint by an infectious agent which produces arthritis.

	People with artificial joints are more at risk than the general population but have slightly different symptoms, are infected with different organisms and require different treatment. Septic arthritis is considered a medical emergency.
Subglottic stenosis	Subglottic stenosis is a congenital or acquired narrowing of the subglottic airway. Although it is relatively rare, it is the third most common congenital airway problem (after laryngomalacia and vocal cord paralysis). Subglottic stenosis can present as a life-threatening airway emergency.
Tracheomalacia	Tracheomalacia is a condition characterized by flaccidity of the tracheal support cartilage which leads to tracheal collapse especially when increased airflow is demanded. The trachea normally dilates slightly during inspiration and narrows slightly during expiration. These processes are exaggerated in tracheomalacia, leading to airway collapse on expiration.
Tuberculosis	Tuberculosis, MTB or TB (short for tubercles bacillus) is a common and in some cases deadly infectious disease caused by various strains of mycobacteria, usually Mycobacterium tuberculosis in humans. Tuberculosis usually attacks the lungs but can also affect other parts of the body. It is spread through the air when people who have an active MTB infection cough, sneeze, or otherwise transmit their saliva through the air.
Gastroesophageal reflux	Gastroesophageal reflux disease (GERD), gastro-oesophageal reflux disease (GORD), gastric reflux disease, or acid reflux disease is defined as chronic symptoms or mucosal damage produced by the abnormal reflux in the oesophagus. This is commonly due to transient or permanent changes in the barrier between the oesophagus and the stomach. This can be due to incompetence of the lower esophageal sphincter, transient lower oesophageal sphincter relaxation, impaired expulsion of gastric reflux from the oesophagus, or a hiatal hernia.
Proton pump	A proton pump is an integral membrane protein that is capable of moving protons across a cell membrane, mitochondrion, or other organelle. In cell respiration, the pump actively transports protons from the matrix of the mitochondrion into the space between the inner and outer mitochondrial membranes. This action creates a concentration gradient across the inner mitochondrial membrane as there are more protons outside the matrix than in.
Vomiting	Vomiting is the forceful expulsion of the contents of one's stomach through the mouth and sometimes the nose.

Vomiting can be caused by a wide variety of conditions; it may present as a specific response to ailments like gastritis or poisoning, or as a non-specific sequela of disorders ranging from brain tumors and elevated intracranial pressure to overexposure to ionizing radiation. The feeling that one is about to vomit is called nausea, which usually precedes, but does not always lead to, vomiting.

Cerebral palsy

Cerebral palsy is an umbrella term encompassing a group of non-progressive, non-contagious motor conditions that cause physical disability in human development, chiefly in the various areas of body movement.

Cerebral refers to the cerebrum, which is the affected area of the brain (although the disorder most likely involves connections between the cortex and other parts of the brain such as the cerebellum), and palsy refers to disorder of movement. Furthermore, 'paralytic disorders' are not cerebral palsy - the condition of quadriplegia, therefore, should not be confused with spastic quadriplegia, nor tardive dyskinesia with dyskinetic cerebral palsy, nor diplegia with spastic diplegia, and so on.

Biliary dyskinesia

Biliary dyskinesia refers to altered tonus of the sphincter of Oddi , disturbance in the coordination of contraction of the biliary ducts, and/or reduction in the speed of emptying of the biliary tree.

Failure of the biliary sphincter can be distinguished from the pancreatic sphincter.

Laparoscopic cholecystectomy has been used to treat the condition.

Binge eating

Binge eating is a pattern of disordered eating which consists of episodes of uncontrollable eating. It is sometimes as a symptom of binge eating disorder or compulsive overeating disorder. During such binges, a person rapidly consumes an excessive amount of food.

Binge eating disorder

Binge eating disorder is the most common eating disorder in the United States affecting 3.5% of females and 2% of males and is prevalent in up to 30% of those seeking weight loss treatment. Although it is not yet classified as a separate eating disorder, it was first described in 1959 by psychiatrist and researcher Albert Stunkard as 'Night Eating Syndrome' (NES), and the term 'Binge Eating Disorder' was coined to describe the same binging-type eating behavior without the exclusive nocturnal component. BED usually leads to obesity although it can occur in normal weight individuals.

Bulimia nervosa

Bulimia nervosa is an eating disorder characterized by binge eating and purging or consuming a large amount of food in a short amount of time, followed by an attempt to rid oneself of the food consumed, usually by purging (vomiting) and/or by laxative, diuretics or excessive exercise. Bulimia nervosa is considered to be less life threatening than anorexia, however the occurrence of bulimia nervosa is higher.

Chapter 3. COMMON PRESENTING SIGNS, SYMPTOMS, DIFFERENTIAL DIAGNOSIS

Cyclic vomiting syndrome	Cyclic vomiting syndrome are recurring attacks of intense nausea, vomiting and sometimes abdominal pain and/or headaches or migraines. Cyclic vomiting usually develops during childhood usually ages 3-7; although it often remits during adolescence, it can persist into adult life. The average age at onset is 3-7 years, but CVS has been seen in infants who are as young as 6 days and in adults who are as old as 73 years.
Eating disorder	Eating disorders refer to a group of conditions defined by abnormal eating habits that may involve either insufficient or excessive food intake to the detriment of an individual's physical and mental health. Bulimia nervosa, anorexia nervosa, and binge eating disorder are the most common specific forms in the United Kingdom. Though primarily thought of as affecting females (an estimated 5-10 million being affected in the U.K)., eating disorders affect males as well Template:An estimated 10 - 15% of people with eating disorders are males (Gorgan, 1999).
Sphincter of Oddi dysfunction	The sphincter of Oddi is a muscular valve that controls the flow of digestive juices (bile and pancreatic juice) through the ampulla of Vater into the first part of the small intestine (duodenum). Sphincter of Oddi dysfunction (SOD) describes the situation when the sphincter does not relax at the appropriate time, due to scarring or spasm. The back-up of juices causes episodes of severe abdominal pain.
Beta-adrenergic agonist	Beta-adrenergic agonists are adrenergic agonists which act upon the beta receptors. β_1 agonists β_1 agonists: stimulates adenylyl cyclase activity; opening of calcium channel. (cardiac stimulants; used to treat cardiogenic shock, acute heart failure, bradyarrhythmias).
Wheezing	A wheeze is a continuous, coarse, whistling sound produced in the respiratory airways during breathing. For wheezes to occur, some part of the respiratory tree must be narrowed or obstructed, or airflow velocity within the respiratory tree must be heightened. wheezing is commonly experienced by persons with a lung disease; the most common cause of recurrent wheezing is asthma attacks.
Biliary atresia	Biliary atresia is a congenital or acquired disease of the liver and one of the principal forms of chronic rejection of a transplanted liver allograft. As a birth defect in newborn infants, it has an occurrence of 1/10,000 to 1/15,000 cases in live births in the United States. In the congenital form, the common bile duct between the liver and the small intestine is blocked or absent.

Hepatitis	Hepatitis is a medical condition defined by the inflammation of the liver and characterized by the presence of inflammatory cells in the tissue of the organ. The name is from the Greek hepar , the root being hepat- , meaning liver, and suffix -itis, meaning 'inflammation' (c. 1727). The condition can be self-limiting (healing on its own) or can progress to fibrosis (scarring) and cirrhosis.
Hepatoblastoma	Hepatoblastoma is an uncommon malignant liver neoplasm occurring in infants and children and composed of tissue resembling fetal or mature liver cells or bile ducts. Affecting 1 in 1.5 million. They are usually present with an abdominal mass.
Hepatocellular carcinoma	Hepatocellular carcinoma is the most common type of liver cancer. Most cases of HCC are secondary to either a viral hepatitis infection (hepatitis B or C) or cirrhosis (alcoholism being the most common cause of hepatic cirrhosis). Compared to other cancers, HCC is quite a rare tumor in the United States.
Liver failure	Liver failure is the inability of the liver to perform its normal synthetic and metabolic function as part of normal physiology. Two forms are recognised, acute and chronic. Acute liver failure is defined as 'the rapid development of hepatocellular dysfunction, specifically coagulopathy and mental status changes (encephalopathy) in a patient without known prior liver disease'.
Infectious hepatitis	Hepatitis A (formerly known as Infectious hepatitis) is an acute infectious disease of the liver caused by the hepatitis A virus (HAV), which is most commonly transmitted by the fecal-oral route via contaminated food or drinking water. Every year, approximately 10 million people worldwide are infected with the virus. The time between infection and the appearance of the symptoms, (the incubation period), is between two and six weeks and the average incubation period is 28 days.
Alagille syndrome	Alagille syndrome is a genetic disorder that affects the liver, heart, kidney, and other systems of the body. Problems associated with the disorder generally become evident in infancy or early childhood. The disorder is inherited in an autosomal dominant pattern, and the estimated prevalence of Alagille syndrome is 1 in every 100,000 live births.
Autoimmune hepatitis	Autoimmune Hepatitis is a disease of the liver that occurs when the body's immune system attacks cells of the liver. Anomalous presentation of human leukocyte antigen (HLA) class II on the surface of hepatocytes, possibly due to genetic predisposition or acute liver infection, causes a cell-mediated immune response against the body's own liver, resulting in autoimmune hepatitis.

Chapter 3. COMMON PRESENTING SIGNS, SYMPTOMS, DIFFERENTIAL DIAGNOSIS

Crigler-Najjar syndrome	Crigler-Najjar syndrome or CNS is a rare disorder affecting the metabolism of bilirubin, a chemical formed from the breakdown of blood. The disorder results in an inherited form of non-hemolytic jaundice, often leading to brain damage in infants. This syndrome is divided into two types: type I and type II, which is sometimes called Arias syndrome.
Cystic fibrosis	Cystic fibrosis is an autosomal recessive genetic disorder affecting most critically the lungs, and also the pancreas, liver, and intestine. It is characterized by abnormal transport of chloride and sodium across an epithelium, leading to thick, viscous secretions. The name cystic fibrosis refers to the characteristic scarring (fibrosis) and cyst formation within the pancreas, first recognized in the 1930s.
Hyperbilirubinemia	Jaundice, also known as icterus (attributive adjective: icteric), is a yellowish discoloration of the skin, the conjunctival membranes over the sclerae (whites of the eyes), and other mucous membranes caused by hyperbilirubinemia. This hyperbilirubinemia subsequently causes increased levels of bilirubin in the extracellular fluids. Typically, the concentration of bilirubin in the plasma must exceed 1.5 mg/dL, three times the usual value of approximately 0.5 mg/dL, for the coloration to be easily visible.
Cardiac output	Cardiac output is the volume of blood being pumped by the heart, in particular by a left or right ventricle in the time interval of one minute. CO may be measured in many ways, for example dm^3/min (1 dm^3 equals 1000 cm^3 or 1 litre). Q is furthermore the combined sum of output from the right ventricle and the output from the left ventricle during the phase of systole of the heart.
Distributive shock	Distributive shock is defined by hypotension and generalized tissular hypoxia. This form of relative hypovolemia is the result of blood vessel dilation. Septic shock is the major cause, but there are other examples as well.
Septic shock	Septic shock is a medical condition as a result of severe infection and sepsis, though the microbe may be systemic or localized to a particular site. It can cause multiple organ dysfunction syndrome (formerly known as multiple organ failure) and death. Its most common victims are children, immunocompromised individuals, and the elderly, as their immune systems cannot deal with the infection as effectively as those of healthy adults.
Stroke volume	In cardiovascular physiology, stroke volume is the volume of blood pumped from one ventricle of the heart with each beat. SV is calculated using measurements of ventricle volumes from an echocardiogram and subtracting the volume of the blood in the ventricle at the end of a beat (called end-systolic volume) from the volume of blood just prior to the beat (called end-diastolic volume).

Distributive	In mathematics, and in particular in abstract algebra, distributivity is a property of binary operations that generalises the distributive law from elementary algebra. For example: $2 \times (1 + 3) = (2 \times 1) + (2 \times 3)$. In the left-hand side of the above equation, the 2 multiplies the sum of 1 and 3; on the right-hand side, it multiplies the 1 and the 3 individually, with the results added afterwards.
Anaphylactic shock	Anaphylactic shock, the most severe type of anaphylaxis, occurs when an allergic response triggers a quick release of large quantities of immunological mediators (histamines, prostaglandins, and leukotrienes) from mast cells, leading to systemic vasodilation (associated with a sudden drop in blood pressure) and edema of bronchial mucosa (resulting in bronchoconstriction and difficulty breathing.) Anaphylactic shock can lead to death in a matter of minutes if left untreated. Due in part to the variety of definitions, an estimated 1.24% to 16.8% of the population of the United States is considered 'at risk' for having an anaphylactic reaction if they are exposed to one or more allergens, especially penicillin and insect stings.
Cardiogenic shock	Cardiogenic shock is based upon an inadequate circulation of blood due to primary failure of the ventricles of the heart to function effectively. Since this is a type of shock there is insufficient perfusion of tissue (i.e. the heart) to meet the required demands for oxygen and nutrients. Cardiogenic shock is a largely irreversible condition and as such is more often fatal than not.
Neurogenic shock	Neurogenic shock is a distributive type of shock resulting in hypotension, occasionally with bradycardia, that is attributed to the disruption of the autonomic pathways within the spinal cord. Hypotension occurs due to decreased systemic vascular resistance resulting in pooling of blood within the extremities lacking sympathetic tone. Bradycardia results from unopposed vagal activity and has been found to be exacerbated by hypoxia and endobronchial suction.

Chapter 3. COMMON PRESENTING SIGNS, SYMPTOMS, DIFFERENTIAL DIAGNOSIS

1. Etiology is the study of causation, or origination.

   The word is most commonly used in medical and philosophical theories, where it is used to refer to the study of why things occur, or even the reasons behind the way that things act, and is used in philosophy, physics, psychology, government, medicine, theology and biology in reference to the causes of various phenomena. An _____ is a myth intended to explain a name or create a mythic history for a place or family.

   a. Etiology
   b. abdominal exam
   c. Etiological myth
   d. Gray platelet syndrome

2. _____ is a heterocyclic aromatic chemical compound with the molecular formula $C_{16}H_{18}N_3SCl$. It has many uses in a range of different fields, such as biology and chemistry. At room temperature it appears as a solid, odorless, dark green powder, that yields a blue solution when dissolved in water.

   a. Nantenine
   b. Physostigmine
   c. Methylene blue
   d. Prednisolone/promethazine

3. _____ literally means joint pain; it is a symptom of injury, infection, illnesses (in particular arthritis) or an allergic reaction to medication.

   According to MeSH, the term '_____' should only be used when the condition is non-inflammatory, and the term 'arthritis' should be used when the condition is inflammatory. Diagnosis and causes

   Diagnosis involves interviewing the patient and performing physical exams.

   a. Asia Pacific League of Associations for Rheumatology
   b. Arthralgia
   c. Overlap syndrome
   d. Blennorrhea

4. An _____ is any localized enlargement or swelling in the human abdomen. Depending on its location, the _____ may be caused by an enlarged liver (hepatomegaly), enlarged spleen (splenomegaly), protruding kidney, a pancreatic mass, a retroperitoneal mass (a mass in the posterior of the peritoneum), an abdominal aortic aneurysm, or various tumours, such as those caused by abdominal carcinomatosis and omental metastasis. The treatments depend on the cause, and may range from watchful waiting to radical surgery.

   a. Acanthosis nigricans
   b. Abdominal mass
   c. Ecchymosis
   d. Elfin facies

5. _____ is defined by an elevated sodium level in the blood. _____ is generally not caused by an excess of sodium, but rather by a relative deficit of free water in the body. For this reason, _____ is often synonymous with the less precise term, dehydration.

    a. Hyperphosphatemia
    b. Hypervolemia
    c. Hypernatremia
    d. Hypocalcaemia

1. c
2. c
3. b
4. b
5. c

You can take the complete Chapter Practice Test

for Chapter 3. COMMON PRESENTING SIGNS, SYMPTOMS, DIFFERENTIAL DIAGNOSIS
on all key terms, persons, places, and concepts.

Online 99 Cents

http://www.epub219.49.13357.3.cram101.com/

Use www.Cram101.com for all your study needs

including Cram101's online interactive problem solving labs in

chemistry, statistics, mathematics, and more.

Mechanical ventilation

Orthostatic intolerance

Syncope

Differential diagnosis

Pathophysiology

Beta-adrenergic agonist

Anorexia nervosa

Atrial fibrillation

Atrial flutter

Wolff-Parkinson-White syndrome

Atrial tachycardia

Heart disease

Rheumatic fever

Sinus tachycardia

Superior vena cava syndrome

22q11.2 deletion syndrome

Dilated cardiomyopathy

Supraventricular tachycardia

Radiation therapy

Chapter 4. CARDIOVASCULAR

_____ | Catheter ablation

_____ | Heart failure

_____ | Ventricular tachycardia

_____ | Etiological myth

_____ | Cardiovascular physiology

_____ | Hypertrophic cardiomyopathy

_____ | Trichomonas vaginalis

_____ | Intensive care

_____ | Palliative care

_____ | Atrial septal defect

_____ | Patent ductus arteriosus

_____ | Ventricular septal defect

_____ | Ductus arteriosus

_____ | Atrioventricular septal defect

_____ | Down syndrome

_____ | Heart defect

_____ | Pulmonic stenosis

_____ | Aortic valve

_____ | Bicuspid aortic valve

CHAPTER OUTLINE: KEY TERMS, PEOPLE, PLACES, CONCEPTS

Mitral valve

Williams syndrome

Lactic acid

Tetralogy of Fallot

Deletion

Venous return

Hyperoxia test

Postpericardiotomy syndrome

Pulmonary hypertension

Bronchopulmonary dysplasia

Cardiomyopathy

Restrictive cardiomyopathy

Chest radiograph

Pericarditis

Prognosis

Myocarditis

Diabetes mellitus

Abdominal mass

Life support

Endocarditis

Metabolic acidosis

Blood pressure

Hypoxic hypoxia

Oxygen saturation

Symptom

Carbon monoxide

Carbon monoxide poisoning

Selective serotonin reuptake inhibitor

Heart rate

Cardiogenic shock

Kawasaki disease

Vascular resistance

Distributive shock

Disease

Septic shock

Histotoxic hypoxia

Mechanical ventilation	In medicine, mechanical ventilation is a method to mechanically assist or replace spontaneous breathing. This may involve a machine called a ventilator or the breathing may be assisted by a physician, respiratory therapist or other suitable person compressing a bag or set of bellows. Traditionally divided into negative-pressure ventilation, where air is essentially sucked into the lungs, or positive pressure ventilation, where air is pushed into the trachea.
Orthostatic intolerance	Orthostatic intolerance is defined as 'the development of symptoms during upright standing relieved by recumbency,' or by sitting back down again. There are many types of orthostatic intolerance. OI can be a subcategory of dysautonomia, a disorder of the autonomic nervous system occurring when an individual stands up.
Syncope	Syncope , the medical term for fainting, is precisely defined as a transient loss of consciousness and postural tone characterized by rapid onset, short duration, and spontaneous recovery due to global cerebral hypoperfusion that most often results from hypotension.
	Many forms of syncope are preceded by a prodromal state that often includes dizziness and loss of vision ('blackout') (temporary), loss of hearing (temporary), loss of pain and feeling (temporary), nausea and abdominal discomfort, weakness, sweating, a feeling of heat, palpitations and other phenomena, which, if they do not progress to loss of consciousness and postural tone are often denoted 'presyncope'. Abdominal discomfort prior to loss of consciousness may be indicative of seizure which should be considered different than syncope.
Differential diagnosis	A differential diagnosis is a systematic diagnostic method used to identify the presence of an entity where multiple alternatives are possible (and the process may be termed differential diagnostic procedure), and may also refer to any of the included candidate alternatives (which may also be termed candidate condition). This method is essentially a process of elimination, or at least, rendering of the probabilities of candidate conditions to negligible levels. In this sense, probabilities are, in fact, imaginative parameters in the mind or hardware of the diagnostician or system, while in reality the target (such as a patient) either has a condition or not with an actual probability of either 0 or 100%.
Pathophysiology	Pathophysiology sample values
	Pathophysiology is the study of the changes of normal mechanical, physical, and biochemical functions, either caused by a disease, or resulting from an abnormal syndrome. More formally, it is the branch of medicine which deals with any disturbances of body functions, caused by disease or prodromal symptoms.
	An alternative definition is 'the study of the biological and physical manifestations of disease as they correlate with the underlying abnormalities and physiological disturbances.'

Chapter 4. CARDIOVASCULAR

Beta-adrenergic agonist	Beta-adrenergic agonists are adrenergic agonists which act upon the beta receptors. β_1 agonists β_1 agonists: stimulates adenylyl cyclase activity; opening of calcium channel. (cardiac stimulants; used to treat cardiogenic shock, acute heart failure, bradyarrhythmias).
Anorexia nervosa	The differential diagnoses of anorexia nervosa (AN) include various medical and psychological conditions which may be misdiagnosed as (AN), in some cases these conditions may be comorbid with anorexia nervosa (AN). The misdiagnosis of AN is not uncommon. In one instance a case of achalasia was misdiagnosed as AN and the patient spent two months confined to a psychiatric hospital.
Atrial fibrillation	Atrial fibrillation is the most common cardiac arrhythmia (irregular heart beat). It may cause no symptoms, but it is often associated with palpitations, fainting, chest pain, or congestive heart failure. However, in some people atrial fibrillation is caused by otherwise idiopathic or benign conditions.
Atrial flutter	Atrial flutter is an abnormal heart rhythm that occurs in the atria of the heart. When it first occurs, it is usually associated with a fast heart rate or tachycardia (beats over 100 per minute), and falls into the category of supra-ventricular tachycardias. While this rhythm occurs most often in individuals with cardiovascular disease (e.g. hypertension, coronary artery disease, and cardiomyopathy) and diabetes, it may occur spontaneously in people with otherwise normal hearts.
Wolff-Parkinson-White syndrome	Wolff-Parkinson-White syndrome is a syndrome of pre-excitation of the ventricles of the heart due to an accessory pathway known as the bundle of Kent. This accessory pathway is an abnormal electrical communication from the atria to the ventricles. WPW is a type of atrioventricular reentrant tachycardia.
Atrial tachycardia	Atrial tachycardia is a type of atrial arrhythmia in which the heart's electrical impulse comes from an ectopic atrial pacemaker rather than from the SA node. Atrial tachycardias are characterized by very regular rates ranging from 140-220 bpm. One form is multifocal atrial tachycardia.
Heart disease	Heart disease is an umbrella term for a variety of diseases affecting the heart. As of 2007, it is the leading cause of death in the United States, England, Canada and Wales, accounting for 25.4% of the total deaths in the United States.

Coronary heart disease refers to the failure of the coronary circulation to supply adequate circulation to cardiac muscle and surrounding tissue. Coronary heart disease is most commonly equated with Coronary artery disease although coronary heart disease can be due to other causes, such as coronary vasospasm.

Rheumatic fever	Rheumatic fever is an inflammatory disease that occurs following a Streptococcus pyogenes infection, such as streptococcal pharyngitis or scarlet fever. Believed to be caused by antibody cross-reactivity that can involve the heart, joints, skin, and brain, the illness typically develops two to three weeks after a streptococcal infection. Acute rheumatic fever commonly appears in children between the ages of 6 and 15, with only 20% of first-time attacks occurring in adults.
Sinus tachycardia	Sinus tachycardia is a heart rhythm with elevated rate of impulses originating from the sinoatrial node, defined as a rate greater than 100 beats/min in an average adult. The normal heart rate in the average adult ranges from 60-100 beats/min. Note that the normal heart rate varies with age, with infants having normal heart rate of 110-150 bpm to the elderly, who have slower normals.
Superior vena cava syndrome	Superior vena cava syndrome or superior vena cava obstruction (SVCO), is usually the result of the direct obstruction of the superior vena cava by malignancies such as compression of the vessel wall by right upper lobe tumors or thymoma and/or mediastinal lymphadenopathy. The most common malignancies that cause SVCS is bronchogenic carcinoma. Cerebral edema is rare, but if it occurs it may be fatal.
22q11.2 deletion syndrome	22q11.2 deletion syndrome, also known as DiGeorge syndrome, DiGeorge anomaly, velo-cardio-facial syndrome, Shprintzen syndrome, conotruncal anomaly face syndrome, Strong syndrome, congenital thymic aplasia, and thymic hypoplasia is a syndrome caused by the deletion of a small piece of chromosome 22. The deletion occurs near the middle of the chromosome at a location designated q11.2 i.e., on the long arm of one of the pair of chromosomes 22. It has a prevalence estimated at 1:4000. The syndrome was described in 1968 by the pediatric endocrinologist Angelo DiGeorge. The features of this syndrome vary widely, even among members of the same family, and affect many parts of the body. Characteristic signs and symptoms may include birth defects such as congenital heart disease, defects in the palate, most commonly related to neuromuscular problems with closure (velo-pharyngeal insufficiency), learning disabilities, mild differences in facial features, and recurrent infections.
Dilated cardiomyopathy	Dilated cardiomyopathy is a condition in which the heart becomes weakened and enlarged and cannot pump blood efficiently. The decreased heart function can affect the lungs, liver, and other body systems.

Chapter 4. CARDIOVASCULAR

Supraventricular tachycardia	Supraventricular tachycardia is a general term that refers to any rapid heart rhythm originating above the ventricular tissue. Supraventricular tachycardias can be contrasted to the potentially more dangerous ventricular tachycardias - rapid rhythms that originate within the ventricular tissue. Although technically an SVT can be due to any supraventricular cause, the term is often used by clinicians to refer to one specific cause of SVT, namely Paroxysmal supraventricular tachycardia.
Radiation therapy	Radiation therapy, radiation oncology, or radiotherapy (in the UK, Canada and Australia), sometimes abbreviated to XRT or DXT, is the medical use of ionizing radiation, generally as part of cancer treatment to control or kill malignant cells. Radiation therapy may be curative in a number of types of cancer if they are localized to one area of the body. It may also be used as part of curative therapy, to prevent tumor recurrence after surgery to remove a primary malignant tumor (for example, early stages of breast cancer).
Catheter ablation	Catheter ablation is an invasive procedure used to remove a faulty electrical pathway from the hearts of those who are prone to developing cardiac arrhythmias such as atrial fibrillation, atrial flutter, supraventricular tachycardias (SVT) and Wolff-Parkinson-White syndrome. It involves advancing several flexible catheters into the patient's blood vessels, usually either in the femoral vein, internal jugular vein, or subclavian vein. The catheters are then advanced towards the heart and high-frequency electrical impulses are used to induce the arrhythmia, and then ablate (destroy) the abnormal tissue that is causing it.
Heart failure	Heart failure often called congestive heart failure or congestive cardiac failure (CCF) is the inability of the heart to provide sufficient pump action to distribute blood flow to meet the needs of the body. Heart failure can cause a number of symptoms including shortness of breath, leg swelling, and exercise intolerance. The condition is diagnosed with echocardiography and blood tests.
Ventricular tachycardia	Ventricular tachycardia is a tachycardia, or fast heart rhythm, that originates in one of the ventricles of the heart. This is a potentially life-threatening arrhythmia because it may lead to ventricular fibrillation, asystole, and sudden death. Ventricular tachycardia can be classified based on its morphology:•Monomorphic ventricular tachycardia means that the appearance of all the beats match each other in each lead of a surface electrocardiogram (ECG).
Etiological myth	Etiology is the study of causation, or origination.

	The word is most commonly used in medical and philosophical theories, where it is used to refer to the study of why things occur, or even the reasons behind the way that things act, and is used in philosophy, physics, psychology, government, medicine, theology and biology in reference to the causes of various phenomena. An etiological myth is a myth intended to explain a name or create a mythic history for a place or family.
Cardiovascular physiology	Cardiovascular physiology is the study of the circulatory system. More specifically, it addresses the physiology of the heart ('cardio') and blood vessels ('vascular').
	These subjects are sometimes addressed separately, under the names cardiac physiology and circulatory physiology.
Hypertrophic cardiomyopathy	Hypertrophic cardiomyopathy is a disease of the myocardium (the muscle of the heart) in which a portion of the myocardium is hypertrophied (thickened) without any obvious cause. It is perhaps most well known as a leading cause of sudden cardiac death in young athletes. The occurrence of hypertrophic cardiomyopathy is a significant cause of sudden unexpected cardiac death in any age group and as a cause of disabling cardiac symptoms.
Trichomonas vaginalis	Trichomonas vaginalis is an anaerobic, flagellated protozoan, a form of microorganism. The parasitic microorganism is the causative agent of trichomoniasis, and is the most common pathogenic protozoan infection of humans in industrialized countries. Infection rates between men and women are the same with women showing symptoms while infections in men are usually asymptomatic.
Intensive care	intensive care medicine or critical care medicine is a branch of medicine concerned with the provision of life support or organ support systems in patients who are critically ill and who usually require intensive monitoring.
	Patients requiring intensive care may require support for hemodynamic instability (hypertension/hypotension), airway or respiratory compromise (such as ventilator support), acute renal failure, potentially lethal cardiac arrhythmias, or the cumulative effects of multiple organ system failure. They may also be admitted for intensive/invasive monitoring, such as the crucial hours after major surgery when deemed too unstable to transfer to a less intensively monitored unit.
Palliative care	Palliative care is an area of healthcare that focuses on relieving and preventing the suffering of patients. Unlike hospice care, palliative medicine is appropriate for patients in all disease stages, including those undergoing treatment for curable illnesses and those living with chronic diseases, as well as patients who are nearing the end of life.

Chapter 4. CARDIOVASCULAR

Atrial septal defect	Atrial septal defect is a form of congenital heart defect that enables blood flow between the left and right atria via the interatrial septum. The interatrial septum is the tissue that divides the right and left atria. Without this septum, or if there is a defect in this septum, it is possible for blood to travel from the left side of the heart to the right side of the heart, or vice versa.
Patent ductus arteriosus	Patent ductus arteriosus is a congenital disorder in the heart wherein a neonate's ductus arteriosus fails to close after birth. Early symptoms are uncommon, but in the first year of life include increased work of breathing and poor weight gain. With age, the PDA may lead to congestive heart failure if left uncorrected.
Ventricular septal defect	A ventricular septal defect is a defect in the ventricular septum, the wall dividing the left and right ventricles of the heart. The ventricular septum consists of an inferior muscular and superior membranous portion and is extensively innervated with conducting cardiomyocytes. The membranous portion, which is close to the atrioventricular node, is most commonly affected in adults and older children in the United States.
Ductus arteriosus	In the developing fetus, the ductus arteriosus also called the ductus Botalli, is a blood vessel connecting the pulmonary artery to the aortic arch. It allows most of the blood from the right ventricle to bypass the fetus's fluid-filled non-functioning lungs. Upon closure at birth, it becomes the ligamentum arteriosum.
Atrioventricular septal defect	Atrioventricular septal defect or atrioventricular canal defect (AVCD), previously known as 'common atrioventricular canal' (CAVC) or 'endocardial cushion defect', is characterized by a deficiency of the atrioventricular septum of the heart. It is caused by an abnormal or inadequate fusion of the superior and inferior endocardial cushions with the mid portion of the atrial septum and the muscular portion of the ventricular septum. A variety of different classifications have been used, but the defects are usefully divided into 'partial' and 'complete' forms.
Down syndrome	Down syndrome, also known as trisomy 21, is a chromosomal condition caused by the presence of all or part of a third copy of chromosome 21. It is named after John Langdon Down, the British physician who described the syndrome in 1866. The condition was clinically described earlier in the 19th century by Jean Etienne Dominique Esquirol in 1838 and Edouard Seguin in 1844. Down syndrome was identified as a chromosome 21 trisomy by Dr. Jérôme Lejeune in 1959. Down syndrome can be identified in a baby at birth, or by prenatal screening.

The CDC estimates that about one of every 691 babies born in the United States each year is born with Down syndrome. Down syndrome occurs in all human populations, and analogous conditions have been found in other species such as chimpanzees.

| Heart defect | A congenital Heart defect (C Heart defect) is a defect in the structure of the heart and great vessels of a newborn. Most Heart defect s either obstruct blood flow in the heart or vessels near it or cause blood to flow through the heart in an abnormal pattern, although other defects affecting heart rhythm (such as long QT syndrome) can also occur. Heart defect s are among the most common birth defects and are the leading cause of birth defect-related deaths. |

| Pulmonic stenosis | Pulmonic stenosis, is a dynamic or fixed obstruction to flow from the right ventricle of the heart to the pulmonary artery. It is usually first diagnosed in childhood. Pulmonic stenosis is usually due to isolated valvular obstruction (Pulmonary valve stenosis), but may be due to subvalvular or supravalvular (Stenosis of pulmonary artery) obstruction. |

| Aortic valve | The aortic valve is one of the valves of the heart. It is normally tricuspid (with three leaflets), although in 1% of the population it is found to be congenitally bicuspid (two leaflets). It lies between the left ventricle and the aorta. |

| Bicuspid aortic valve | A bicuspid aortic valve is most commonly a congenital condition of the aortic valve where two of the aortic valvular leaflets fuse during development resulting in a valve that is bicuspid instead of the normal tricuspid configuration. Normally the only cardiac valve that is bicuspid is the mitral valve (bicuspid valve) which is situated between the left atrium and left ventricle. Cardiac valves play a crucial role in ensuring the unidirectional flow of blood from the atrium to the ventricles, or the ventricle to the aorta or pulmonary trunk. |

| Mitral valve | The mitral valve is a dual-flap valve in the heart that lies between the left atrium (LA) and the left ventricle (LV). The mitral valve and the tricuspid valve are known collectively as the atrioventricular valves because they lie between the atria and the ventricles of the heart and control the flow of blood.

During diastole, a normally-functioning mitral valve opens as a result of increased pressure from the left atrium as it fills with blood (preloading). |

| Williams syndrome | Williams syndrome is a rare neurodevelopmental disorder characterized by a distinctive, 'elfin' facial appearance, along with a low nasal bridge; an unusually cheerful demeanor and ease with strangers; developmental delay coupled with strong language skills; and cardiovascular problems, such as supravalvular aortic stenosis and transient hypercalcaemia.

It is caused by a deletion of about 26 genes from the long arm of chromosome 7. |

The syndrome was first identified in 1961 by Dr. J. C. P. Williams of New Zealand and has an estimated prevalence of 1 in 7,500 to 1 in 20,000 births.

Signs and symptoms

The most common symptoms of Williams syndrome are mental disability, heart defects, and unusual facial features.

Lactic acid	Lactic acid, is a chemical compound that plays a role in various biochemical processes and was first isolated in 1780 by the Swedish chemist Carl Wilhelm Scheele. Lactic acid is a carboxylic acid with the chemical formula $C_3H_6O_3$. It has a hydroxyl group adjacent to the carboxyl group, making it an alpha hydroxy acid (AHA).
Tetralogy of Fallot	Tetralogy of Fallot is a congenital heart defect which is classically understood to involve four anatomical abnormalities (although only three of them are always present). It is the most common cyanotic heart defect, and the most common cause of blue baby syndrome. It was described in 1672 by Niels Stensen, in 1773 by Edward Sandifort, and in 1888 by the French physician Étienne-Louis Arthur Fallot, after whom it is named.
Deletion	In genetics, a deletion (also called gene deletion, deficiency, or deletion mutation) (sign: Δ) is a mutation (a genetic aberration) in which a part of a chromosome or a sequence of DNA is missing. Deletion is the loss of genetic material. Any number of nucleotides can be deleted, from a single base to an entire piece of chromosome.
Venous return	Venous return is the rate of blood flow back to the heart. It normally limits cardiac output. Superimposition of the cardiac function curve and venous return curve is used in one hemodynamic model. Venous return (VR) is the flow of blood back to the heart. Under steady-state conditions, venous return must equal cardiac output (CO) when averaged over time because the cardiovascular system is essentially a closed loop. Otherwise, blood would accumulate in either the systemic or pulmonary circulations. Although cardiac output and venous return are interdependent, each can be independently regulated.
Hyperoxia test	A hyperoxia test is a test that is performed--usually on an infant-- to determine whether the patient's cyanosis is due to lung disease or a problem with blood circulation. It is performed by measuring the arterial blood gases of the patient while he breathes room air, then re-measuring the blood gases after the patient has breathed 100% oxygen for 10 minutes.

Postpericardiotomy syndrome	Postpericardiotomy syndrome is a medical syndrome referring to an immune phenomenon that occurs days to months (usually 1-6 weeks) after surgical incision of the pericardium . PPS can also be caused after a trauma, a puncture of the cardiac or pleural structures (such as a bullet or stab wound), after percutaneous coronary intervention (such as stent placement after a myocardial infarction or heart attack), or due to pacemaker or pacemaker wire placement. Signs & Symptoms

The typical signs of post-pericartiotomy syndrome include fever, pleuritis (with possible pleural effusion), pericarditis (with possible pericardial effusion), occasional but rare pulmonary infiltrates, and fatigue. |
Pulmonary hypertension	In medicine, pulmonary hypertension is an increase in blood pressure in the pulmonary artery, pulmonary vein, or pulmonary capillaries, together known as the lung vasculature, leading to shortness of breath, dizziness, fainting, and other symptoms, all of which are exacerbated by exertion. Pulmonary hypertension can be a severe disease with a markedly decreased exercise tolerance and heart failure. It was first identified by Dr. Ernst von Romberg in 1891. According to the most recent classification, it can be one of five different types: arterial, venous, hypoxic, thromboembolic or miscellaneous.
Bronchopulmonary dysplasia	Bronchopulmonary dysplasia is a chronic lung disorder that is most common among children who were born prematurely, with low birthweights and who received prolonged mechanical ventilation to treat respiratory distress syndrome. The classic diagnosis of BPD may be assigned at 28 days of life if the following criteria are met (Bureau of Maternal and Child Health, 1989): (1) Positive pressure ventilation during the first 2 weeks of life for a minimum of 3 days.(2) Clinical signs of abnormal respiratory function.(3) Requirements for supplemental oxygen for longer than 28 days of age to maintain PaO2 above 50 mm Hg.(4) Chest radiograph with diffuse abnormal findings characteristic of BPD.
Cardiomyopathy	Cardiomyopathy is the measurable deterioration of the function of the myocardium (the heart muscle) for any reason, usually leading to heart failure; common symptoms are dyspnea (breathlessness) and peripheral edema (swelling of the legs). People with cardiomyopathy are often at risk of dangerous forms of irregular heart beat and sudden cardiac death. The most common form of cardiomyopathy is dilated cardiomyopathy.
Restrictive cardiomyopathy	Restrictive cardiomyopathy (a.k.a. Obliterative cardiomyopathy, once known as 'constrictive cardiomyopathy') is a form of cardiomyopathy in which the walls are rigid, and the heart is restricted from stretching and filling with blood properly.

It is the least common of Goodwin's three original subtypes of cardiomyopathy, which includes hypertrophic and dilated as well as restrictive. |

Chapter 4. CARDIOVASCULAR

Chest radiograph	In medicine, a chest radiograph, commonly called a chest X-ray (CXR), is a projection radiograph of the chest used to diagnose conditions affecting the chest, its contents, and nearby structures. Chest radiographs are among the most common films taken, being diagnostic of many conditions. Like all methods of radiography, chest radiography employs ionizing radiation in the form of X-rays to generate images of the chest.
Pericarditis	Pericarditis is an inflammation of the pericardium (the fibrous sac surrounding the heart). A characteristic chest pain is often present. The causes of pericarditis are varied, including viral infections of the pericardium, idiopathic causes, uremic pericarditis, bacterial infections of the pericardium (e.g., Mycobacterium tuberculosis), post-infarct pericarditis or Dressler's pericarditis.
Prognosis	Prognosis is a medical term to describe the likely outcome of an illness. When applied to large populations, prognostic estimates can be very accurate: for example the statement '45% of patients with severe septic shock will die within 28 days' can be made with some confidence, because previous research found that this proportion of patients died. However, it is much harder to translate this into a prognosis for an individual patient: additional information is needed to determine whether a patient belongs to the 45% who will succumb, or to the 55% who survive.
Myocarditis	Myocarditis is inflammation of heart muscle (myocardium). Myocarditis is most often due to infection by common viruses, such as parvovirus B19, less commonly nonviral pathogens such as Borrelia burgdorferi (Lyme disease) or Trypanosoma cruzi, or as a hypersensitivity response to drugs. The definition of myocarditis varies, but the central feature is an infection of the heart, with an inflammatory infiltrate, and damage to the heart muscle, without the blockage of coronary arteries that define a heart attack (myocardial infarction) or other common noninfectious causes.
Diabetes mellitus	Diabetes mellitus, often simply referred to as diabetes, is a group of metabolic diseases in which a person has high blood sugar, either because the body does not produce enough insulin, or because cells do not respond to the insulin that is produced. This high blood sugar produces the classical symptoms of polyuria (frequent urination), polydipsia (increased thirst) and polyphagia (increased hunger).

Abdominal mass	An abdominal mass is any localized enlargement or swelling in the human abdomen. Depending on its location, the abdominal mass may be caused by an enlarged liver (hepatomegaly), enlarged spleen (splenomegaly), protruding kidney, a pancreatic mass, a retroperitoneal mass (a mass in the posterior of the peritoneum), an abdominal aortic aneurysm, or various tumours, such as those caused by abdominal carcinomatosis and omental metastasis. The treatments depend on the cause, and may range from watchful waiting to radical surgery.
Life support	Life support in medicine is a broad term that applies to any therapy used to sustain a patient's life while they are critically ill or injured, as part of intensive-care medicine. There are many therapies and techniques that may be used by clinicians to achieve the goal of sustaining life. Some examples include:•Feeding tube•Total parenteral nutrition•Mechanical ventilation•Heart/Lung bypass•Urinary catheterization•Dialysis•Cardiopulmonary resuscitation•Defibrillation•Artificial pacemaker These techniques are applied most commonly in the Emergency Department, Intensive Care Unit and, Operating Rooms.
Endocarditis	Endocarditis is an inflammation of the inner layer of the heart, the endocardium. It usually involves the heart valves (native or prosthetic valves). Other structures that may be involved include the interventricular septum, the chordae tendineae, the mural endocardium, or even on intracardiac devices.
Metabolic acidosis	In medicine, metabolic acidosis is a condition that occurs when the body produces too much acid or when the kidneys are not removing enough acid from the body. If unchecked, metabolic acidosis leads to acidemia, i.e., blood pH is low (less than 7.35) due to increased production of hydrogen by the body or the inability of the body to form bicarbonate (HCO_3^-) in the kidney. Its causes are diverse, and its consequences can be serious, including coma and death.
Blood pressure	Blood pressure is the pressure exerted by circulating blood upon the walls of blood vessels, and is one of the principal vital signs. When used without further specification, 'blood pressure' usually refers to the arterial pressure of the systemic circulation. During each heartbeat, blood pressure varies between a maximum (systolic) and a minimum (diastolic) pressure.
Hypoxic hypoxia	Hypoxic hypoxia is a result of insufficient oxygen available to the lungs. A blocked airway, a drowning or a reduction in partial pressure (high altitude above 10,000 feet) are obvious examples of how lungs can be deprived of oxygen. Some medical examples are abnormal pulmonary function or respiratory obstruction, or a right-to-left shunt in the heart.
Oxygen saturation	Oxygen saturation is dissolved or carried in a given medium. It can be measured with a dissolved oxygen probe such as an oxygen sensor or an optode in liquid media, usually water.

	The standard unit is milligrams per litre, or mgL^{-1}
	Oxygen saturation can be measured regionally and non-invasively.
Symptom	A symptom is a departure from normal function or feeling which is noticed by a patient, indicating the presence of disease or abnormality. A symptom is subjective, observed by the patient, and not measured.
	A symptom may not be a malady, for example symptoms of pregnancy.
Carbon monoxide	Carbon monoxide also called carbonous oxide, is a colorless, odorless, and tasteless gas that is slightly lighter than air. It can be toxic to humans and animals when encountered in higher concentrations, although it is also produced in normal animal metabolism in low quantities, and is thought to have some normal biological functions. In the atmosphere however, it is short lived and spatially variable, since it combines with oxygen to form carbon dioxide and ozone.
Carbon monoxide poisoning	Carbon monoxide poisoning occurs after enough inhalation of carbon monoxide (CO). Carbon monoxide is a toxic gas, but, being colorless, odorless, tasteless, and initially non-irritating, it is very difficult for people to detect. Carbon monoxide is a product of incomplete combustion of organic matter due to insufficient oxygen supply to enable complete oxidation to carbon dioxide (CO_2).
Selective serotonin reuptake inhibitor	Selective serotonin reuptake inhibitors or serotonin-specific reuptake inhibitor are a class of compounds typically used as antidepressants in the treatment of depression, anxiety disorders, and some personality disorders. They are also typically effective and used in treating some cases of insomnia.
	Selective serotonin reuptake inhibitors are believed to increase the extracellular level of the neurotransmitter serotonin by inhibiting its reuptake into the presynaptic cell, increasing the level of serotonin in the synaptic cleft available to bind to the postsynaptic receptor.
Heart rate	Heart rate is the number of heartbeats per unit of time, typically expressed as beats per minute (bpm). Heart rate can vary as the body's need to absorb oxygen and excrete carbon dioxide changes, such as during exercise or sleep.
	The measurement of heart rate is used by medical professionals to assist in the diagnosis and tracking of medical conditions.
Cardiogenic shock	Cardiogenic shock is based upon an inadequate circulation of blood due to primary failure of the ventricles of the heart to function effectively.

Since this is a type of shock there is insufficient perfusion of tissue (i.e. the heart) to meet the required demands for oxygen and nutrients. Cardiogenic shock is a largely irreversible condition and as such is more often fatal than not.

Kawasaki disease	Kawasaki disease also known as Kawasaki syndrome, lymph node syndrome and mucocutaneous lymph node syndrome, is an autoimmune disease in which the medium-sized blood vessels throughout the body become inflamed. It is largely seen in children under five years of age. It affects many organ systems, mainly those including the blood vessels, skin, mucous membranes and lymph nodes; however its rare but most serious effect is on the heart where it can cause fatal coronary artery aneurysms in untreated children.
Vascular resistance	Vascular resistance is a term used to define the resistance to flow that must be overcome to push blood through the circulatory system. The resistance offered by the peripheral circulation is known as the systemic vascular resistance while the resistance offered by the vasculature of the lungs is known as the pulmonary vascular resistance. The systemic vascular resistance may also be referred to as the total peripheral resistance.
Distributive shock	Distributive shock is defined by hypotension and generalized tissular hypoxia. This form of relative hypovolemia is the result of blood vessel dilation. Septic shock is the major cause, but there are other examples as well.
Disease	A disease is an abnormal condition affecting the body of an organism. It is often construed to be a medical condition associated with specific symptoms and signs. It may be caused by external factors, such as infectious disease, or it may be caused by internal dysfunctions, such as autoimmune diseases.
Septic shock	Septic shock is a medical condition as a result of severe infection and sepsis, though the microbe may be systemic or localized to a particular site. It can cause multiple organ dysfunction syndrome (formerly known as multiple organ failure) and death. Its most common victims are children, immunocompromised individuals, and the elderly, as their immune systems cannot deal with the infection as effectively as those of healthy adults.
Histotoxic hypoxia	Histotoxic hypoxia is the inability of cells to take up or utilize oxygen from the bloodstream, despite physiologically normal delivery of oxygen to such cells and tissues. Histotoxic hypoxia results from tissue poisoning, such as that caused by alcohol, narcotics, cyanide (which acts by inhibiting cytochrome oxidase), and certain other poisons like hydrogen sulfide (byproduct of sewage and used in leather tanning).

Chapter 4. CARDIOVASCULAR

1. _____ sample values

_____ is the study of the changes of normal mechanical, physical, and biochemical functions, either caused by a disease, or resulting from an abnormal syndrome. More formally, it is the branch of medicine which deals with any disturbances of body functions, caused by disease or prodromal symptoms.

An alternative definition is 'the study of the biological and physical manifestations of disease as they correlate with the underlying abnormalities and physiological disturbances.'

The study of pathology and the study of _____ often involves substantial overlap in diseases and processes, but pathology emphasizes direct observations, while _____ emphasizes quantifiable measurements.

a. Pathophysiology of chronic fatigue syndrome
b. Pathophysiology
c. Gliosis
d. Health Sciences Descriptors

2. A _____ is a systematic diagnostic method used to identify the presence of an entity where multiple alternatives are possible (and the process may be termed differential diagnostic procedure), and may also refer to any of the included candidate alternatives (which may also be termed candidate condition). This method is essentially a process of elimination, or at least, rendering of the probabilities of candidate conditions to negligible levels. In this sense, probabilities are, in fact, imaginative parameters in the mind or hardware of the diagnostician or system, while in reality the target (such as a patient) either has a condition or not with an actual probability of either 0 or 100%.

a. Hospital emergency codes
b. Fremitus
c. Differential diagnosis
d. Health Sciences Descriptors

3. _____, the medical term for fainting, is precisely defined as a transient loss of consciousness and postural tone characterized by rapid onset, short duration, and spontaneous recovery due to global cerebral hypoperfusion that most often results from hypotension.

Many forms of syncope are preceded by a prodromal state that often includes dizziness and loss of vision ('blackout') (temporary), loss of hearing (temporary), loss of pain and feeling (temporary), nausea and abdominal discomfort, weakness, sweating, a feeling of heat, palpitations and other phenomena, which, if they do not progress to loss of consciousness and postural tone are often denoted 'presyncope'. Abdominal discomfort prior to loss of consciousness may be indicative of seizure which should be considered different than syncope.

a. Vertigo
b. Medical ventilator
c. Syncope
d. Nebulizer

4. . _____ is a congenital disorder in the heart wherein a neonate's ductus arteriosus fails to close after birth.

Early symptoms are uncommon, but in the first year of life include increased work of breathing and poor weight gain. With age, the PDA may lead to congestive heart failure if left uncorrected.

a. Patent ductus arteriosus
b. Transposition of the great vessels
c. Ostium primum atrial septal defect
d. Overriding aorta

5. _____, also known as DiGeorge syndrome, DiGeorge anomaly, velo-cardio-facial syndrome, Shprintzen syndrome, conotruncal anomaly face syndrome, Strong syndrome, congenital thymic aplasia, and thymic hypoplasia is a syndrome caused by the deletion of a small piece of chromosome 22. The deletion occurs near the middle of the chromosome at a location designated q11.2 i.e., on the long arm of one of the pair of chromosomes 22. It has a prevalence estimated at 1:4000. The syndrome was described in 1968 by the pediatric endocrinologist Angelo DiGeorge.

The features of this syndrome vary widely, even among members of the same family, and affect many parts of the body. Characteristic signs and symptoms may include birth defects such as congenital heart disease, defects in the palate, most commonly related to neuromuscular problems with closure (velo-pharyngeal insufficiency), learning disabilities, mild differences in facial features, and recurrent infections.

a. Precordial catch syndrome
b. Long QT syndrome
c. 22q11.2 deletion syndrome
d. 3-M syndrome

1. b
2. c
3. c
4. a
5. c

You can take the complete Chapter Practice Test

for Chapter 4. CARDIOVASCULAR
on all key terms, persons, places, and concepts.

Online 99 Cents

http://www.epub219.49.13357.4.cram101.com/

Use www.Cram101.com for all your study needs

including Cram101's online interactive problem solving labs in

chemistry, statistics, mathematics, and more.

Chapter 5. PULMONARY DISEASE

Chest pain

Dyspnea

Respiratory disease

Aplastic anemia

Bradypnea

Cheyne-Stokes respiration

Kussmaul breathing

Pectus carinatum

Pectus excavatum

Periodic breathing

Tachypnea

Palpation

Physical examination

Grunting

Snoring

Skull

Skull fracture

Terminal sedation

Pulmonary hypertension

CHAPTER OUTLINE: KEY TERMS, PEOPLE, PLACES, CONCEPTS

Vocal cords

Vocal cord dysfunction

Asthma

Bronchopulmonary dysplasia

Heart disease

Rheumatic fever

Sickle-cell disease

Cerebral palsy

Kyphoscoliosis

Thalassemia

Pathophysiology

Prevalence

Lupus erythematosus

Systemic lupus erythematosus

Risk factor

Methylmalonic acidemia

Oxygen therapy

Medication

Ipratropium bromide

	Activation syndrome
	Intensive care
	Status asthmaticus
	Mechanical ventilation
	Respiratory failure
	Cystic fibrosis
	Haemophilus influenzae
	Pseudomonas aeruginosa
	Staphylococcus aureus
	Chest physiotherapy
	Parenteral nutrition
	Factor IX
	Factor VII
	Gastroesophageal reflux
	Cardiac arrest
	Pulmonary arteries
	Cardiopulmonary resuscitation
	Foreign body
	Differential diagnosis

Chapter 5. PULMONARY DISEASE

CHAPTER OUTLINE: KEY TERMS, PEOPLE, PLACES, CONCEPTS

_____ | Chylothorax

_____ | Pleural effusion

_____ | Etiological myth

_____ | Tuberculosis

_____ | Chest radiograph

_____ | Computed tomography

_____ | Lyme disease

_____ | Abdominal mass

_____ | Alveolar gas equation

_____ | Arterial blood

_____ | Pulse oximetry

_____ | Blood gas

_____ | Nitric oxide

_____ | Life support

_____ | Sleep apnea

_____ | Gallbladder disease

_____ | Gas exchange

_____ | Hypopnea

_____ | Consequence

Chapter 5. PULMONARY DISEASE

Muscular dystrophies

Prognosis

Acetylcholinesterase inhibitor

Restrictive lung disease

Muscle biopsy

Motor neuron

Arnold-Chiari malformation

Prader-Willi syndrome

Obesity hypoventilation syndrome

CHAPTER HIGHLIGHTS & NOTES: KEY TERMS, PEOPLE, PLACES, CONCEPTS

Chest pain	Chest pain may be a symptom of a number of serious conditions and is generally considered a medical emergency. Even though it may be determined that the pain is non-cardiac in origin, this is often a diagnosis of exclusion made after ruling out more serious causes of the pain.
	Causes of chest pain range from non-serious to serious to life threatening.
Dyspnea	Dyspnea is the subjective symptom of breathlessness.
	It is a normal symptom of heavy exertion but becomes pathological if it occurs in unexpected situations. In 85% of cases it is due to either asthma, pneumonia, cardiac ischemia, interstitial lung disease, congestive heart failure, chronic obstructive pulmonary disease, or psychogenic causes.

Respiratory disease	Respiratory disease is a medical term that encompasses pathological conditions affecting the organs and tissues that make gas exchange possible in higher organisms, and includes conditions of the upper respiratory tract, trachea, bronchi, bronchioles, alveoli, pleura and pleural cavity, and the nerves and muscles of breathing. Respiratory diseases range from mild and self-limiting, such as the common cold, to life-threatening entities like bacterial pneumonia, pulmonary embolism, and lung cancer. The study of respiratory disease is known as pulmonology.
Aplastic anemia	Aplastic anemia is a condition where bone marrow does not produce sufficient new cells to replenish blood cells. The condition, as the name indicates, involves both aplasia and anemia. Typically, anemia refers to low red blood cell counts, but aplastic anemia patients have lower counts of all three blood cell types: red blood cells, white blood cells, and platelets, termed pancytopenia.
Bradypnea	Bradypnea refers to an abnormally slow breathing rate. The rate at which bradypnea is diagnosed depends upon the age of the patient. Age ranges and bradypnea•Age 0-1 year < 30 breaths per minute•Age 1-3 years < 25 breaths per minute•Age 3-12 years < 20 breaths per minute•Age 12-50 years < 12 breaths per minute•Age 50 and up < 3 breaths per minute.
Cheyne-Stokes respiration	Cheyne-Stokes respiration is an abnormal pattern of breathing characterized by progressively deeper and sometimes faster breathing, followed by a gradual decrease that results in a temporary stop in breathing called an apnea. The pattern repeats, with each cycle usually taking 30 seconds to 2 minutes. It is an oscillation of ventilation between apnea and hyperpnea with a crescendo-decrescendo pattern, and is associated with changing serum partial pressures of oxygen and carbon dioxide.
Kussmaul breathing	Kussmaul breathing is a deep and labored breathing pattern often associated with severe metabolic acidosis, particularly diabetic ketoacidosis (DKA) but also renal failure. It is a form of hyperventilation, which is any breathing pattern that reduces carbon dioxide in the blood due to increased rate or depth of respiration. In metabolic acidosis, breathing is first rapid and shallow but as acidosis worsens, breathing gradually becomes deep, labored and gasping.
Pectus carinatum	Pectus carinatum, (L carinatus, equiv. to carin(a) keel), also called pigeon chest, is a deformity of the chest characterized by a protrusion of the sternum and ribs. It is the opposite of pectus excavatum.

Chapter 5. PULMONARY DISEASE

Pectus excavatum	Pectus excavatum is the most common congenital deformity of the anterior wall of the chest, in which several ribs and the sternum grow abnormally. This produces a caved-in or sunken appearance of the chest. It can either be present at birth or not develop until puberty.
Periodic breathing	Periodic breathing is an abnormal pattern of breathing characterized by oscillation of ventilation between hyperpnea and hypopnea (not hyperpnea and Apnea as in Cheyne-Stokes respiration) with a crescendo-decrescendo pattern in the depth of respirations, to compensate for changing serum partial pressures of oxygen and carbon dioxide. Cheyne-Stokes respiration and periodic breathing are known together as Central sleep apnoea syndrome (CSAS).
Tachypnea	Tachypnea means rapid breathing. Any rate between 12-20 breaths per minute is normal. Tachypnea is a respiration rate greater than 20 breaths per minute.
Palpation	Palpation is used as part of a physical examination in which an object is felt (usually with the hands of a healthcare practitioner) to determine its size, shape, firmness, or location. Palpation should not be confused with palpitation, which is an awareness of the beating of the heart. Palpation is used by various therapists such as medical doctors, practitioners of chiropractic, osteopathic medicine, physical therapists, occupational therapists, and massage therapists, to assess the texture of a patient's tissue (such as swelling or muscle tone), to locate the spatial coordinates of particular anatomical landmarks (e.g., to assess range and quality of joint motion), and assess tenderness through tissue deformation (e.g. provoking pain with pressure or stretching).
Physical examination	A physical examination, medical examination, or clinical examination (more popularly known as a check-up or medical) is the process by which a doctor investigates the body of a patient for signs of disease. It generally follows the taking of the medical history -- an account of the symptoms as experienced by the patient. Together with the medical history, the physical examination aids in determining the correct diagnosis and devising the treatment plan.
Grunting	Grunting in tennis refers to the loud noise, sometimes described as 'shrieking' or 'screaming', made by some players during their strokes. It is prominent in women's tennis but also exists in men's tennis. Many players and fans find it to be quite obnoxious above a certain sound level.
Snoring	Snoring is the vibration of respiratory structures and the resulting sound, due to obstructed air movement during breathing while sleeping. In some cases the sound may be soft, but in other cases, it can be loud and unpleasant. Snoring during sleep may be a sign, or first alarm, of obstructive sleep apnea (OSA).

Skull	The skull is a bony structure in the head of many animals that supports the structures of the face and forms a cavity for the brain. The skull is composed of two parts: the cranium and the mandible. A skull without a mandible is only a cranium.
Skull fracture	Skull fracture is the term used to describe a break in one or more of the eight bones which form the cranial portion of the skull usually occurring as a result of blunt force trauma. If the force of the impact is excessive the bone may fracture at or near the site of the impact and may cause damage to the underlying physical structures contained within the skull such as the membranes, blood vessels, and brain, even in the absence of a fracture. While an uncomplicated skull fracture can occur without associated physical or neurological damage and is in itself usually not clinically significant, a fracture in healthy bone indicates that a substantial amount of force has been applied and increases the possibility of associated injury.
Terminal sedation	In medicine, specifically in end-of-life care, terminal sedation is the palliative practice of relieving distress in a terminally ill person in the last hours or days of a dying patient's life, usually by means of a continuous intravenous or subcutaneous infusion of a sedative drug. This is a option of last resort for patients whose symptoms cannot be controlled by any other means. This should be differentiated from euthanasia as the goal of palliative sedation is to control symptoms through sedation but not shorten the patient's life, while in euthanasia the goal is to shorten life to relieve symptoms.
Pulmonary hypertension	In medicine, pulmonary hypertension is an increase in blood pressure in the pulmonary artery, pulmonary vein, or pulmonary capillaries, together known as the lung vasculature, leading to shortness of breath, dizziness, fainting, and other symptoms, all of which are exacerbated by exertion. Pulmonary hypertension can be a severe disease with a markedly decreased exercise tolerance and heart failure. It was first identified by Dr. Ernst von Romberg in 1891. According to the most recent classification, it can be one of five different types: arterial, venous, hypoxic, thromboembolic or miscellaneous.
Vocal cords	The vocal folds, also known commonly as Vocal cords, are composed of twin infoldings of mucous membrane stretched horizontally across the larynx. They vibrate, modulating the flow of air being expelled from the lungs during phonation. Open during inhalation, closed when holding one's breath, and vibrating for speech or singing , the folds are controlled via the vagus nerve.

Chapter 5. PULMONARY DISEASE

Vocal cord dysfunction	Vocal cord dysfunction is a condition that affects the vocal folds, commonly referred to as the vocal cords, which is characterized by full or partial vocal fold closure that usually occurs during inhalation for short periods of time; however, it can occur during both inhalation and exhalation.. This closure may cause airflow obstruction; however, rarely results in reduction of oxygen saturation. Symptoms can include shortness of breath dyspnea, wheezing, coughing, tightness in the throat, skin discoloration due to oxygen deprivation, noise during inhalation stridor, and in severe cases, loss of consciousness.
Asthma	Asthma is the common chronic inflammatory disease of the airways characterized by variable and recurring symptoms, reversible airflow obstruction, and bronchospasm. Symptoms include wheezing, coughing, chest tightness, and shortness of breath. Asthma is clinically classified according to the frequency of symptoms, forced expiratory volume in 1 second (FEV1), and peak expiratory flow rate.
Bronchopulmonary dysplasia	Bronchopulmonary dysplasia is a chronic lung disorder that is most common among children who were born prematurely, with low birthweights and who received prolonged mechanical ventilation to treat respiratory distress syndrome. The classic diagnosis of BPD may be assigned at 28 days of life if the following criteria are met (Bureau of Maternal and Child Health, 1989): (1) Positive pressure ventilation during the first 2 weeks of life for a minimum of 3 days.(2) Clinical signs of abnormal respiratory function.(3) Requirements for supplemental oxygen for longer than 28 days of age to maintain PaO2 above 50 mm Hg.(4) Chest radiograph with diffuse abnormal findings characteristic of BPD.
Heart disease	Heart disease is an umbrella term for a variety of diseases affecting the heart. As of 2007, it is the leading cause of death in the United States, England, Canada and Wales, accounting for 25.4% of the total deaths in the United States. Coronary heart disease refers to the failure of the coronary circulation to supply adequate circulation to cardiac muscle and surrounding tissue. Coronary heart disease is most commonly equated with Coronary artery disease although coronary heart disease can be due to other causes, such as coronary vasospasm.
Rheumatic fever	Rheumatic fever is an inflammatory disease that occurs following a Streptococcus pyogenes infection, such as streptococcal pharyngitis or scarlet fever. Believed to be caused by antibody cross-reactivity that can involve the heart, joints, skin, and brain, the illness typically develops two to three weeks after a streptococcal infection. Acute rheumatic fever commonly appears in children between the ages of 6 and 15, with only 20% of first-time attacks occurring in adults.

Sickle-cell disease	Sickle-cell disease or sickle-cell anaemia or drepanocytosis, is an autosomal recessive genetic blood disorder with overdominance, characterized by red blood cells that assume an abnormal, rigid, sickle shape. Sickling decreases the cells' flexibility and results in a risk of various complications. The sickling occurs because of a mutation in the hemoglobin gene.
Cerebral palsy	Cerebral palsy is an umbrella term encompassing a group of non-progressive, non-contagious motor conditions that cause physical disability in human development, chiefly in the various areas of body movement. Cerebral refers to the cerebrum, which is the affected area of the brain (although the disorder most likely involves connections between the cortex and other parts of the brain such as the cerebellum), and palsy refers to disorder of movement. Furthermore, 'paralytic disorders' are not cerebral palsy - the condition of quadriplegia, therefore, should not be confused with spastic quadriplegia, nor tardive dyskinesia with dyskinetic cerebral palsy, nor diplegia with spastic diplegia, and so on.
Kyphoscoliosis	Kyphoscoliosis describes an abnormal curvature of the spine in both a coronal and sagittal plane. It is a combination of kyphosis and scoliosis. Kyphoscoliosis is a musculoskeletal disorder causing chronic underventilation of the lungs and may be one of the major causes of pulmonary hypertension.
Thalassemia	Thalassemia is a group of inherited autosomal recessive blood disorders that originated in the Mediterranean region. In thalassemia the genetic defect, which could be either mutation or deletion, results in reduced rate of synthesis or no synthesis of one of the globin chains that make up hemoglobin. This can cause the formation of abnormal hemoglobin molecules, thus causing anemia, the characteristic presenting symptom of the thalassemias.
Pathophysiology	Pathophysiology sample values Pathophysiology is the study of the changes of normal mechanical, physical, and biochemical functions, either caused by a disease, or resulting from an abnormal syndrome. More formally, it is the branch of medicine which deals with any disturbances of body functions, caused by disease or prodromal symptoms. An alternative definition is 'the study of the biological and physical manifestations of disease as they correlate with the underlying abnormalities and physiological disturbances.' The study of pathology and the study of pathophysiology often involves substantial overlap in diseases and processes, but pathology emphasizes direct observations, while pathophysiology emphasizes quantifiable measurements.

Chapter 5. PULMONARY DISEASE

Prevalence	In epidemiology, the prevalence of a health-related state (typically disease, but also other things like smoking or seatbelt use) in a statistical population is defined as the total number of cases of the risk factor in the population at a given time, or the total number of cases in the population, divided by the number of individuals in the population. It is used as an estimate of how common a disease is within a population over a certain period of time. It helps physicians or other health professionals understand the probability of certain diagnoses and is routinely used by epidemiologists, health care providers, government agencies and insurers.
Lupus erythematosus	Lupus erythematosus is a category for a collection of diseases with similar underlying problems with immunity (autoimmune disease). Symptoms of these diseases can affect many different body systems, including joints, skin, kidneys, blood cells, heart, and lungs. Four main types of lupus exist: systemic lupus erythematosus, discoid lupus erythematosus, drug-induced lupus erythematosus, and neonatal lupus erythematosus.
Systemic lupus erythematosus	Systemic lupus erythematosus often abbreviated to SLE or lupus, is a systemic autoimmune disease that can affect any part of the body. As occurs in other autoimmune diseases, the immune system attacks the body's cells and tissue, resulting in inflammation and tissue damage. It is a Type III hypersensitivity reaction caused by antibody-immune complex formation.
Risk factor	In epidemiology, a risk factor is a variable associated with an increased risk of disease or infection. Sometimes, determinant is also used, being a variable associated with either increased or decreased risk. Risk factors or determinants are correlational and not necessarily causal, because correlation does not prove causation.
Methylmalonic acidemia	Methylmalonic acidemia also called methylmalonic aciduria, is an autosomal recessive metabolic disorder. It is a classical type of organic acidemia. Methylmalonic acidemia stems from several genotypes, all forms of the disorder usually diagnosed in the early neonatal period, presenting progressive encephalopathy, and secondary hyperammonemia.
Oxygen therapy	Oxygen therapy is the administration of oxygen as a medical intervention, which can be for a variety of purposes in both chronic and acute patient care. Oxygen is essential for cell metabolism, and in turn, tissue oxygenation is essential for all normal physiological functions. Room air only contains 21% oxygen, and increasing the fraction of oxygen in the breathing gas increases the amount of oxygen in the blood.

Medication	A pharmaceutical drug, also referred to as medicine, medication or medicament, can be loosely defined as any chemical substance intended for use in the medical diagnosis, cure, treatment, or prevention of disease. medications can be classified in various ways, such as by chemical properties, mode or route of administration, biological system affected, or therapeutic effects. An elaborate and widely used classification system is the Anatomical Therapeutic Chemical Classification System (ATC system).
Ipratropium bromide	Ipratropium bromide is an anticholinergic drug used for the treatment of chronic obstructive pulmonary disease and acute asthma. It blocks the muscarinic acetylcholine receptors in the smooth muscles of the bronchi in the lungs, opening the bronchi. Ipratropium is administered by inhalation for the treatment of chronic obstructive pulmonary disease (COPD).
Activation syndrome	Activation syndrome is a form of sometimes suicidal or homicidal stimulation or agitation that can occur in response to some psychoactive drugs. A study of paroxetine found that 21 out of 93 (23 percent) of youth taking Paxil reported manic-like symptoms which included hostility, emotional lability and nervousness. Pfizer has denied that sertraline can cause such effects.
Intensive care	intensive care medicine or critical care medicine is a branch of medicine concerned with the provision of life support or organ support systems in patients who are critically ill and who usually require intensive monitoring. Patients requiring intensive care may require support for hemodynamic instability (hypertension/hypotension), airway or respiratory compromise (such as ventilator support), acute renal failure, potentially lethal cardiac arrhythmias, or the cumulative effects of multiple organ system failure. They may also be admitted for intensive/invasive monitoring, such as the crucial hours after major surgery when deemed too unstable to transfer to a less intensively monitored unit.
Status asthmaticus	Status asthmaticus is an acute exacerbation of asthma that does not respond to standard treatments of bronchodilators and steroids. Symptoms include chest tightness, rapidly progressive dyspnea (shortness of breath), dry cough, use of accessory muscles, labored breathing and extreme wheezing. It is a life-threatening episode of airway obstruction considered a medical emergency.
Mechanical ventilation	In medicine, mechanical ventilation is a method to mechanically assist or replace spontaneous breathing. This may involve a machine called a ventilator or the breathing may be assisted by a physician, respiratory therapist or other suitable person compressing a bag or set of bellows.

Chapter 5. PULMONARY DISEASE

Respiratory failure	The term respiratory failure, in medicine, is used to describe inadequate gas exchange by the respiratory system, with the result that arterial oxygen and/or carbon dioxide levels cannot be maintained within their normal ranges. A drop in blood oxygenation is known as hypoxemia; a rise in arterial carbon dioxide levels is called hypercapnia. The normal reference values are: oxygen PaO_2 greater than 80 mmHg (11 kPa), and carbon dioxide $PaCO_2$ less than 45 mmHg (6.0 kPa).
Cystic fibrosis	Cystic fibrosis is an autosomal recessive genetic disorder affecting most critically the lungs, and also the pancreas, liver, and intestine. It is characterized by abnormal transport of chloride and sodium across an epithelium, leading to thick, viscous secretions.
	The name cystic fibrosis refers to the characteristic scarring (fibrosis) and cyst formation within the pancreas, first recognized in the 1930s.
Haemophilus influenzae	Haemophilus influenzae, formerly called Pfeiffer's bacillus or Bacillus influenzae, Gram-negative, rod-shaped bacterium first described in 1892 by Richard Pfeiffer during an influenza pandemic. A member of the Pasteurellaceae family, it is generally aerobic, but can grow as a facultative anaerobe. H. influenzae was mistakenly considered to be the cause of influenza until 1933, when the viral etiology of the flu became apparent.
Pseudomonas aeruginosa	Pseudomonas aeruginosa is a common bacterium which can cause disease in animals and humans. It is found in soil, water, skin flora and most man-made environments throughout the world. It thrives not only in normal atmospheres, but also with little oxygen, and has thus colonised many natural and artificial environments.
Staphylococcus aureus	Staphylococcus aureus is a bacterial species named from Greek σταφυλ?κοκκος meaning the 'golden grape-cluster berry'. Also known as 'golden staph' and Oro staphira, it is a facultative anaerobic Gram-positive coccal bacterium. It is frequently found as part of the normal skin flora on the skin and nasal passages.
Chest physiotherapy	Chest physiotherapy is a broad, non-specific term used to describe treatments generally performed by physiotherapists (in Canada) and respiratory therapists whereby breathing is improved by the indirect removal of mucus from the breathing passages of a patient. Other terms used in Australia include respiratory or cardiothoracic physiotherapy.
	Techniques include clapping or percussion: the therapist lightly claps the patient's chest, back, and area under the arms.
Parenteral nutrition	Parenteral nutrition is feeding a person intravenously, bypassing the usual process of eating and digestion. The person receives nutritional formulae that contain nutrients such as glucose, amino acids, lipids and added vitamins and dietary minerals.

Factor IX	Factor IX (EC 3.4.21.22) is one of the serine proteases of the coagulation system; it belongs to peptidase family S1. Deficiency of this protein causes hemophilia B. It was discovered in 1952 after a young boy named Stephen Christmas was found to be lacking this exact factor, leading to hemophilia..
	Factor IX is produced as a zymogen, an inactive precursor. It is processed to remove the signal peptide, glycosylated and then cleaved by factor XIa (of the contact pathway) or factor VIIa (of the tissue factor pathway) to produce a two-chain form where the chains are linked by a disulfide bridge.
Factor VII	Factor VII is one of the proteins that causes blood to clot in the coagulation cascade. It is an enzyme (EC 3.4.21.21) of the serine protease class. A recombinant form of human factor VIIa (NovoSeven, eptacog alfa [activated]) has U.S. Food and Drug Administration approval for uncontrolled bleeding in hemophilia patients.
Gastroesophageal reflux	Gastroesophageal reflux disease (GERD), gastro-oesophageal reflux disease (GORD), gastric reflux disease, or acid reflux disease is defined as chronic symptoms or mucosal damage produced by the abnormal reflux in the oesophagus.
	This is commonly due to transient or permanent changes in the barrier between the oesophagus and the stomach. This can be due to incompetence of the lower esophageal sphincter, transient lower oesophageal sphincter relaxation, impaired expulsion of gastric reflux from the oesophagus, or a hiatal hernia.
Cardiac arrest	Cardiac arrest, (also known as cardiopulmonary arrest or circulatory arrest) is the cessation of normal circulation of the blood due to failure of the heart to contract effectively. Medical personnel can refer to an unexpected cardiac arrest as a sudden cardiac arrest or SCA.
	A cardiac arrest is different from (but may be caused by) a heart attack, where blood flow to the muscle of the heart is impaired.
	Arrested blood circulation prevents delivery of oxygen to the body.
Pulmonary arteries	The pulmonary arteries carry blood from heart to the lungs. They are the only arteries (other than umbilical arteries in the fetus) that carry deoxygenated blood.
	In the human heart, the pulmonary trunk (pulmonary artery or main pulmonary artery) begins at the base of the right ventricle.

Chapter 5. PULMONARY DISEASE

Cardiopulmonary resuscitation	Cardiopulmonary resuscitation is an emergency procedure which is performed in an effort to manually preserve intact brain function until further measures are taken to restore spontaneous blood circulation and breathing in a person in cardiac arrest. It is indicated in those who are unresponsive with no breathing or abnormal breathing, for example agonal respirations. It may be performed both in and outside of a hospital.
Foreign body	A foreign body is any object originating outside the body. In machinery, it can mean any unwanted intruding object. Most references to foreign bodies involve propulsion through natural orifices into hollow organs.
Differential diagnosis	A differential diagnosis is a systematic diagnostic method used to identify the presence of an entity where multiple alternatives are possible (and the process may be termed differential diagnostic procedure), and may also refer to any of the included candidate alternatives (which may also be termed candidate condition). This method is essentially a process of elimination, or at least, rendering of the probabilities of candidate conditions to negligible levels. In this sense, probabilities are, in fact, imaginative parameters in the mind or hardware of the diagnostician or system, while in reality the target (such as a patient) either has a condition or not with an actual probability of either 0 or 100%.
Chylothorax	A chylothorax is a type of pleural effusion. It results from lymphatic fluid (chyle) accumulating in the pleural cavity. Its cause is usually leakage from the thoracic duct or one of the main lymphatic vessels that drain to it.
Pleural effusion	Pleural effusion is excess fluid that accumulates between the two pleural layers, the fluid-filled space that surrounds the lungs. Excessive amounts of such fluid can impair breathing by limiting the expansion of the lungs during ventilation. Pleural fluid is secreted by the parietal layer of the pleura and reabsorbed by the visceral layer of the pleura.
Etiological myth	Etiology is the study of causation, or origination. The word is most commonly used in medical and philosophical theories, where it is used to refer to the study of why things occur, or even the reasons behind the way that things act, and is used in philosophy, physics, psychology, government, medicine, theology and biology in reference to the causes of various phenomena. An etiological myth is a myth intended to explain a name or create a mythic history for a place or family.

Tuberculosis	Tuberculosis, MTB or TB (short for tubercles bacillus) is a common and in some cases deadly infectious disease caused by various strains of mycobacteria, usually Mycobacterium tuberculosis in humans. Tuberculosis usually attacks the lungs but can also affect other parts of the body. It is spread through the air when people who have an active MTB infection cough, sneeze, or otherwise transmit their saliva through the air.
Chest radiograph	In medicine, a chest radiograph, commonly called a chest X-ray (CXR), is a projection radiograph of the chest used to diagnose conditions affecting the chest, its contents, and nearby structures. Chest radiographs are among the most common films taken, being diagnostic of many conditions.
	Like all methods of radiography, chest radiography employs ionizing radiation in the form of X-rays to generate images of the chest.
Computed tomography	Computed tomography is a medical imaging method employing tomography created by computer processing. Digital geometry processing is used to generate a three-dimensional image of the inside of an object from a large series of two-dimensional X-ray images taken around a single axis of rotation.
	Computed tomography produces a volume of data which can be manipulated, through a process known as 'windowing', in order to demonstrate various bodily structures based on their ability to block the X-ray/Röntgen beam.
Lyme disease	Lyme disease, is an emerging infectious disease caused by at least three species of bacteria belonging to the genus Borrelia. Borrelia burgdorferi sensu stricto is the main cause of Lyme disease in the United States, whereas Borrelia afzelii and Borrelia garinii cause most European cases. he town of Lyme, Connecticut, USA, where a number of cases were identified in 1975. Although Allen Steere realized that Lyme disease was a tick-borne disease in 1978, the cause of the disease remained a mystery until 1981, when B. burgdorferi was identified by Willy Burgdorfer.
Abdominal mass	An abdominal mass is any localized enlargement or swelling in the human abdomen. Depending on its location, the abdominal mass may be caused by an enlarged liver (hepatomegaly), enlarged spleen (splenomegaly), protruding kidney, a pancreatic mass, a retroperitoneal mass (a mass in the posterior of the peritoneum), an abdominal aortic aneurysm, or various tumours, such as those caused by abdominal carcinomatosis and omental metastasis. The treatments depend on the cause, and may range from watchful waiting to radical surgery.

Chapter 5. PULMONARY DISEASE

Alveolar gas equation	The alveolar partial pressure of oxygen (pO_2) is required to calculate both the alveolar-arterial gradient of oxygen and the amount of right-to-left cardiac shunt, which are both clinically useful quantities. However it is not practicable to take a sample of gas from the alveoli in order to directly measure the partial pressure of oxygen. The Alveolar gas equation allows the calculation of the alveolar partial pressure of oxygen from data that is practically measurable.
Arterial blood	Arterial blood is the oxygenated blood in the circulatory system found in the lungs, the left chambers of the heart, and in the arteries. It is bright red in color, while venous blood is dark red in color (but looks purple through the opaque skin). It is the contralateral term to venous blood.
Pulse oximetry	Pulse oximetry is a non-invasive method allowing the monitoring of the oxygenation of a patient's hemoglobin. A sensor is placed on a thin part of the patient's body, usually a fingertip or earlobe, or in the case of an infant, across a foot. Light of two different wavelengths is passed through the patient to a photodetector.
Blood gas	Blood gas is a term used to describe a laboratory test of blood where the purpose is primarily to measure ventilation and oxygenation. The source is generally noted by an added word to the beginning; arterial blood gases come from arteries, venous blood gases come from veins and capillary blood gases come from capillaries. •pH -- The acidity or basicity of the blood.•PaCO2 -- The partial pressure of carbon dioxide in the blood.•PaO2 -- The partial pressure of oxygen in the blood.•HCO3 -- The level of bicarbonate in the blood.•BE -- The base-excess of bicarbonate in the blood.Purposes for testing •Acidosis•Diabetic ketoacidosis•Lactic acidosis•Metabolic acidosis•Respiratory acidosis•Respiratory alkalosisAbnormal results Abnormal results may be due to lung, kidney, or metabolic diseases.
Nitric oxide	Nitric oxide or nitrogen monoxide (systematic name) is a chemical compound with chemical formula Nitric oxide. This gas is an important signaling molecule in the body of mammals, including humans, and is an extremely important intermediate in the chemical industry. It is also an air pollutant produced by cigarette smoke, automobile engines and power plants. Nitric oxide is an important messenger molecule involved in many physiological and pathological processes within the mammalian body both beneficial and detrimental.
Life support	Life support in medicine is a broad term that applies to any therapy used to sustain a patient's life while they are critically ill or injured, as part of intensive-care medicine. There are many therapies and techniques that may be used by clinicians to achieve the goal of sustaining life.

	Some examples include:•Feeding tube•Total parenteral nutrition•Mechanical ventilation•Heart/Lung bypass•Urinary catheterization•Dialysis•Cardiopulmonary resuscitation•Defibrillation•Artificial pacemaker These techniques are applied most commonly in the Emergency Department, Intensive Care Unit and, Operating Rooms.
Sleep apnea	Sleep apnea is a sleep disorder characterized by abnormal pauses in breathing or instances of abnormally low breathing, during sleep. Each pause in breathing, called an apnea, can last from a few seconds to minutes, and may occur 5 to 30 times or more an hour. Similarly, each abnormally low breathing event is called a hypopnea.
Gallbladder disease	Gallbladder diseases are diseases involving the gallbladder. Gallstones may develop in the gallbladder as well as elsewhere in the biliary tract. If gallstones in the gallbladder are symptomatic and cannot be dissolved by medication or broken into small pieces by ultrasonic waves, surgical removal of the gallbladder, known as cholecystectomy, may be indicated.
Gas exchange	Gas exchange is a process in biology where gases contained in an organism and environment transfer or exchange. In human gas-exchange, gases contained in the blood of human bodies exchange with gases contained in the atmosphere. Human gas-exchange occurs in the lungs.
Hypopnea	Hypopnea is a medical term for a disorder which involves episodes of overly shallow breathing or an abnormally low respiratory rate. This differs from apnea in that there remains some flow of air. Hypopnea events may happen while asleep or while awake.
Consequence	Consequence, or a Consequence is the concept of a resulting effect Plural form · Consequences , a parlour game · Consequences (Buffy the Vampire Slayer), an episode of Buffy the Vampire Slayer · Consequences (New York Contemporary Five album), 1963 · Consequences (Dave Burrell album) · Consequences (Endwell album) · Consequences (Godley & Creme album) · Consequences (Kipling story), a short story by Rudyard Kipling · Consequences (Cather story), a short story by Willa Cather · Consequences (Torchwood), a novel based on the television series Torchwood · Consequences · Consequences (8 Simple Rules episode) · Consequences Creed, a professional wrestler
Muscular dystrophies	Muscular dystrophy refers to a group of hereditary muscle diseases that weaken the muscles that move the human body.

muscular dystrophies are characterized by progressive skeletal muscle weakness, defects in muscle proteins, and the death of muscle cells and tissue. Nine diseases including Duchenne, Becker, limb girdle, congenital, facioscapulohumeral, myotonic, oculopharyngeal, distal, and Emery-Dreifuss are always classified as muscular dystrophy but there are more than 100 diseases in total with similarities to muscular dystrophy.

Prognosis	Prognosis is a medical term to describe the likely outcome of an illness. When applied to large populations, prognostic estimates can be very accurate: for example the statement '45% of patients with severe septic shock will die within 28 days' can be made with some confidence, because previous research found that this proportion of patients died. However, it is much harder to translate this into a prognosis for an individual patient: additional information is needed to determine whether a patient belongs to the 45% who will succumb, or to the 55% who survive.
Acetylcholinesterase inhibitor	An acetylcholinesterase inhibitor or anti-cholinesterase is a chemical that inhibits the cholinesterase enzyme from breaking down acetylcholine, increasing both the level and duration of action of the neurotransmitter acetylcholine. Uses Acetylcholinesterase inhibitors:•Occur naturally as venoms and poisons•Are used as weapons in the form of nerve agents•Are used medicinally: •To treat myasthenia gravis. In myasthenia gravis, they are used to increase neuromuscular transmission.•To treat Glaucoma•To treat Alzheimer's disease•To treat Lewy Body Dementia•As an antidote to anticholinergic poisoning
Restrictive lung disease	Restrictive lung diseases are a category of extrapulmonary, pleural, or parenchymal respiratory diseases that restrict lung expansion, resulting in a decreased lung volume, an increased work of breathing, and inadequate ventilation and/or oxygenation. Pulmonary function test demonstrates a decrease in the forced vital capacity. In disorders that are intrinsic to the lung parenchyma, the underlying process is usually pulmonary fibrosis (scarring of the lung).
Muscle biopsy	In medicine, a muscle biopsy is a procedure in which a piece of muscle tissue is removed from an organism and examined microscopically. A biopsy needle is usually inserted into a muscle, wherein a small amount of tissue remains. Alternatively, an 'open biopsy' can be performed by obtaining the muscle tissue through a small surgical incision.
Motor neuron	In vertebrates, the term motor neuron classically applies to neurons located in the central nervous system (or CNS) that project their axons outside the CNS and directly or indirectly control muscles.

The motor neuron is often associated with efferent neuron, primary neuron, or alpha motor neurons.

Anatomy and physiology

According to their targets, motor neurons are classified into three broad categories:

Somatic motor neurons, which directly innervate skeletal muscles, involved in locomotion (such as the muscles of the limbs, abdominal, and intercostal muscles).

Arnold-Chiari malformation	Arnold-Chiari malformation is a malformation of the brain. It consists of a downward displacement of the cerebellar tonsils through the foramen magnum, sometimes causing hydrocephalus as a result of obstruction of cerebrospinal fluid (CSF) outflow . The cerebrospinal fluid outflow is caused by phase difference in outflow and influx of blood in the vasculature of the brain.
Prader-Willi syndrome	Prader-Willi syndrome is a very rare genetic disorder, in which seven genes on chromosome 15 are missing or unexpressed (chromosome 15q partial deletion) on the paternal chromosome. It was first described in 1956 by Andrea Prader, Heinrich Willi, Alexis Labhart, Andrew Ziegler, and Guido Fanconi of Switzerland. The incidence of PWS is between 1 in 10,000 and 1 in 15,000 live births.
Obesity hypoventilation syndrome	Obesity hypoventilation syndrome is a condition in which severely overweight people fail to breathe rapidly enough or deeply enough, resulting in low blood oxygen levels and high blood carbon dioxide (CO_2) levels. Many people with this condition also frequently stop breathing altogether for short periods of time during sleep (obstructive sleep apnea), resulting in many partial awakenings during the night, which leads to continual sleepiness during the day. The disease puts strain on the heart, which eventually may lead to the symptoms of heart failure, such as leg swelling and various other related symptoms.

Chapter 5. PULMONARY DISEASE

1. _____ may be a symptom of a number of serious conditions and is generally considered a medical emergency. Even though it may be determined that the pain is non-cardiac in origin, this is often a diagnosis of exclusion made after ruling out more serious causes of the pain.

   Causes of _____ range from non-serious to serious to life threatening.

   a. Coccydynia
   b. Complex regional pain syndrome
   c. Condylar resorption
   d. Chest pain

2. _____ refers to an abnormally slow breathing rate. The rate at which _____ is diagnosed depends upon the age of the patient.

   Age ranges and _____•Age 0-1 year < 30 breaths per minute•Age 1-3 years < 25 breaths per minute•Age 3-12 years < 20 breaths per minute•Age 12-50 years < 12 breaths per minute•Age 50 and up < 3 breaths per minute.

   a. Bradypnea
   b. Hypoproteinemia
   c. hemoglobinuria
   d. Bacteriophage

3. _____ is the common chronic inflammatory disease of the airways characterized by variable and recurring symptoms, reversible airflow obstruction, and bronchospasm. Symptoms include wheezing, coughing, chest tightness, and shortness of breath. _____ is clinically classified according to the frequency of symptoms, forced expiratory volume in 1 second (FEV1), and peak expiratory flow rate.

   a. Asthmagen
   b. Asthma
   c. Exhaled nitric oxide
   d. Inhaler

4. _____ is the vibration of respiratory structures and the resulting sound, due to obstructed air movement during breathing while sleeping. In some cases the sound may be soft, but in other cases, it can be loud and unpleasant. _____ during sleep may be a sign, or first alarm, of obstructive sleep apnea (OSA).

   a. Somniloquy
   b. Somnology
   c. Stanford Protocol
   d. Snoring

5. . The _____ carry blood from heart to the lungs. They are the only arteries (other than umbilical arteries in the fetus) that carry deoxygenated blood.

In the human heart, the pulmonary trunk (pulmonary artery or main pulmonary artery) begins at the base of the right ventricle.

a. Posterior intercostal arteries
b. Subcostal arteries
c. Accessory breasts
d. Pulmonary arteries

1. d
2. a
3. b
4. d
5. d

You can take the complete Chapter Practice Test

for Chapter 5. PULMONARY DISEASE
on all key terms, persons, places, and concepts.

Online 99 Cents

http://www.epub219.49.13357.5.cram101.com/

Use www.Cram101.com for all your study needs

including Cram101's online interactive problem solving labs in

chemistry, statistics, mathematics, and more.

CHAPTER OUTLINE: KEY TERMS, PEOPLE, PLACES, CONCEPTS

Lumbar puncture

Cerebrospinal fluid

Cerebrovascular disease

Gastrointestinal bleeding

Terminal sedation

Computed tomography

Abdominal mass

Physiology

Electrophysiology

Evidence-based medicine

Absence seizure

Atonic seizure

Drop attack

Grand mal seizures

Seizure

Status epilepticus

Tonic-clonic seizures

Febrile seizure

Automatism

Chapter 6. NEUROLOGIC
CHAPTER OUTLINE: KEY TERMS, PEOPLE, PLACES, CONCEPTS

Complex partial seizure

Hypsarrhythmia

Isovaleric acidemia

Juvenile myoclonic epilepsy

Partial seizure

Etiological myth

Prognosis

Sickle-cell disease

Heart disease

Subarachnoid hemorrhage

Venous thrombosis

Magnesium sulfate

Hypotonia

Spinal muscular atrophies

Differential diagnosis

Nervous system

Peripheral nervous system

Botulism

Clostridium botulinum

Chapter 6. NEUROLOGIC

CHAPTER OUTLINE: KEY TERMS, PEOPLE, PLACES, CONCEPTS

Congenital myasthenic syndrome

Muscle biopsy

Muscular dystrophies

Myasthenia gravis

Myotonic dystrophy

Riley-Day Syndrome

Health care

Motor neuron

Neuromuscular junction

Transverse myelitis

Becker muscular dystrophy

Congenital myopathy

Duchenne muscular dystrophy

Zellweger syndrome

Lactic acid

Confusion

Delirium

Hallucination

Obtundation

Chapter 6. NEUROLOGIC

Stupor

Vegetative state

Heart failure

Mental state

Local anesthetic

Locked-in syndrome

Minimally conscious state

Regional analgesia

Akinetic mutism

Brain death

Coma scale

Physical examination

Cheyne-Stokes respiration

Corn syrup

Corneal reflex

Neuroimaging

Flumazenil

Intracranial pressure

Opioid overdose

CHAPTER OUTLINE: KEY TERMS, PEOPLE, PLACES, CONCEPTS

	Palliative care
	Epidemiology
	Methylmalonic acidemia
	Acute disseminated encephalomyelitis
	Multiple sclerosis

CHAPTER HIGHLIGHTS & NOTES: KEY TERMS, PEOPLE, PLACES, CONCEPTS

| Lumbar puncture | A lumbar puncture is a diagnostic and at times therapeutic procedure that is performed in order to collect a sample of cerebrospinal fluid (CSF) for biochemical, microbiological, and cytological analysis, or very rarely as a treatment ('therapeutic lumbar puncture') to relieve increased intracranial pressure.

The most common purpose for a lumbar puncture is to collect cerebrospinal fluid in a case of suspected meningitis, since there is no other reliable tool with which meningitis, a life-threatening but highly treatable condition, can be excluded. Young infants commonly require lumbar puncture as a part of the routine workup for fever without a source, as they have a much higher risk of meningitis than older persons and do not reliably show signs of meningeal irritation (meningismus). |
| --- | --- |
| Cerebrospinal fluid | Cerebrospinal fluid Liquor cerebrospinalis, is a clear, colorless, bodily fluid, that occupies the subarachnoid space and the ventricular system around and inside the brain and spinal cord.

The CSF occupies the space between the arachnoid mater (the middle layer of the brain cover, meninges) and the pia mater (the layer of the meninges closest to the brain). It constitutes the content of all intra-cerebral (inside the brain, cerebrum) ventricles, cisterns, and sulci, as well as the central canal of the spinal cord. |
| Cerebrovascular disease | Cerebrovascular disease is a group of brain dysfunctions related to disease of the blood vessels supplying the brain. |

Chapter 6. NEUROLOGIC

Hypertension is the most important cause; it damages the blood vessel lining, endothelium, exposing the underlying collagen where platelets aggregate to initiate a repairing process which is not always complete and perfect. Sustained hypertension permanently changes the architecture of the blood vessels making them narrow, stiff, deformed, uneven and more vulnerable to fluctuations in blood pressure.

Gastrointestinal bleeding	Gastrointestinal bleeding, from the pharynx to the rectum. It has diverse causes, and a medical history, as well as physical examination, generally distinguishes between the main forms. The degree of bleeding can range from nearly undetectable to acute, massive, life-threatening bleeding.
Terminal sedation	In medicine, specifically in end-of-life care, terminal sedation is the palliative practice of relieving distress in a terminally ill person in the last hours or days of a dying patient's life, usually by means of a continuous intravenous or subcutaneous infusion of a sedative drug. This is a option of last resort for patients whose symptoms cannot be controlled by any other means. This should be differentiated from euthanasia as the goal of palliative sedation is to control symptoms through sedation but not shorten the patient's life, while in euthanasia the goal is to shorten life to relieve symptoms.
Computed tomography	Computed tomography is a medical imaging method employing tomography created by computer processing. Digital geometry processing is used to generate a three-dimensional image of the inside of an object from a large series of two-dimensional X-ray images taken around a single axis of rotation.

Computed tomography produces a volume of data which can be manipulated, through a process known as 'windowing', in order to demonstrate various bodily structures based on their ability to block the X-ray/Röntgen beam. |
| Abdominal mass | An abdominal mass is any localized enlargement or swelling in the human abdomen. Depending on its location, the abdominal mass may be caused by an enlarged liver (hepatomegaly), enlarged spleen (splenomegaly), protruding kidney, a pancreatic mass, a retroperitoneal mass (a mass in the posterior of the peritoneum), an abdominal aortic aneurysm, or various tumours, such as those caused by abdominal carcinomatosis and omental metastasis. The treatments depend on the cause, and may range from watchful waiting to radical surgery. |
| Physiology | Physiology is the science of the function of living systems. This includes how organisms, organ systems, organs, cells, and bio-molecules carry out the chemical or physical functions that exist in a living system. The highest honor awarded in physiology is the Nobel Prize in Physiology or Medicine, awarded since 1901 by the Royal Swedish Academy of Sciences. |

Electrophysiology	Electrophysiology is the study of the electrical properties of biological cells and tissues. It involves measurements of voltage change or electric current on a wide variety of scales from single ion channel proteins to whole organs like the heart. In neuroscience, it includes measurements of the electrical activity of neurons, and particularly action potential activity.
Evidence-based medicine	Evidence-based medicine or evidence-based practice (EBP) aims to apply the best available evidence gained from the scientific method to clinical decision making. It seeks to assess the strength of the evidence of risks and benefits of treatments (including lack of treatment) and diagnostic tests. This helps clinicians understand whether or not a treatment will do more good than harm.
Absence seizure	Absence seizures are one of several kinds of seizures. These seizures are sometimes referred to as petit mal seizures .

Absence seizures are brief (usually less than 20 seconds), generalized epileptic seizures of sudden onset and termination. |
| Atonic seizure | Atonic seizures (also called drop seizures, akinetic seizures or drop attacks), are a type of seizure that consist of a brief lapse in muscle tone that are caused by temporary alterations in brain function. The seizures are brief - usually less than fifteen seconds. They begin in childhood and may persist into adulthood. |
| Drop attack | Drop attacks are sudden spontaneous falls while standing or walking, followed by a very swift recovery, within seconds or minutes.

Drop attacks are typically seen in elderly patients, and the most common cause is carotid sinus hypersensitivity, resulting in either short periods of reversible asystole, or in marked drop in blood pressure in response to carotid sinus stimulation. |

Chapter 6. NEUROLOGIC

	Other causes include the following:•vascular - transient ischemic attack, cerebrovascular accident, dissection, occlusion, hemorrhage •intracranial hematoma•posterior circulation infarction, emboli, vasospasm•bilateral anterior circulation occlusion•migraine accompagnee - develop over 1hr with assoc paresthesia, HA•basilar artery insuff - older pt with no LOC, transient loss of LE tone•epilepsyparoxysmal •neurally mediated syncope - 75% of all causes•Atonic seizure•Lennox-Gastaut syndrome - atonic, myoclonic, GTC typically in neuro abnormal pt•Juvenile Myoclonic Epilepsy - fall with myoclonus•cataplexy associated with narcolepsy•periodic paralyses•complex partial seizure•breath holding spells - associate pallor/cyanosis, emotional aspect•pure autonomic failure (Riley Day, long standing DM)•episodic ataxia•Panayiotopoulos syndrome•degenerative •postural instability with Parkinsons•structural •chronic odontoid instability•spinal cord trauma with transient paraplegia•brainstem mass•metabolic •hypoglycemia, hypocalcemia, Hypomagnesemia•toxins, drugs - cocaine, sedatives, antihistamine, TCA•cardiac •prolonged QT, tachycardia, bradycardia, sick sinus syndrome, arrhythmia, IHSS. AS•hypovolemia•psychiatric •malingering, conversion, panic, anxiety•labyrinth hydrops: an overflow of endolymph in ear labyrinth causes distortions and breaks; see also Ménière's syndromeDiagnosis •important if there was an inciting event (NMS, breatholding, postural), any LOC, and presence of postictal pd•initially get glucose, EKG, pregnancy test, Utox, CT head, lytes•later consider EEG, echocardiogram, MRI, tilt test.
Grand mal seizures	Tonic-clonic seizures are a type of generalized seizure that affects the entire brain. Formerly known as Grand mal seizures or gran mal seizures, these terms are now discouraged and rarely used in a clinical setting. Tonic-clonic seizures are the seizure type most commonly associated with epilepsy and seizures in general, though it is a misconception that they are the only type.
Seizure	An epileptic Seizure, occasionally referred to as a fit, is defined as a transient symptom of 'abnormal excessive or synchronous neuronal activity in the brain'. The outward effect can be as dramatic as a wild thrashing movement (tonic-clonic Seizure) or as mild as a brief loss of awareness. It can manifest as an alteration in mental state, tonic or clonic movements, convulsions, and various other psychic symptoms (such as déjà vu or jamais vu).
Status epilepticus	Status epilepticus is a life-threatening condition in which the brain is in a state of persistent seizure. Definitions vary, but traditionally it is defined as one continuous unremitting seizure lasting longer than 30 minutes, or recurrent seizures without regaining consciousness between seizures for greater than 30 minutes. Treatment is, however, generally started after the seizure has lasted 5 minutes.
Tonic-clonic seizures	Tonic-clonic seizures are a type of generalized seizure that affects the entire brain. Formerly known as grand mal seizures or gran mal seizures, these terms are now discouraged and rarely used in a clinical setting.

Febrile seizure	A febrile seizure, is a convulsion associated with a significant rise in body temperature. They most commonly occur in children between the ages of 6 months to 6 years and are twice as common in boys as in girls. The direct cause of a febrile seizure is not known; however, it is normally precipitated by a recent upper respiratory infection or gastroenteritis.
Automatism	Automatism, in toxicology, refers to a tendency to take a drug over and over again, forgetting each time that one has already taken the dose. This can lead to a cumulative overdose. A particular example is barbiturates which were once commonly used as hypnotic (sleep inducing) drugs.
Complex partial seizure	A complex partial seizure is an epileptic seizure that is limited to one cerebral hemisphere and causes impairment of awareness or responsiveness. Presentation Complex partial seizures are often preceded by a seizure aura. The seizure aura is a simple partial seizure.
Hypsarrhythmia	Hypsarrhythmia is an abnormal interictal pattern, consisting of high amplitude and irregular waves and spikes in a background of chaotic and disorganized activity seen on electroencephalogram (EEG), frequently encountered in an infant diagnosed with infantile spasms, although it can be found in other conditions. In simpler terms, it is a very chaotic and disorganized brain electrical activity with no recognizable pattern, whereas a normal EEG shows clear separation between each signal and visible pattern. Gibbs and Gibbs described hypsarrhythmia in 1952 as '...random high voltage waves and spikes.
Isovaleric acidemia	Isovaleric acidemia, is a rare autosomal recessive metabolic disorder which disrupts or prevents normal metabolism of the branched-chain amino acid leucine. It is a classical type of organic acidemia. A characteristic feature of isovaleric acidemia is a distinctive odor of sweaty feet.
Juvenile myoclonic epilepsy	Juvenile myoclonic epilepsy also known as Janz syndrome, is a fairly common form of idiopathic generalized epilepsy, representing 5-10% of all epilepsies. This disorder typically first manifests itself between the ages of 12 and 18 with myoclonus occurring early in the morning. Most patients also have tonic-clonic seizures and many also have absence seizures.

Chapter 6. NEUROLOGIC

Partial seizure	Partial seizures (also called focal seizures and localized seizures) are seizures which affect only a part of the brain at onset, and are split into two main categories; simple partial seizures and complex partial seizures. A simple partial seizure will often be a precursor to a larger seizure such as a complex partial seizure, or a tonic-clonic seizure. When this is the case, the simple partial seizure is usually called an aura.
Etiological myth	Etiology is the study of causation, or origination. The word is most commonly used in medical and philosophical theories, where it is used to refer to the study of why things occur, or even the reasons behind the way that things act, and is used in philosophy, physics, psychology, government, medicine, theology and biology in reference to the causes of various phenomena. An etiological myth is a myth intended to explain a name or create a mythic history for a place or family.
Prognosis	Prognosis is a medical term to describe the likely outcome of an illness. When applied to large populations, prognostic estimates can be very accurate: for example the statement '45% of patients with severe septic shock will die within 28 days' can be made with some confidence, because previous research found that this proportion of patients died. However, it is much harder to translate this into a prognosis for an individual patient: additional information is needed to determine whether a patient belongs to the 45% who will succumb, or to the 55% who survive.
Sickle-cell disease	Sickle-cell disease or sickle-cell anaemia or drepanocytosis, is an autosomal recessive genetic blood disorder with overdominance, characterized by red blood cells that assume an abnormal, rigid, sickle shape. Sickling decreases the cells' flexibility and results in a risk of various complications. The sickling occurs because of a mutation in the hemoglobin gene.
Heart disease	Heart disease is an umbrella term for a variety of diseases affecting the heart. As of 2007, it is the leading cause of death in the United States, England, Canada and Wales, accounting for 25.4% of the total deaths in the United States. Coronary heart disease refers to the failure of the coronary circulation to supply adequate circulation to cardiac muscle and surrounding tissue. Coronary heart disease is most commonly equated with Coronary artery disease although coronary heart disease can be due to other causes, such as coronary vasospasm.
Subarachnoid hemorrhage	A subarachnoid hemorrhage or subarachnoid haemorrhage in British English, is bleeding into the subarachnoid space--the area between the arachnoid membrane and the pia mater surrounding the brain.

	This may occur spontaneously, usually from a ruptured cerebral aneurysm, or may result from head injury.
	Symptoms of SAH include a severe headache with a rapid onset ('thunderclap headache'), vomiting, confusion or a lowered level of consciousness, and sometimes seizures.
Venous thrombosis	A venous thrombosis is a blood clot (thrombus) that forms within a vein. Thrombosis is a medical term for a blood clot occurring inside a blood vessel. A classical venous thrombosis is deep vein thrombosis (DVT), which can break off (embolize), and become a life-threatening pulmonary embolism (PE).
Magnesium sulfate	Magnesium sulfate is an inorganic salt (chemical compound) containing magnesium, sulfur and oxygen, with the formula $MgSO_4$. It is often encountered as the heptahydrate sulfate mineral epsomite ($MgSO_4 \cdot 7H_2O$), commonly called Epsom salt England, where the salt was produced from the springs that arise where the porous chalk of the North Downs meets non-porous London clay. Epsom salt occurs naturally as a pure mineral.
Hypotonia	Hypotonia is a state of low muscle tone (the amount of tension or resistance to movement in a muscle), often involving reduced muscle strength. Hypotonia is not a specific medical disorder, but a potential manifestation of many different diseases and disorders that affect motor nerve control by the brain or muscle strength. Recognizing hypotonia, even in early infancy, is usually relatively straightforward, but diagnosing the underlying cause can be difficult and often unsuccessful.
Spinal muscular atrophies	Spinal Muscular Atrophies are a genetically and clinically heterogeneous group of disorders characterized by degeneration and loss of anterior horn cells in the spinal cord, leading to degeneration of motor neurons, resulting in muscle weakness and atrophy. The clinical spectrum of spinal muscular atrophies ranges from early infant death to normal adult life with only mild weakness.
	Patients often require comprehensive medical care involving multiple disciplines, including pediatric pulmonology, pediatric neurology, pediatric orthopedic surgery, lower extremity and spinal orthoses, pediatric critical care, and physical therapy, occupational therapy, respiratory therapy, and clinical nutrition.
Differential diagnosis	A differential diagnosis is a systematic diagnostic method used to identify the presence of an entity where multiple alternatives are possible (and the process may be termed differential diagnostic procedure), and may also refer to any of the included candidate alternatives (which may also be termed candidate condition). This method is essentially a process of elimination, or at least, rendering of the probabilities of candidate conditions to negligible levels.

Chapter 6. NEUROLOGIC

Nervous system	The nervous system is an organ system containing a network of specialized cells called neurons that coordinate the actions of an animal and transmit signals between different parts of its body. In most animals the nervous system consists of two parts, central and peripheral. The central nervous system of vertebrates (such as humans) contains the brain, spinal cord, and retina.
Peripheral nervous system	The peripheral nervous system consists of the nerves and ganglia outside of the brain and spinal cord. The main function of the PNS is to connect the central nervous system (CNS) to the limbs and organs. Unlike the CNS, the PNS is not protected by the bone of spine and skull, or by the blood-brain barrier, leaving it exposed to toxins and mechanical injuries.
Botulism	Botulism is a protein produced under anaerobic conditions by the bacterium Clostridium botulinum, and affecting a wide range of mammals, birds and fish. The toxin enters the human body in one of three ways: by colonization of the digestive tract by the bacterium in children (infant botulism) or adults (adult intestinal toxemia), by ingestion of toxin from foods or by contamination of a wound by the bacterium (wound botulism). Person to person transmission of botulism does not occur.
Clostridium botulinum	Clostridium botulinum is a Gram-positive, rod-shaped bacterium that produces several toxins. The best known are its neurotoxins, subdivided in types A-G, that cause the flaccid muscular paralysis seen in botulism. It is also the main paralytic agent in botox.
Congenital myasthenic syndrome	Congenital myasthenic syndrome is an inherited neuromuscular disorder caused by defects of several types at the neuromuscular junction. The effects of the disease are similar to Lambert-Eaton syndrome and Myasthenia gravis, the difference being that CMS is not an autoimmune disorder. The types of CMS are classified into three categories: presynaptic, postsynaptic, and synaptic.
Muscle biopsy	In medicine, a muscle biopsy is a procedure in which a piece of muscle tissue is removed from an organism and examined microscopically. A biopsy needle is usually inserted into a muscle, wherein a small amount of tissue remains. Alternatively, an 'open biopsy' can be performed by obtaining the muscle tissue through a small surgical incision.
Muscular dystrophies	Muscular dystrophy refers to a group of hereditary muscle diseases that weaken the muscles that move the human body. muscular dystrophies are characterized by progressive skeletal muscle weakness, defects in muscle proteins, and the death of muscle cells and tissue.

Myasthenia gravis	Myasthenia gravis is an autoimmune neuromuscular disease leading to fluctuating muscle weakness and fatiguability. It is an autoimmune disorder, in which weakness is caused by circulating antibodies that block acetylcholine receptors at the postsynaptic neuromuscular junction, inhibiting the excitatory effects of the neurotransmitter acetylcholine on nicotinic receptors throughout neuromuscular junctions. Myasthenia is treated medically with acetylcholinesterase inhibitors or immunosuppressants, and, in selected cases, thymectomy.
Myotonic dystrophy	Myotonic dystrophy is a chronic, slowly progressing, highly variable, inherited multisystemic disease. It is characterized by wasting of the muscles (muscular dystrophy), cataracts, heart conduction defects, endocrine changes, and myotonia. Two types of adult onset myotonic dystrophy exist.
Riley-Day Syndrome	Familial dysautonomia (FD, sometimes called Riley-Day syndrome) is a disorder of the autonomic nervous system which affects the development and survival of sensory, sympathetic and some parasympathetic neurons in the autonomic and sensory nervous system resulting in variable symptoms including: insensitivity to pain, inability to produce tears, poor growth, and labile blood pressure (episodic hypertension and postural hypotension). People with FD have frequent vomiting crises, pneumonia, problems with speech and movement, difficulty swallowing, inappropriate perception of heat, pain, and taste, as well as unstable blood pressure and gastrointestinal dysmotility. FD does not affect intelligence.
Health care	Health care is the diagnosis, treatment, and prevention of disease, illness, injury, and other physical and mental impairments in humans. Health care is delivered by practitioners in medicine, chiropractic, dentistry, nursing, pharmacy, allied health, and other care providers. It refers to the work done in providing primary care, secondary care and tertiary care, as well as in public health.
Motor neuron	In vertebrates, the term motor neuron classically applies to neurons located in the central nervous system (or CNS) that project their axons outside the CNS and directly or indirectly control muscles. The motor neuron is often associated with efferent neuron, primary neuron, or alpha motor neurons.

Anatomy and physiology

According to their targets, motor neurons are classified into three broad categories:

Somatic motor neurons, which directly innervate skeletal muscles, involved in locomotion (such as the muscles of the limbs, abdominal, and intercostal muscles).

Chapter 6. NEUROLOGIC

Neuromuscular junction	A neuromuscular junction is the synapse or junction of the axon terminal of a motor neuron with the motor end plate, the highly-excitable region of muscle fiber plasma membrane responsible for initiation of action potentials across the muscle's surface, ultimately causing the muscle to contract. In vertebrates, the signal passes through the neuromuscular junction via the neurotransmitter acetylcholine. The neuromuscular junction is the location where the neuron activates muscle to contract.
Transverse myelitis	Transverse myelitis is a neurological disorder caused by an inflammatory process of the spinal cord, and can cause axonal demyelination. The name is derived from Greek myelón referring to the 'spinal cord', and the suffix -itis, which denotes inflammation. Transverse implies that the inflammation is across the thickness of the spinal cord.
Becker muscular dystrophy	Becker muscular dystrophy is an X-linked recessive inherited disorder characterized by slowly progressive muscle weakness of the legs and pelvis. It is a type of dystrophinopathy, which includes a spectrum of muscle diseases in which there is insufficient dystrophin produced in the muscle cells, resulting in instability in the structure of muscle cell membrane. This is caused by mutations in the dystrophin gene, which encodes the protein dystrophin.
Congenital myopathy	Congenital myopathy is a term for any muscle disorder present at birth. By this definition the congenital myopathies could include hundreds of distinct neuromuscular syndromes and disorders. Congenital myopathies do not show evidence for either a progressive dystrophic process (i.e., muscle death) or inflammation, but instead characteristic microscopic changes are seen in association with reduced contractile ability of the muscles.
Duchenne muscular dystrophy	Duchenne muscular dystrophy is a recessive X-linked form of muscular dystrophy, which results in muscle degeneration, difficulty walking, breathing, and death. The incidence is 1 in 3,000. Females and males are affected, though females are rarely affected and are more often carriers. The disorder is caused by a mutation in the dystrophin gene, located in humans on the X chromosome (Xp21).
Zellweger syndrome	Zellweger syndrome, is a rare congenital disorder, characterized by the reduction or absence of functional peroxisomes in the cells of an individual. It is one of a family of disorders called leukodystrophies. Zellweger syndrome is named after Hans Zellweger, a former professor of Pediatrics and Genetics at the University of Iowa who researched this disorder.
Lactic acid	Lactic acid, is a chemical compound that plays a role in various biochemical processes and was first isolated in 1780 by the Swedish chemist Carl Wilhelm Scheele. Lactic acid is a carboxylic acid with the chemical formula $C_3H_6O_3$.

Confusion	Confusion of a pathological degree, usually refers to loss of orientation (ability to place oneself correctly in the world by time, location, and personal identity) and often memory (ability to correctly recall previous events or learn new material). Confusion as such is not synonymous with inability to focus attention, although severe inability to focus attention can cause, or greatly contribute to, Confusion. Together, Confusion and inability to focus attention (both of which affect judgment) are the twin symptoms of a loss or lack of normal brain function (mentation).
Delirium	Delirium is a common and severe neuropsychiatric syndrome with core features of acute onset and fluctuating course, attentional deficits and generalized severe disorganization of behavior. It typically involves other cognitive deficits, changes in arousal (hyperactive, hypoactive, or mixed), perceptual deficits, altered sleep-wake cycle, and psychotic features such as hallucinations and delusions. It is often caused by a disease process outside the brain, such as infection (urinary tract infection, pneumonia) or drug effects, particularly anticholinergics or other CNS depressants (benzodiazepines and opioids).
Hallucination	A hallucination, in the broadest sense of the word, is a perception in the absence of a stimulus. In a stricter sense, hallucinations are defined as perceptions in a conscious and awake state in the absence of external stimuli which have qualities of real perception, in that they are vivid, substantial, and located in external objective space. The latter definition distinguishes hallucinations from the related phenomena of dreaming, which does not involve wakefulness; illusion, which involves distorted or misinterpreted real perception; imagery, which does not mimic real perception and is under voluntary control; and pseudohallucination, which does not mimic real perception, but is not under voluntary control.
Obtundation	Obtundation refers to less than full mental capacity in a medical patient, typically as a result of a medical condition or trauma. The root word, obtund, means 'dulled or less sharp'.
Stupor	Stupor is the lack of critical cognitive function and level of consciousness wherein a sufferer is almost entirely unresponsive and only responds to base stimuli such as pain. A person is also rigid and mute and only appears to be conscious as the eyes are open and follow surrounding objects (Gelder, Mayou and Geddes 2005). The word derives from the Latin stupure, meaning insensible.
Vegetative state	A persistent Vegetative state is a condition of patients with severe brain damage who were in a coma, but then progressed to a state of wakefulness without detectable awareness. It is a diagnosis of some uncertainty in that it deals with a syndrome. It is classified as a Permanent Vegetative state after approximately 1 year of being in a Persistent Vegetative state which is called so after 4 weeks in a Vegetative state.

Chapter 6. NEUROLOGIC

Heart failure	Heart failure often called congestive heart failure or congestive cardiac failure (CCF) is the inability of the heart to provide sufficient pump action to distribute blood flow to meet the needs of the body. Heart failure can cause a number of symptoms including shortness of breath, leg swelling, and exercise intolerance. The condition is diagnosed with echocardiography and blood tests.
Mental state	· In psychology, Mental state is an indication of a person's mental health. · Relaxed in Flow (psychology), a Relaxed Mental state of arousal, flow, over-learned self-control and relaxation. · In the philosophy of mind, a Mental state is the kind of state or process that is unique to thinking and feeling beings. These can be representational states, see propositional attitude, or qualitative states, see qualia.
Local anesthetic	A local anesthetic is a drug that causes reversible local anesthesia, generally for the aim of having local analgesic effect, that is, inducing absence of pain sensation, although other local senses are often affected as well. Also, when it is used on specific nerve pathways (nerve block), paralysis (loss of muscle power) can be achieved as well. Clinical local anesthetics belong to one of two classes: aminoamide and aminoester local anesthetics.
Locked-in syndrome	Locked-in syndrome is a condition in which a patient is aware and awake but cannot move or communicate verbally due to complete paralysis of nearly all voluntary muscles in the body except for the eyes. Total locked-in syndrome is a version of locked-in syndrome where the eyes are paralyzed as well. The term for this disorder was coined by Fred Plum and Jerome Posner in 1966. Locked-in syndrome is also known as cerebromedullospinal disconnection, de-efferented state, pseudocoma, and ventral pontine syndrome.
Minimally conscious state	Minimally Conscious State is a disorder of consciousness distinct from Persistent vegetative state and Locked-in syndrome. Unlike persistent vegetative state, patients with MCS have partial preservation of conscious awareness. MCS is a relatively new category of disorders of consciousness.
Regional analgesia	Regional analgesia blocks passage of pain impulses through a nerve by depositing an analgesic drug close to the nerve trunk, cutting off sensory innervation to the region it supplies. The drug is normally injected at a site where the nerve is unprotected by bone.
Akinetic mutism	Akinetic mutism is a medical term describing patients tending neither to move (akinesia)nor speak (mutism). It is the result of severe frontal lobe injury in which the pattern of inhibitory control is one of increasing passivity and gradually decreasing speech and motion.

Brain death	Brain death is the irreversible end of all brain activity (including involuntary activity necessary to sustain life) due to total necrosis of the cerebral neurons following loss of brain oxygenation. It should not be confused with a persistent vegetative state. Patients classified as brain dead can have their organs surgically removed for organ donation.
Coma scale	A Coma scale is a system to assess the severity of coma. There are several such systems: The Glasgow Coma Scale is neurological scale which aims to give a reliable, objective way of recording the conscious state of a person, for initial as well as continuing assessment. A patient is assessed against the criteria of the scale, and the resulting points give a patient score between 3 (indicating deep unconsciousness) and either 14 (original scale) or 15 (the more widely used modified or revised scale).
Physical examination	A physical examination, medical examination, or clinical examination (more popularly known as a check-up or medical) is the process by which a doctor investigates the body of a patient for signs of disease. It generally follows the taking of the medical history -- an account of the symptoms as experienced by the patient. Together with the medical history, the physical examination aids in determining the correct diagnosis and devising the treatment plan.
Cheyne-Stokes respiration	Cheyne-Stokes respiration is an abnormal pattern of breathing characterized by progressively deeper and sometimes faster breathing, followed by a gradual decrease that results in a temporary stop in breathing called an apnea. The pattern repeats, with each cycle usually taking 30 seconds to 2 minutes. It is an oscillation of ventilation between apnea and hyperpnea with a crescendo-decrescendo pattern, and is associated with changing serum partial pressures of oxygen and carbon dioxide.
Corn syrup	Corn syrup is a food syrup, which is made from the starch of corn or 'maize' (U.K). and which is composed mainly of glucose. Corn syrup is used in foods to soften texture, add volume, prevent crystallization of sugar, and enhance flavour.
Corneal reflex	The corneal reflex, is an involuntary blinking of the eyelids elicited by stimulation (such as touching or a foreign body) of the cornea, or bright light, though could result from any peripheral stimulus. Stimulation should elicit both a direct and consensual response (response of the opposite eye). The reflex consumes a rapid rate of 0.1 second.
Neuroimaging	Neuroimaging includes the use of various techniques to either directly or indirectly image the structure, function/pharmacology of the brain. It is a relatively new discipline within medicine and neurosciencepsychology. Physicians who specialize in the performance and interpretation of neuroimaging in the clinical setting are neuroradiologists.

Chapter 6. NEUROLOGIC

Flumazenil	Flumazenil is a benzodiazepine antagonist available for injection only, and the only benzodiazepine receptor antagonist on the market today. It was first introduced in 1987 by Hoffmann-La Roche under the trade name Anexate, but only approved by the FDA on December 20, 1991. Some years ago an oral preparation was under development, though it had low bio-availability and was thus abandoned. There is hope that oral flumazenil or other benzodiazepine antagonists such as B-carbolines will be developed in the future.
Intracranial pressure	Intracranial pressure is the pressure inside the skull and thus in the brain tissue and cerebrospinal fluid (CSF). The body has various mechanisms by which it keeps the ICP stable, with CSF pressures varying by about 1 mmHg in normal adults through shifts in production and absorption of CSF. CSF pressure has been shown to be influenced by abrupt changes in intrathoracic pressure during coughing (intraabdominal pressure), valsalva (Queckenstedt's maneuver), and communication with the vasculature (venous and arterial systems). ICP is measured in millimeters of mercury (mmHg) and, at rest, is normally 7-15 mmHg for a supine adult, and becomes negative (averaging −10 mmHg) in the vertical position.
Opioid overdose	An opioid overdose is an acute condition due to excessive use of narcotics. It should not be confused with opioid dependency. Opiate overdose symptoms and signs include: decreased level of consciousness and pinpoint pupil except with meperidine (Demerol) where one sees dilated pupils, known as pinpoint pupils.
Palliative care	Palliative care is an area of healthcare that focuses on relieving and preventing the suffering of patients. Unlike hospice care, palliative medicine is appropriate for patients in all disease stages, including those undergoing treatment for curable illnesses and those living with chronic diseases, as well as patients who are nearing the end of life. Palliative medicine utilizes a multidisciplinary approach to patient care, relying on input from physicians, pharmacists, nurses, chaplains, social workers, psychologists, and other allied health professionals in formulating a plan of care to relieve suffering in all areas of a patient's life.
Epidemiology	Epidemiology is the study of the distribution and patterns of health-events, health-characteristics and their causes or influences in well-defined populations. It is the cornerstone method of public health research and practice, and helps inform policy decisions and evidence-based medicine by identifying risk factors for disease and targets for preventive medicine and public policies. Epidemiologists are involved in the design of studies, collection and statistical analysis of data, and interpretation and dissemination of results (including peer review and occasional systematic review).

Methylmalonic acidemia	Methylmalonic acidemia also called methylmalonic aciduria, is an autosomal recessive metabolic disorder. It is a classical type of organic acidemia.
	Methylmalonic acidemia stems from several genotypes, all forms of the disorder usually diagnosed in the early neonatal period, presenting progressive encephalopathy, and secondary hyperammonemia.
Acute disseminated encephalomyelitis	Acute disseminated encephalomyelitis is an immune mediated disease of the brain. It usually occurs following a viral infection but may appear following vaccination, bacterial or parasitic infection, or even appear spontaneously. As it involves autoimmune demyelination, it is similar to multiple sclerosis, and is considered part of the Multiple sclerosis borderline diseases.
Multiple sclerosis	Multiple sclerosis is a disease in which the fatty myelin sheaths around the axons of the brain and spinal cord are damaged, leading to demyelination and scarring as well as a broad spectrum of signs and symptoms. Disease onset usually occurs in young adults, and it is more common in females. It has a prevalence that ranges between 2 and 150 per 100,000. Multiple sclerosis was first described in 1868 by Jean-Martin Charcot.

CHAPTER QUIZ: KEY TERMS, PEOPLE, PLACES, CONCEPTS

1. Etiology is the study of causation, or origination.

   The word is most commonly used in medical and philosophical theories, where it is used to refer to the study of why things occur, or even the reasons behind the way that things act, and is used in philosophy, physics, psychology, government, medicine, theology and biology in reference to the causes of various phenomena. An _____ is a myth intended to explain a name or create a mythic history for a place or family.

   a. Etiology
   b. abdominal exam
   c. Etiological myth
   d. Platypnea

2. . _____ is an X-linked recessive inherited disorder characterized by slowly progressive muscle weakness of the legs and pelvis.

   It is a type of dystrophinopathy, which includes a spectrum of muscle diseases in which there is insufficient dystrophin produced in the muscle cells, resulting in instability in the structure of muscle cell membrane. This is caused by mutations in the dystrophin gene, which encodes the protein dystrophin.

   a. Bacteriophage
   b. Becker muscular dystrophy

Chapter 6. NEUROLOGIC

Visit Cram101.com for full Practice Exams

c. Patch clamp

d. Peristimulus time histogram

3. _____ also known as Janz syndrome, is a fairly common form of idiopathic generalized epilepsy, representing 5-10% of all epilepsies. This disorder typically first manifests itself between the ages of 12 and 18 with myoclonus occurring early in the morning. Most patients also have tonic-clonic seizures and many also have absence seizures.

a. Juvenile myoclonic epilepsy

b. Neurological disorder

c. Balance disorder

d. Basilar invagination

4. _____ is a protein produced under anaerobic conditions by the bacterium Clostridium botulinum, and affecting a wide range of mammals, birds and fish.

The toxin enters the human body in one of three ways: by colonization of the digestive tract by the bacterium in children (infant _____) or adults (adult intestinal toxemia), by ingestion of toxin from foods or by contamination of a wound by the bacterium (wound _____). Person to person transmission of _____ does not occur.

a. Chikungunya

b. Botulism

c. Coxiella burnetii

d. Defoliation bacilli bomb

5. _____s (also called focal seizures and localized seizures) are seizures which affect only a part of the brain at onset, and are split into two main categories; simple _____s and complex _____s.

A simple _____ will often be a precursor to a larger seizure such as a complex _____, or a tonic-clonic seizure. When this is the case, the simple _____ is usually called an aura.

a. Partial seizure

b. Pel-Ebstein fever

c. Perspiration

d. Platypnea

1. c
2. b
3. a
4. b
5. a

You can take the complete Chapter Practice Test

for Chapter 6. NEUROLOGIC
on all key terms, persons, places, and concepts.

Online 99 Cents

http://www.epub219.49.13357.6.cram101.com/

Use www.Cram101.com for all your study needs

including Cram101's online interactive problem solving labs in

chemistry, statistics, mathematics, and more.

Chapter 7. GASTROENTEROLOGY

CHAPTER OUTLINE: KEY TERMS, PEOPLE, PLACES, CONCEPTS

	Abdominal pain
	Functional gastrointestinal disorder
	Physical examination
	Cyclic vomiting syndrome
	Polyethylene glycol
	Trichomonas vaginalis
	Irritable bowel syndrome
	Gastrointestinal bleeding
	Hematemesis
	Melena
	Pathophysiology
	Apt-Downey test
	Upper gastrointestinal bleeding
	Risk factor
	Bain-marie
	Computed tomography
	Esophageal varices
	Helicobacter pylori
	Mallory-Weiss syndrome

Portal hypertension

Symptom

Anal fissure

Cerebrospinal fluid

Lower gastrointestinal bleeding

Milk allergy

Hemolytic anemia

Proton pump

Differential diagnosis

Gastroesophageal reflux

Hemolytic-uremic syndrome

Encopresis

Constipation

Anorectal manometry

Magnesium citrate

Mineral oil

Activation syndrome

Patient education

Gastroesophageal reflux disease

	Cerebral palsy
	Esophageal pH monitoring
	Gastrointestinal series
	Prognosis
	Ulcerative colitis
	Imaging
	Inflammatory bowel disease
	Abdominal mass
	Barium
	Capsule endoscopy
	Endoscopy
	Palliative care
	Terminal sedation
	Parenteral nutrition
	Cystic fibrosis
	Hepatitis
	Etiological myth
	ACE inhibitor
	Liver failure

Cerebral edema

Hepatic encephalopathy

Glucose transporter

Prevention

ERCP

Magnetic resonance cholangiopancreatography

Pancreatitis

Conversion disorder

CHAPTER HIGHLIGHTS & NOTES: KEY TERMS, PEOPLE, PLACES, CONCEPTS

Abdominal pain	Abdominal pain can be one of the symptoms associated with transient disorders or serious disease. Making a definitive diagnosis of the cause of abdominal pain can be difficult, because many diseases can result in this symptom. Abdominal pain is a common problem.
Functional gastrointestinal disorder	Functional gastrointestinal disorder include a number of separate idiopathic disorders which affect different part of the gastrointestinal tract. •Functional esophageal disorders •Functional heartburn•Functional chest pain of presumed esophageal origin•Functional dysphagia•Globus pharyngis•Functional colonic disease •Functional constipation•Functional rectal painDiagnosis The Rome process has helped to define the functional gastrointestinal disorders. Successively, the Rome I, Rome II and the Rome III meetings have proposed a consensual classification system and terminology, as recommended by the Rome Coordinating Committee.
Physical examination	A physical examination, medical examination, or clinical examination (more popularly known as a check-up or medical) is the process by which a doctor investigates the body of a patient for signs of disease.

	It generally follows the taking of the medical history -- an account of the symptoms as experienced by the patient. Together with the medical history, the physical examination aids in determining the correct diagnosis and devising the treatment plan.
Cyclic vomiting syndrome	Cyclic vomiting syndrome are recurring attacks of intense nausea, vomiting and sometimes abdominal pain and/or headaches or migraines. Cyclic vomiting usually develops during childhood usually ages 3-7; although it often remits during adolescence, it can persist into adult life. The average age at onset is 3-7 years, but CVS has been seen in infants who are as young as 6 days and in adults who are as old as 73 years.
Polyethylene glycol	Polyethylene glycol is a polyether compound with many applications from industrial manufacturing to medicine. The structure of PEG is (note the repeated element in parentheses):$HO-CH_2-(CH_2-O-CH_2-)_n-CH_2-OH$ PEG is also known as polyethylene oxide (PEO) or polyoxyethylene (POE), depending on its molecular weight, and under the tradename Carbowax. Available forms and nomenclature PEG, PEO, or POE refers to an oligomer or polymer of ethylene oxide.
Trichomonas vaginalis	Trichomonas vaginalis is an anaerobic, flagellated protozoan, a form of microorganism. The parasitic microorganism is the causative agent of trichomoniasis, and is the most common pathogenic protozoan infection of humans in industrialized countries. Infection rates between men and women are the same with women showing symptoms while infections in men are usually asymptomatic.
Irritable bowel syndrome	Irritable bowel syndrome is a symptom-based diagnosis characterized by chronic abdominal pain, discomfort, bloating, and alteration of bowel habits. As a functional bowel disorder, IBS has no known organic cause. Diarrhea or constipation may predominate, or they may alternate (classified as IBS-D, IBS-C or IBS-A, respectively).
Gastrointestinal bleeding	Gastrointestinal bleeding, from the pharynx to the rectum. It has diverse causes, and a medical history, as well as physical examination, generally distinguishes between the main forms. The degree of bleeding can range from nearly undetectable to acute, massive, life-threatening bleeding.
Hematemesis	Hematemesis is the vomiting of blood. The source is generally the upper gastrointestinal tract. Patients can easily confuse it with hemoptysis (coughing up blood), although the latter is more common.

Chapter 7. GASTROENTEROLOGY

Melena	In medicine, Melena or melaena refers to the black, 'tarry' feces that are associated with gastrointestinal hemorrhage. The black color is caused by oxidation of the iron in hemoglobin during its passage through the ileum and colon.
	Bleeding originating from the lower GI tract (such as the sigmoid colon and rectum) is generally associated with the passage of bright red blood, or hematochezia, particularly when brisk.
Pathophysiology	Pathophysiology sample values
	Pathophysiology is the study of the changes of normal mechanical, physical, and biochemical functions, either caused by a disease, or resulting from an abnormal syndrome. More formally, it is the branch of medicine which deals with any disturbances of body functions, caused by disease or prodromal symptoms.
	An alternative definition is 'the study of the biological and physical manifestations of disease as they correlate with the underlying abnormalities and physiological disturbances.'
	The study of pathology and the study of pathophysiology often involves substantial overlap in diseases and processes, but pathology emphasizes direct observations, while pathophysiology emphasizes quantifiable measurements.
Apt-Downey test	The Apt-Downey test is used to help differentiate between maternal and baby blood.
	The blood is placed in a test tube; sterile water is added to hemolyze the RBCs, yielding free hemoglobin.
	This solution then is mixed with 1% sodium hydroxide.
Upper gastrointestinal bleeding	Upper gastrointestinal (GI) bleeding refers to hemorrhage in the upper gastrointestinal tract. The anatomic cut-off for upper GI bleeding is the ligament of Treitz, which connects the fourth portion of the duodenum to the diaphragm near the splenic flexure of the colon.
	Upper GI bleeds are considered medical emergencies, and require admission to hospital for urgent diagnosis and management. Due to advances in medications and endoscopy, upper GI hemorrhage is now usually treated without surgery. Presentation
	Patients with upper GI hemorrhage often present with hematemesis, coffee ground vomiting, melena, or hematochezia (maroon coloured stool) if the hemorrhage is severe. The presentation of bleeding depends on the amount and location of hemorrhage.

Patients may also present with complications of anemia, including chest pain, syncope, fatigue and shortness of breath.

The physical examination performed by the physician concentrates on the following things:•Vital signs, in order to determine the severity of bleeding and the timing of intervention•Abdominal and rectal examination, in order to determine possible causes of hemorrhage•Assessment for portal hypertension and stigmata of chronic liver disease in order to determine if the bleeding is from a variceal source.

Laboratory findings include anemia, coagulopathy, and an elevated BUN-to-creatinine ratio. Causes

A number of medications increase the risk of bleeding including NSAIDs and SSRIs. SSRIs double the rate of upper gastrointestinal bleeding.

Risk factor	In epidemiology, a risk factor is a variable associated with an increased risk of disease or infection. Sometimes, determinant is also used, being a variable associated with either increased or decreased risk. Risk factors or determinants are correlational and not necessarily causal, because correlation does not prove causation.
Bain-marie	A bain-marie is a French term for a piece of equipment used in science, industry, and cooking to heat materials gently and gradually to fixed temperatures, or to keep materials warm over a period of time. The bain-marie comes in a wide variety of shapes, sizes, and types, but traditionally is a wide, cylindrical, usually metal container made of three or four basic parts: a handle, an outer container that holds the working-liquid, an inner (or upper), smaller container that fits inside the outer one and which holds the material to be heated or cooked, and sometimes a base underneath. Under the outer container of the bain-marie is a heat source.
Computed tomography	Computed tomography is a medical imaging method employing tomography created by computer processing. Digital geometry processing is used to generate a three-dimensional image of the inside of an object from a large series of two-dimensional X-ray images taken around a single axis of rotation. Computed tomography produces a volume of data which can be manipulated, through a process known as 'windowing', in order to demonstrate various bodily structures based on their ability to block the X-ray/R

Chapter 7. GASTROENTEROLOGY

Esophageal varices	In medicine (gastroenterology), esophageal varices are extremely dilated sub-mucosal veins in the lower third of the esophagus. They are most often a consequence of portal hypertension, commonly due to cirrhosis; patients with esophageal varices have a strong tendency to develop bleeding. Esophageal varices are diagnosed with endoscopy.
Helicobacter pylori	Helicobacter pylori previously named Campylobacter pyloridis, is a Gram-negative, microaerophilic bacterium found in the stomach. It was identified in 1982 by Barry Marshall and Robin Warren, who found that it was present in patients with chronic gastritis and gastric ulcers, conditions that were not previously believed to have a microbial cause. It is also linked to the development of duodenal ulcers and stomach cancer.
Mallory-Weiss syndrome	Mallory-Weiss syndrome refers to bleeding from tears (a Mallory-Weiss tear) in the mucosa at the junction of the stomach and esophagus, usually caused by severe retching, coughing, or vomiting. It is often associated with alcoholism and eating disorders and there is some evidence that presence of a hiatal hernia is a predisposing condition. Mallory-Weiss syndrome often presents as an episode of vomiting up blood (hematemesis) after violent retching or vomiting, but may also be noticed as old blood in the stool (melena), and a history of retching may be absent.
Portal hypertension	In medicine, portal hypertension is hypertension (high blood pressure) in the portal vein and its tributaries. It is often defined as a portal pressure gradient (the difference in pressure between the portal vein and the hepatic veins) of 10 mmHg or greater. Causes can be divided into prehepatic, intrahepatic, and posthepatic.
Symptom	A symptom is a departure from normal function or feeling which is noticed by a patient, indicating the presence of disease or abnormality. A symptom is subjective, observed by the patient, and not measured. A symptom may not be a malady, for example symptoms of pregnancy.
Anal fissure	An anal fissure is a break or tear in the skin of the anal canal. Anal fissures may be noticed by bright red anal bleeding on the toilet paper, sometimes in the toilet. If acute they may cause severe periodic pain after defecation but with chronic fissures pain intensity is often less.

CHAPTER HIGHLIGHTS & NOTES: KEY TERMS, PEOPLE, PLACES, CONCEPTS

Cerebrospinal fluid	Cerebrospinal fluid Liquor cerebrospinalis, is a clear, colorless, bodily fluid, that occupies the subarachnoid space and the ventricular system around and inside the brain and spinal cord. The CSF occupies the space between the arachnoid mater (the middle layer of the brain cover, meninges) and the pia mater (the layer of the meninges closest to the brain). It constitutes the content of all intra-cerebral (inside the brain, cerebrum) ventricles, cisterns, and sulci, as well as the central canal of the spinal cord.
Lower gastrointestinal bleeding	Lower gastrointestinal bleeding, commonly abbreviated LGIB, refers to any form of bleeding in the lower gastrointestinal tract. LGIB is a common ailment seen at emergency departments. It presents less commonly than upper gastrointestinal bleeding (UGIB).
Milk allergy	A milk allergy is a food allergy, an adverse immune reaction to one or more of the constituents of milk from any animal (most commonly alpha S1-casein, a protein in cow's milk). This milk-induced allergic reaction can involve anaphylaxis, a potentially life-threatening condition. It is important to note that a milk allergy is a separate and distinct condition from lactose intolerance.
Hemolytic anemia	Hemolytic anemia is a form of anemia due to hemolysis, the abnormal breakdown of red blood cells (RBCs), either in the blood vessels (intravascular hemolysis) or elsewhere in the human body (extravascular). It has numerous possible causes, ranging from relatively harmless to life-threatening. The general classification of hemolytic anemia is either inherited or acquired.
Proton pump	A proton pump is an integral membrane protein that is capable of moving protons across a cell membrane, mitochondrion, or other organelle. In cell respiration, the pump actively transports protons from the matrix of the mitochondrion into the space between the inner and outer mitochondrial membranes. This action creates a concentration gradient across the inner mitochondrial membrane as there are more protons outside the matrix than in.
Differential diagnosis	A differential diagnosis is a systematic diagnostic method used to identify the presence of an entity where multiple alternatives are possible (and the process may be termed differential diagnostic procedure), and may also refer to any of the included candidate alternatives (which may also be termed candidate condition). This method is essentially a process of elimination, or at least, rendering of the probabilities of candidate conditions to negligible levels. In this sense, probabilities are, in fact, imaginative parameters in the mind or hardware of the diagnostician or system, while in reality the target (such as a patient) either has a condition or not with an actual probability of either 0 or 100%.

Chapter 7. GASTROENTEROLOGY

Gastroesophageal reflux	Gastroesophageal reflux disease (GERD), gastro-oesophageal reflux disease (GORD), gastric reflux disease, or acid reflux disease is defined as chronic symptoms or mucosal damage produced by the abnormal reflux in the oesophagus. This is commonly due to transient or permanent changes in the barrier between the oesophagus and the stomach. This can be due to incompetence of the lower esophageal sphincter, transient lower oesophageal sphincter relaxation, impaired expulsion of gastric reflux from the oesophagus, or a hiatal hernia.
Hemolytic-uremic syndrome	Hemolytic-uremic syndrome , abbreviated HUS, is a disease characterized by hemolytic anemia (anemia caused by destruction of red blood cells), acute kidney failure (uremia) and a low platelet count (thrombocytopenia). It predominantly, but not exclusively, affects children. Most cases are preceded by an episode of infectious, sometimes bloody, diarrhea caused by E. coli O157:H7, which is acquired as a foodborne illness or from a contaminated water supply.
Encopresis	Encopresis (from the Greek κοπρος (kopros, dung), also known as paradoxical diarrhea) is involuntary fecal soiling in adults and children who have usually already been toilet trained. Persons with encopresis often leak stool into their undergarments. The estimated prevalence of encopresis in four-year-olds is between one and three percent.
Constipation	Constipation refers to bowel movements that are infrequent or hard to pass. Constipation is a common cause of painful defecation. Severe constipation includes obstipation (failure to pass stools or gas) and fecal impaction .
Anorectal manometry	Anorectal manometry is a technique used to measure contractility in the anus and rectum. It may be used to assist in the diagnosis of Hirschprung disease.
Magnesium citrate	Magnesium citrate, a magnesium preparation in salt form with citric acid, is a chemical agent used medicinally as a saline laxative and to completely empty the bowel prior to a major surgery or colonoscopy. It is available without a prescription, both as a generic or under the brand name Citromag or Citroma. It is also used as a magnesium supplement in pills.
Mineral oil	A mineral oil is any of various colorless, odorless, light mixtures of alkanes in the C15 to C40 range from a non-vegetable (mineral) source, particularly a distillate of petroleum. The name mineral oil by itself is imprecise, having been used to label many specific oils over the past few centuries. Other names, similarly imprecise, include white oil, liquid paraffin, and liquid petroleum.

Activation syndrome	Activation syndrome is a form of sometimes suicidal or homicidal stimulation or agitation that can occur in response to some psychoactive drugs. A study of paroxetine found that 21 out of 93 (23 percent) of youth taking Paxil reported manic-like symptoms which included hostility, emotional lability and nervousness. Pfizer has denied that sertraline can cause such effects.
Patient education	Patient education is the process by which health professionals and others impart information to patients that will alter their health behaviors or improve their health status. Education providers may include: physicians, pharmacists, registered dietitians, nurses, hospital discharge planners, medical social workers, psychologists, disease or disability advocacy groups, special interest groups, and pharmaceutical companies.

Health education is also a tool used by managed care plans, and may include both general preventive education or health promotion and disease or condition specific education. |
| Gastroesophageal reflux disease | Gastroesophageal reflux disease gastro-oesophageal reflux disease (GORD), gastric reflux disease, or acid reflux disease is a chronic symptom of mucosal damage caused by stomach acid coming up from the stomach into the esophagus.

GERD is usually caused by changes in the barrier between the stomach and the esophagus, including abnormal relaxation of the lower esophageal sphincter, which normally holds the top of the stomach closed; impaired expulsion of gastric reflux from the esophagus, or a hiatal hernia. These changes may be permanent or temporary ('transient'). |
| Cerebral palsy | Cerebral palsy is an umbrella term encompassing a group of non-progressive, non-contagious motor conditions that cause physical disability in human development, chiefly in the various areas of body movement.

Cerebral refers to the cerebrum, which is the affected area of the brain (although the disorder most likely involves connections between the cortex and other parts of the brain such as the cerebellum), and palsy refers to disorder of movement. Furthermore, 'paralytic disorders' are not cerebral palsy - the condition of quadriplegia, therefore, should not be confused with spastic quadriplegia, nor tardive dyskinesia with dyskinetic cerebral palsy, nor diplegia with spastic diplegia, and so on. |
| Esophageal pH monitoring | Esophageal pH monitoring is the current gold standard for diagnosis of gastroesophageal reflux disease (GERD). It provides direct physiologic measurement of acid in the esophagus and is the most objective method to document reflux disease, assess the severity of the disease and monitor the response of the disease to medical or surgical treatment. It can also be used in diagnosing laryngopharyngeal reflux. |

Chapter 7. GASTROENTEROLOGY

Gastrointestinal series	A Gastrointestinal series is a radiologic examination of the upper and/or lower gastrointestinal tract. · Upper GI series · Lower GI series
Prognosis	Prognosis is a medical term to describe the likely outcome of an illness. When applied to large populations, prognostic estimates can be very accurate: for example the statement '45% of patients with severe septic shock will die within 28 days' can be made with some confidence, because previous research found that this proportion of patients died. However, it is much harder to translate this into a prognosis for an individual patient: additional information is needed to determine whether a patient belongs to the 45% who will succumb, or to the 55% who survive.
Ulcerative colitis	Ulcerative colitis is a form of inflammatory bowel disease (IBD). Ulcerative colitis is a form of colitis, a disease of the colon (large intestine), that includes characteristic ulcers, or open sores. The main symptom of active disease is usually constant diarrhea mixed with blood, of gradual onset.
Imaging	Imaging is the representation or reproduction of an object's outward form; especially a visual representation (i.e., the formation of an image). · Chemical Imaging, the simultaneous measurement of spectra and pictures · Creation of a disk image, a file which contains the exact content of a non-volatile computer data storage medium.
Inflammatory bowel disease	In medicine, inflammatory bowel disease is a group of inflammatory conditions of the colon and small intestine. The major types of IBD are Crohn's disease and ulcerative colitis. The main forms of IBD are Crohn's disease and ulcerative colitis (UC).
Abdominal mass	An abdominal mass is any localized enlargement or swelling in the human abdomen. Depending on its location, the abdominal mass may be caused by an enlarged liver (hepatomegaly), enlarged spleen (splenomegaly), protruding kidney, a pancreatic mass, a retroperitoneal mass (a mass in the posterior of the peritoneum), an abdominal aortic aneurysm, or various tumours, such as those caused by abdominal carcinomatosis and omental metastasis. The treatments depend on the cause, and may range from watchful waiting to radical surgery.
Barium	Barium is a chemical element with the symbol Ba and atomic number 56. It is the fifth element in Group 2, a soft silvery metallic alkaline earth metal.

	Barium is never found in nature as a free element, due to its high chemical reactivity. Its oxide is historically known as baryta, but this oxide (in a similar way to calcium oxide, or quicklime) must be artificially produced since it reacts avidly with water and carbon dioxide, and is not found as a mineral.
Capsule endoscopy	Capsule endoscopy is a way to record images of the digestive tract for use in medicine. The capsule is the size and shape of a pill and contains a tiny camera. After a patient swallows the capsule, it takes pictures of the inside of the gastrointestinal tract.
Endoscopy	Endoscopy, an instrument used to examine the interior of a hollow organ or cavity of the body. Unlike most other medical imaging devices, endoscopes are inserted directly into the organ. Endoscopy can also refer to using a borescope in technical situations where direct line of-sight observation is not feasible.
Palliative care	Palliative care is an area of healthcare that focuses on relieving and preventing the suffering of patients. Unlike hospice care, palliative medicine is appropriate for patients in all disease stages, including those undergoing treatment for curable illnesses and those living with chronic diseases, as well as patients who are nearing the end of life. Palliative medicine utilizes a multidisciplinary approach to patient care, relying on input from physicians, pharmacists, nurses, chaplains, social workers, psychologists, and other allied health professionals in formulating a plan of care to relieve suffering in all areas of a patient's life.
Terminal sedation	In medicine, specifically in end-of-life care, terminal sedation is the palliative practice of relieving distress in a terminally ill person in the last hours or days of a dying patient's life, usually by means of a continuous intravenous or subcutaneous infusion of a sedative drug. This is a option of last resort for patients whose symptoms cannot be controlled by any other means. This should be differentiated from euthanasia as the goal of palliative sedation is to control symptoms through sedation but not shorten the patient's life, while in euthanasia the goal is to shorten life to relieve symptoms.
Parenteral nutrition	Parenteral nutrition is feeding a person intravenously, bypassing the usual process of eating and digestion. The person receives nutritional formulae that contain nutrients such as glucose, amino acids, lipids and added vitamins and dietary minerals. It is called total parenteral nutrition or total nutrient admixture (TNA) when no food is given by other routes.
Cystic fibrosis	Cystic fibrosis is an autosomal recessive genetic disorder affecting most critically the lungs, and also the pancreas, liver, and intestine. It is characterized by abnormal transport of chloride and sodium across an epithelium, leading to thick, viscous secretions.

Chapter 7. GASTROENTEROLOGY

Hepatitis	Hepatitis is a medical condition defined by the inflammation of the liver and characterized by the presence of inflammatory cells in the tissue of the organ. The name is from the Greek hepar , the root being hepat- , meaning liver, and suffix -itis, meaning 'inflammation' (c. 1727). The condition can be self-limiting (healing on its own) or can progress to fibrosis (scarring) and cirrhosis.
Etiological myth	Etiology is the study of causation, or origination. The word is most commonly used in medical and philosophical theories, where it is used to refer to the study of why things occur, or even the reasons behind the way that things act, and is used in philosophy, physics, psychology, government, medicine, theology and biology in reference to the causes of various phenomena. An etiological myth is a myth intended to explain a name or create a mythic history for a place or family.
ACE inhibitor	ACE inhibitors are a group of drugs used primarily for the treatment of hypertension (high blood pressure) and congestive heart failure. Originally synthesized from compounds found in pit viper venom, they inhibit angiotensin-converting enzyme (ACE), a component of the blood pressure-regulating renin-angiotensin system.
Liver failure	Liver failure is the inability of the liver to perform its normal synthetic and metabolic function as part of normal physiology. Two forms are recognised, acute and chronic. Acute liver failure is defined as 'the rapid development of hepatocellular dysfunction, specifically coagulopathy and mental status changes (encephalopathy) in a patient without known prior liver disease'.
Cerebral edema	Cerebral edema or cerebral Å"dema is an excess accumulation of water in the intracellular and/or extracellular spaces of the brain. Four types of Cerebral edema have been distinguished: Due to a breakdown of tight endothelial junctions which make up the blood-brain barrier (BBB). This allows normally excluded intravascular proteins and fluid to penetrate into cerebral parenchymal extracellular space.
Hepatic encephalopathy	Hepatic encephalopathy is the occurrence of confusion, altered level of consciousness and coma as a result of liver failure. In the advanced stages it is called hepatic coma or coma hepaticum. It may ultimately lead to death.
Glucose transporter	Glucose transporters (GLUT or SLC2A family) are a family of membrane proteins found in most mammalian cells.

	Structure
	Glucose transporters are integral membrane proteins that contain 12 membrane-spanning helices with both the amino and carboxyl termini exposed on the cytoplasmic side of the plasma membrane. Glucose transporter proteins transport glucose and related hexoses according to a model of alternate conformation, which predicts that the transporter exposes a single substrate binding site toward either the outside or the inside of the cell.
Prevention	Prevention refers to:
	· Preventive medicine · Hazard Prevention, the process of risk study and elimination and mitigation in emergency management · Risk Prevention · Risk management · Preventive maintenance · Crime Prevention
	· Prevention, an album by Scottish band De Rosa · Prevention a magazine about health in the United States · Prevent (company), a textile company from Slovenia
ERCP	Endoscopic retrograde cholangiopancreatography (ERCP) is a technique that combines the use of endoscopy and fluoroscopy to diagnose and treat certain problems of the biliary or pancreatic ductal systems. Through the endoscope, the physician can see the inside of the stomach and duodenum, and inject dyes into the ducts in the biliary tree and pancreas so they can be seen on x-rays.
	ERCP is used primarily to diagnose and treat conditions of the bile ducts, including gallstones, inflammatory strictures (scars), leaks , and cancer.
Magnetic resonance cholangiopancreatogr aphy	Magnetic resonance cholangiopancreatography is a medical imaging technique that uses magnetic resonance imaging to visualise the biliary and pancreatic ducts in a non-invasive manner. This procedure can be used to determine if gallstones are lodged in any of the ducts surrounding the gallbladder.
	It was introduced in 1991.
Pancreatitis	Pancreatitis is inflammation of the pancreas. It occurs when pancreatic enzymes (especially trypsin) that digest food are activated in the pancreas instead of the small intestine. It may be acute - beginning suddenly and lasting a few days, or chronic - occurring over many years.
Conversion disorder	Conversion disorder is where patients suffer apparently neurological symptoms, such as numbness, blindness, paralysis, or fits, but without a neurological cause.

Chapter 7. GASTROENTEROLOGY

It is thought that these problems arise in response to difficulties in the patient's life, and conversion is considered a psychiatric disorder in the Diagnostic and Statistical Manual of Mental Disorders fourth edition (DSM-IV).

Formerly known as 'hysteria', the disorder has arguably been known for millennia, though it came to greatest prominence at the end of the 19th century, when the neurologists Jean-Martin Charcot and Sigmund Freud and psychiatrist Pierre Janet focused their studies on the subject.

1. _____ gastro-oesophageal reflux disease (GORD), gastric reflux disease, or acid reflux disease is a chronic symptom of mucosal damage caused by stomach acid coming up from the stomach into the esophagus.

   GERD is usually caused by changes in the barrier between the stomach and the esophagus, including abnormal relaxation of the lower esophageal sphincter, which normally holds the top of the stomach closed; impaired expulsion of gastric reflux from the esophagus, or a hiatal hernia. These changes may be permanent or temporary ('transient').

   a. Genu valgum
   b. Hemorrhoid
   c. Gastroesophageal reflux disease
   d. Hypertriglyceridemia

2. _____ can be one of the symptoms associated with transient disorders or serious disease. Making a definitive diagnosis of the cause of _____ can be difficult, because many diseases can result in this symptom. _____ is a common problem.

   a. Irritable bowel syndrome
   b. Ischemia
   c. abdominal exam
   d. Abdominal pain

3. . In medicine, specifically in end-of-life care, _____ is the palliative practice of relieving distress in a terminally ill person in the last hours or days of a dying patient's life, usually by means of a continuous intravenous or subcutaneous infusion of a sedative drug. This is a option of last resort for patients whose symptoms cannot be controlled by any other means. This should be differentiated from euthanasia as the goal of palliative sedation is to control symptoms through sedation but not shorten the patient's life, while in euthanasia the goal is to shorten life to relieve symptoms.

   a. Terminal sedation
   b. Voluntary euthanasia
   c. Whose Life Is It Anyway?

Chapter 7. GASTROENTEROLOGY

4. _____ previously named Campylobacter pyloridis, is a Gram-negative, microaerophilic bacterium found in the stomach. It was identified in 1982 by Barry Marshall and Robin Warren, who found that it was present in patients with chronic gastritis and gastric ulcers, conditions that were not previously believed to have a microbial cause. It is also linked to the development of duodenal ulcers and stomach cancer.

a. Helicobacter pylori
b. Lactagen
c. Lactulose
d. Laminarid

5. _____ is a symptom-based diagnosis characterized by chronic abdominal pain, discomfort, bloating, and alteration of bowel habits. As a functional bowel disorder, IBS has no known organic cause. Diarrhea or constipation may predominate, or they may alternate (classified as IBS-D, IBS-C or IBS-A, respectively).

a. Ischemia
b. Sodium dodecyl sulfate
c. Irritable bowel syndrome
d. Sorbitol

1. c
2. d
3. a
4. a
5. c

You can take the complete Chapter Practice Test

for Chapter 7. GASTROENTEROLOGY
on all key terms, persons, places, and concepts.

Online 99 Cents

http://www.epub219.49.13357.7.cram101.com/

Use www.Cram101.com for all your study needs

including Cram101's online interactive problem solving labs in

chemistry, statistics, mathematics, and more.

Chapter 8. HEMATOLOGY-ONCOLOGY

CHAPTER OUTLINE: KEY TERMS, PEOPLE, PLACES, CONCEPTS

Anemia

Sickle-cell disease

Dactylitis

ACE inhibitor

Nitric oxide

Pain assessment

Patient-controlled analgesia

Nurse practitioner

Palliative care

Regional analgesia

Avascular necrosis

Gastrointestinal bleeding

Protease inhibitor

Osteomyelitis

Parenteral nutrition

Glucose-6-phosphate dehydrogenase

Cardiopulmonary resuscitation

Glucose-6-phosphate dehydrogenase deficiency

Sickle-cell

CHAPTER OUTLINE: KEY TERMS, PEOPLE, PLACES, CONCEPTS

Autoimmune hemolytic anemia

Hemolytic anemia

Cystic fibrosis

Hemolytic-uremic syndrome

Pathogenesis

Thrombocytopenic purpura

Thrombotic thrombocytopenic purpura

Diamond-Blackfan anemia

Fanconi anemia

Kearns-Sayre syndrome

Pearson syndrome

Transient erythroblastopenia of childhood

Pathophysiology

Blood transfusion

Bone marrow

Aplastic anemia

Factor IX

Factor VII

Von Willebrand factor

Diabetes insipidus

Idiopathic thrombocytopenic purpura

Subtyping

Von Willebrand disease

Venous thrombosis

Abdominal mass

Risk factor

Factor V

Nerve injury

Erythrocytapheresis

Exchange transfusion

Tumor lysis syndrome

Bisphosphonate

Superior vena cava syndrome

Hyperparathyroidism

Spina bifida

Neonatal sepsis

Physical examination

Spinal cord

CHAPTER OUTLINE: KEY TERMS, PEOPLE, PLACES, CONCEPTS

_____ Spinal cord compression

_____ Idiopathic intracranial hypertension

_____ Respiratory distress

_____ Stem cell

_____ Transfusion reaction

CHAPTER HIGHLIGHTS & NOTES: KEY TERMS, PEOPLE, PLACES, CONCEPTS

Anemia	Anemia is a decrease in number of red blood cells (RBCs) or less than the normal quantity of hemoglobin in the blood. However, it can include decreased oxygen-binding ability of each hemoglobin molecule due to deformity or lack in numerical development as in some other types of hemoglobin deficiency.
Sickle-cell disease	Sickle-cell disease or sickle-cell anaemia or drepanocytosis, is an autosomal recessive genetic blood disorder with overdominance, characterized by red blood cells that assume an abnormal, rigid, sickle shape. Sickling decreases the cells' flexibility and results in a risk of various complications. The sickling occurs because of a mutation in the hemoglobin gene.
Dactylitis	Dactylitis is inflammation of an entire digit (a finger or toe), and can be painful. The word dactyl comes from the Greek word 'daktylos' meaning 'finger'. In its medical term, it refers to both the fingers and the toes.
ACE inhibitor	ACE inhibitors are a group of drugs used primarily for the treatment of hypertension (high blood pressure) and congestive heart failure. Originally synthesized from compounds found in pit viper venom, they inhibit angiotensin-converting enzyme (ACE), a component of the blood pressure-regulating renin-angiotensin system.
Nitric oxide	Nitric oxide or nitrogen monoxide (systematic name) is a chemical compound with chemical formula Nitric oxide.

	This gas is an important signaling molecule in the body of mammals, including humans, and is an extremely important intermediate in the chemical industry. It is also an air pollutant produced by cigarette smoke, automobile engines and power plants. Nitric oxide is an important messenger molecule involved in many physiological and pathological processes within the mammalian body both beneficial and detrimental.
Pain assessment	Pain is often regarded as the fifth vital sign in regard to healthcare because it is accepted now in healthcare that pain, like other vital signs, is an objective sensation rather than subjective. As a result nurses are trained and expected to assess pain. Pain assessment and re-assessment after administration of analgesics or pain management is regulated in healthcare facilities by accreditation bodies, like the Joint Commission.
Patient-controlled analgesia	Patient-controlled analgesia is any method of allowing a person in pain to administer their own pain relief. The infusion is programmable by the prescriber. If it is programmed and functioning as intended, the machine is unlikely to deliver an overdose of medication.
Nurse practitioner	A Nurse Practitioner is an Advanced Practice Nurse (APN) who has completed graduate-level education (either a Master's or a Doctoral degree). Additional APN roles include the Certified Registered Nurse Anesthetist (CRNA)s, CNMs, and CNSs. All Nurse Practitioners are Registered Nurses who have completed extensive additional education, training, and have a dramatically expanded scope of practice over the traditional RN role.
Palliative care	Palliative care is an area of healthcare that focuses on relieving and preventing the suffering of patients. Unlike hospice care, palliative medicine is appropriate for patients in all disease stages, including those undergoing treatment for curable illnesses and those living with chronic diseases, as well as patients who are nearing the end of life. Palliative medicine utilizes a multidisciplinary approach to patient care, relying on input from physicians, pharmacists, nurses, chaplains, social workers, psychologists, and other allied health professionals in formulating a plan of care to relieve suffering in all areas of a patient's life.
Regional analgesia	Regional analgesia blocks passage of pain impulses through a nerve by depositing an analgesic drug close to the nerve trunk, cutting off sensory innervation to the region it supplies. The drug is normally injected at a site where the nerve is unprotected by bone.
Avascular necrosis	Avascular necrosis is a disease where there is cellular death (necrosis) of bone components due to interruption of the blood supply. Without blood, the bone tissue dies and the bone collapses. If avascular necrosis involves the bones of a joint, it often leads to destruction of the joint articular surfaces .

Gastrointestinal bleeding	Gastrointestinal bleeding, from the pharynx to the rectum. It has diverse causes, and a medical history, as well as physical examination, generally distinguishes between the main forms. The degree of bleeding can range from nearly undetectable to acute, massive, life-threatening bleeding.
Protease inhibitor	Protease inhibitors are a class of drugs used to treat or prevent infection by viruses, including HIV and Hepatitis C. Protease inhibitors prevent viral replication by inhibiting the activity of proteases, e.g.HIV-1 protease, enzymes used by the viruses to cleave nascent proteins for final assembly of new virons.
	Protease inhibitors have been developed or are presently undergoing testing for treating various viruses:•HIV/AIDS: antiretroviral protease inhibitors (saquinavir, ritonavir, indinavir, nelfinavir, amprenavir etc).•Hepatitis C: experimental agents: BILN 2061 (All clinical trials of BILN 2061 have been suspended due to cardiac issues), VX 950 (trade name Telaprevir), or SCH 503034
	Given the specificity of the target of these drugs there is the risk, as in antibiotics, of the development of drug-resistant mutated viruses. To reduce this risk it is common to use several different drugs together that are each aimed at different targets.
Osteomyelitis	Osteomyelitis simply means an infection of the bone or bone marrow. It can be usefully subclassified on the basis of the causative organism (pyogenic bacteria or mycobacteria), the route, duration and anatomic location of the infection.
	In general, microorganisms may infect bone through one or more of three basic methods: via the bloodstream, contiguously from local areas of infection (as in cellulitis), or penetrating trauma, including iatrogenic causes such as joint replacements or internal fixation of fractures or root-canaled teeth.
Parenteral nutrition	Parenteral nutrition is feeding a person intravenously, bypassing the usual process of eating and digestion. The person receives nutritional formulae that contain nutrients such as glucose, amino acids, lipids and added vitamins and dietary minerals. It is called total parenteral nutrition or total nutrient admixture (TNA) when no food is given by other routes.
Glucose-6-phosphate dehydrogenase	Glucose-6-phosphate dehydrogenase is a cytosolic enzyme in the pentose phosphate pathway , a metabolic pathway that supplies reducing energy to cells (such as erythrocytes) by maintaining the level of the co-enzyme nicotinamide adenine dinucleotide phosphate (NADPH). The NADPH in turn maintains the level of glutathione in these cells that helps protect the red blood cells against oxidative damage. Of greater quantitative importance is the production of NADPH for tissues actively engaged in biosynthesis of fatty acids and/or isoprenoids, such as the liver, mammary glands, adipose tissue, and the adrenal glands.

Chapter 8. HEMATOLOGY-ONCOLOGY

Cardiopulmonary resuscitation	Cardiopulmonary resuscitation is an emergency procedure which is performed in an effort to manually preserve intact brain function until further measures are taken to restore spontaneous blood circulation and breathing in a person in cardiac arrest. It is indicated in those who are unresponsive with no breathing or abnormal breathing, for example agonal respirations. It may be performed both in and outside of a hospital.
Glucose-6-phosphate dehydrogenase deficiency	Glucose-6-phosphate dehydrogenase deficiency is an X-linked recessive hereditary disease characterised by abnormally low levels of glucose-6-phosphate dehydrogenase , a metabolic enzyme involved in the pentose phosphate pathway, especially important in red blood cell metabolism. Individuals with the disease may exhibit nonimmune hemolytic anemia in response to a number of causes, most commonly infection or exposure to certain medications or chemicals. G6PD deficiency is closely linked to favism, a disorder characterized by a hemolytic reaction to consumption of broad beans, with a name derived from the Italian name of the broad bean (fava).
Sickle-cell	Sickle-cell disease is a life-long blood disorder characterized by red blood cells that assume an abnormal, rigid, sickle shape. Sickling decreases the cells' flexibility and results in a risk of various complications. The sickling occurs because of a mutation in the hemoglobin gene.
Autoimmune hemolytic anemia	Autoimmune hemolytic anemia occurs when antibodies directed against the person's own red blood cells (RBCs) cause them to burst (lyse), leading to insufficient plasma concentration. The lifetime of the RBCs is reduced from the normal 100-120 days to just a few days in serious cases. The intracellular components of the RBCs are released into the circulating blood and into tissues, leading to some of the characteristic symptoms of this condition.
Hemolytic anemia	Hemolytic anemia is a form of anemia due to hemolysis, the abnormal breakdown of red blood cells (RBCs), either in the blood vessels (intravascular hemolysis) or elsewhere in the human body (extravascular). It has numerous possible causes, ranging from relatively harmless to life-threatening. The general classification of hemolytic anemia is either inherited or acquired.
Cystic fibrosis	Cystic fibrosis is an autosomal recessive genetic disorder affecting most critically the lungs, and also the pancreas, liver, and intestine. It is characterized by abnormal transport of chloride and sodium across an epithelium, leading to thick, viscous secretions. The name cystic fibrosis refers to the characteristic scarring (fibrosis) and cyst formation within the pancreas, first recognized in the 1930s.
Hemolytic-uremic syndrome	Hemolytic-uremic syndrome , abbreviated HUS, is a disease characterized by hemolytic anemia (anemia caused by destruction of red blood cells), acute kidney failure (uremia) and a low platelet count (thrombocytopenia). It predominantly, but not exclusively, affects children. Most cases are preceded by an episode of infectious, sometimes bloody, diarrhea caused by E.

Pathogenesis	The pathogenesis of a disease is the mechanism by which the disease is caused. The term can also be used to describe the origin and development of the disease and whether it is acute, chronic or recurrent. The word comes from the Greek pathos, 'disease', and genesis, 'creation'.
Thrombocytopenic purpura	Thrombocytopenic purpura are purpura associated with a reduction in circulating blood platelets which can result from a variety of causes. By tradition, the term idiopathic thrombocytopenic purpura is used when the cause is idiopathic. However, most cases are now considered to be immune-mediated.
Thrombotic thrombocytopenic purpura	Thrombotic thrombocytopenic purpura is a rare disorder of the blood-coagulation system, causing extensive microscopic clots to form in the small blood vessels throughout the body. These small blood clots, called thromboses, can damage many organs including the kidneys, heart and brain. In the era before effective treatment with plasma exchange, the fatality rate was about 90%.
Diamond-Blackfan anemia	Diamond-Blackfan anemia (DBA) is a congenital erythroid aplasia that usually presents in infancy. DBA patients have low red blood cell counts (anemia). The rest of their blood cells (the platelets and the white blood cells) are normal.
Fanconi anemia	Fanconi anemia is a genetic disease with an incidence of 1 per 350,000 births, with a higher frequency in Ashkenazi Jews and Afrikaners in South Africa. FA is the result of a genetic defect in a cluster of proteins responsible for DNA repair. As a result, the majority of FA patients develop cancer, most often acute myelogenous leukemia, and 90% develop bone marrow failure (the inability to produce blood cells) by age 40. About 60-75% of FA patients have congenital defects, commonly short stature, abnormalities of the skin, arms, head, eyes, kidneys, and ears, and developmental disabilities. Around 75% of FA patients have some form of endocrine problem, with varying degrees of severity.
Kearns-Sayre syndrome	Kearns-Sayre syndrome also known as oculocraniosomatic disease or Oculocraniosomatic neuromuscular disease with ragged red fibers is a mitochondrial myopathy with a typical onset is before 20 years of age. Kearns-Sayre syndromeS is a more severe syndromic variant of chronic progressive external ophthalmoplegia, a syndrome that is characterized by isolated involvement of the muscles controlling eye-lid movement (levator palpebrae, orbicularis oculi), and those controlling eye movement (extra-ocular muscles). This results in ptosis and ophthalmoplegia respectively.
Pearson syndrome	Pearson syndrome is a mitochondrial disease characterized by sideroblastic anemia and exocrine pancreas dysfunction.

	Other clinical features are failure to thrive, pancreatic fibrosis with insulin-dependent diabetes and exocrine pancreatic deficiency, muscle and neurologic impairment, and, frequently, early death. It is usually fatal in infancy.
Transient erythroblastopenia of childhood	Transient erythroblastopenia of childhood is a slowly developing anemia of early childhood characterized by gradual onset of pallor. Individuals with Transient erythroblastopenia of childhood have a median age of presentation of 18-26 months; however, the disorder may occur in infants younger than 6 months and in children as old as age 10 years. Because of the gradual onset of the anemia, children are often healthier than expected from their low hemoglobin levels.
Pathophysiology	Pathophysiology sample values Pathophysiology is the study of the changes of normal mechanical, physical, and biochemical functions, either caused by a disease, or resulting from an abnormal syndrome. More formally, it is the branch of medicine which deals with any disturbances of body functions, caused by disease or prodromal symptoms. An alternative definition is 'the study of the biological and physical manifestations of disease as they correlate with the underlying abnormalities and physiological disturbances.' The study of pathology and the study of pathophysiology often involves substantial overlap in diseases and processes, but pathology emphasizes direct observations, while pathophysiology emphasizes quantifiable measurements.
Blood transfusion	Blood transfusion is the process of receiving blood products into one's circulation intravenously. Transfusions are used in a variety of medical conditions to replace lost components of the blood. Early transfusions used whole blood, but modern medical practice commonly uses only components of the blood, such as red blood cells, white blood cells, plasma, clotting factors, and platelets.
Bone marrow	Bone marrow is the flexible tissue found in the interior of bones. In humans, red blood cells are produced in the heads of long bones, in a process known as hematopoesis. On average, bone marrow constitutes 4% of the total body mass of humans; in an adult weighing 65 kilograms (140 lb), bone marrow accounts for approximately 2.6 kilograms (5.7 lb).
Aplastic anemia	Aplastic anemia is a condition where bone marrow does not produce sufficient new cells to replenish blood cells. The condition, as the name indicates, involves both aplasia and anemia.

Factor IX	Factor IX (EC 3.4.21.22) is one of the serine proteases of the coagulation system; it belongs to peptidase family S1. Deficiency of this protein causes hemophilia B. It was discovered in 1952 after a young boy named Stephen Christmas was found to be lacking this exact factor, leading to hemophilia.. Factor IX is produced as a zymogen, an inactive precursor. It is processed to remove the signal peptide, glycosylated and then cleaved by factor XIa (of the contact pathway) or factor VIIa (of the tissue factor pathway) to produce a two-chain form where the chains are linked by a disulfide bridge.
Factor VII	Factor VII is one of the proteins that causes blood to clot in the coagulation cascade. It is an enzyme (EC 3.4.21.21) of the serine protease class. A recombinant form of human factor VIIa (NovoSeven, eptacog alfa [activated]) has U.S. Food and Drug Administration approval for uncontrolled bleeding in hemophilia patients.
Von Willebrand factor	Von Willebrand factor is a blood glycoprotein involved in hemostasis. It is deficient or defective in von Willebrand disease and is involved in a large number of other diseases, including thrombotic thrombocytopenic purpura, Heyde's syndrome, and possibly hemolytic-uremic syndrome. Increased plasma levels in a large number of cardiovascular, neoplastic and connective tissue diseases are presumed to arise from adverse changes to the endothelium, and may contribute to an increased risk of thrombosis.
Diabetes insipidus	Diabetes insipidus is a condition characterized by excessive thirst and excretion of large amounts of severely diluted urine, with reduction of fluid intake having no effect on the concentration of the urine. There are several different types of DI, each with a different cause. The most common type in humans is central DI, caused by a deficiency of arginine vasopressin (AVP), also known as antidiuretic hormone (ADH).
Idiopathic thrombocytopenic purpura	Idiopathic thrombocytopenic purpura is the condition of having an abnormally low platelet count (thrombocytopenia) of unknown cause (idiopathic). As most incidents of ITP appear to be related to the production of antibodies against platelets, immune thrombocytopenic purpura or immune thrombocytopenia are terms also used to describe this condition. Often ITP is asymptomatic (devoid of obvious symptoms) and can be discovered incidentally, but a very low platelet count can lead to an increased risk of bleeding and purpura.
Subtyping	In programming language theory, subtyping or subtype polymorphism is a form of type polymorphism in which a subtype is a datatype that is related to another datatype (the supertype) by some notion of substitutability, meaning that program constructs, typically subroutines or functions, written to operate on elements of the supertype can also operate on elements of the subtype. If S is a subtype of T, the subtyping relation is often written S <: T, to mean that any term of type S can be safely used in a context where a term of type T is expected.

Chapter 8. HEMATOLOGY-ONCOLOGY

Von Willebrand disease	Von Willebrand disease (vWD) is the most common hereditary coagulation abnormality described in humans, although it can also be acquired as a result of other medical conditions. It arises from a qualitative or quantitative deficiency of von Willebrand factor (vWF), a multimeric protein that is required for platelet adhesion. It is known to affect humans and dogs.
Venous thrombosis	A venous thrombosis is a blood clot (thrombus) that forms within a vein. Thrombosis is a medical term for a blood clot occurring inside a blood vessel. A classical venous thrombosis is deep vein thrombosis (DVT), which can break off (embolize), and become a life-threatening pulmonary embolism (PE).
Abdominal mass	An abdominal mass is any localized enlargement or swelling in the human abdomen. Depending on its location, the abdominal mass may be caused by an enlarged liver (hepatomegaly), enlarged spleen (splenomegaly), protruding kidney, a pancreatic mass, a retroperitoneal mass (a mass in the posterior of the peritoneum), an abdominal aortic aneurysm, or various tumours, such as those caused by abdominal carcinomatosis and omental metastasis. The treatments depend on the cause, and may range from watchful waiting to radical surgery.
Risk factor	In epidemiology, a risk factor is a variable associated with an increased risk of disease or infection. Sometimes, determinant is also used, being a variable associated with either increased or decreased risk.
	Risk factors or determinants are correlational and not necessarily causal, because correlation does not prove causation.
Factor V	Factor V is a protein of the coagulation system, rarely referred to as proaccelerin or labile factor. In contrast to most other coagulation factors, it is not enzymatically active but functions as a cofactor. Deficiency leads to predisposition for hemorrhage, while some mutations (most notably factor V Leiden) predispose for thrombosis.
Nerve injury	Nerve injury is injury to nervous tissue. There is no single classification system that can describe all the many variations of nerve injury. Most systems attempt to correlate the degree of injury with symptoms, pathology and prognosis.
Erythrocytapheresis	Erythrocytapheresis is an apheresis procedure by which erythrocytes (red blood cells) are separated from whole blood. It is an extracorporeal blood separation method whereby whole blood is extracted from a donor or patient, the red blood cells are separated, and the remaining blood is returned to circulation. Overview

Exchange transfusion	An exchange transfusion is a medical treatment in which apheresis is used to remove one person's red blood cells or platelets and replace them with transfused blood products. Exchange transfusion is used in the treatment of a number of diseases, including:•Sickle cell disease•Thrombotic thrombocytopenic purpura (TTP)•Hemolytic disease of the newbornDescription An exchange transfusion requires that the patient's blood can be removed and replaced. In most cases, this involves placing one or more thin tubes, called catheters, into a blood vessel.
Tumor lysis syndrome	In medicine (oncology and hematology), tumor lysis syndrome is a group of metabolic complications that can occur after treatment of cancer, usually lymphomas and leukemias, and sometimes even without treatment. These complications are caused by the break-down products of dying cancer cells and include hyperkalemia, hyperphosphatemia, hyperuricemia and hyperuricosuria, hypocalcemia, and consequent acute uric acid nephropathy and acute renal failure. The most common tumors associated with this syndrome are poorly differentiated lymphomas, such as Burkitt's lymphoma, and leukemias, such as acute lymphoblastic leukemia (ALL) and acute myeloid leukemia (AML).
Bisphosphonate	Bisphosphonates (also called diphosphonates) are a class of drugs that prevent the loss of bone mass, used to treat osteoporosis and similar diseases. They are called bisphosphonates because they have two phosphonate (PO_3) groups and are similar in structure to pyrophosphate. Evidence shows that they reduce the risk of osteoporotic fracture in those who have had previous fractures.
Superior vena cava syndrome	Superior vena cava syndrome or superior vena cava obstruction (SVCO), is usually the result of the direct obstruction of the superior vena cava by malignancies such as compression of the vessel wall by right upper lobe tumors or thymoma and/or mediastinal lymphadenopathy. The most common malignancies that cause SVCS is bronchogenic carcinoma. Cerebral edema is rare, but if it occurs it may be fatal.
Hyperparathyroidism	Hyperparathyroidism is overactivity of the parathyroid glands resulting in excess production of parathyroid hormone (PTH). The parathyroid hormone regulates calcium and phosphate levels and helps to maintain these levels. Excessive PTH secretion may be due to problems in the glands themselves, in which case it is referred to as primary hyperparathyroidism and which leads to hypercalcemia (raised calcium levels).

Chapter 8. HEMATOLOGY-ONCOLOGY

Spina bifida	Spina bifida is a developmental congenital disorder caused by the incomplete closing of the embryonic neural tube. Some vertebrae overlying the spinal cord are not fully formed and remain unfused and open. If the opening is large enough, this allows a portion of the spinal cord to protrude through the opening in the bones.
Neonatal sepsis	In common clinical usage, neonatal sepsis specifically refers to the presence of a bacterial blood stream infection (BSI) (such as meningitis, pneumonia, pyelonephritis, or gastroenteritis) in the setting of fever. Criteria with regards to hemodynamic compromise or respiratory failure are not useful clinically because these symptoms often do not arise in neonates until death is imminent and unpreventable. It is difficult to clinically exclude sepsis in newborns less than 90 days old that have fever (defined as a temperature > 38°C (100.4°F).
Physical examination	A physical examination, medical examination, or clinical examination (more popularly known as a check-up or medical) is the process by which a doctor investigates the body of a patient for signs of disease. It generally follows the taking of the medical history -- an account of the symptoms as experienced by the patient. Together with the medical history, the physical examination aids in determining the correct diagnosis and devising the treatment plan.
Spinal cord	The Spinal cord is a long, thin, tubular bundle of nervous tissue and support cells that extends from the brain. The brain and Spinal cord together make up the central nervous system. The Spinal cord extends down to the space in between the first and second lumbar vertebrae.
Spinal cord compression	Spinal cord compression develops when the spinal cord is compressed by bone fragments from a vertebral fracture, a tumor, abscess, ruptured intervertebral disc or other lesion. It is regarded as a medical emergency independent of its cause, and requires swift diagnosis and treatment to prevent long-term disability due to irreversible spinal cord injury. Symptoms suggestive of cord compression are back pain, a dermatome of increased sensation, paralysis of limbs below the level of compression, decreased sensation below the level of compression, urinary and fecal incontinence and/or urinary retention.
Idiopathic intracranial hypertension	Idiopathic intracranial hypertension sometimes called by the older names benign intracranial hypertension (BIH) or pseudotumor cerebri (PTC), is a neurological disorder that is characterized by increased intracranial pressure (pressure around the brain) in the absence of a tumor or other diseases. The main symptoms are headache, nausea and vomiting, as well as pulsatile tinnitus (buzzing in the ears synchronous with the pulse), double vision and other visual symptoms. If untreated, it may lead to swelling of the optic disc in the eye, which can progress to vision loss.

Respiratory distress	Respiratory distress is a medical term that refers to both difficulty in breathing, and to the psychological experience associated with such difficulty, even if there is no physiological basis for experiencing such distress. The physical presentation of respiratory distress is generally referred to as labored breathing,s while the sensation of respiratory distress is called shortness of breath or dyspnea. Respiratory distress occurs in connection with various physical ailments, such as acute respiratory distress syndrome, a serious reaction to various forms of injuries to the lung, and infant respiratory distress syndrome, a syndrome in premature infants caused by developmental insufficiency of surfactant production and structural immaturity in the lungs.
Stem cell	Stem cells are biological cells found in all multicellular organisms, that can divide (through mitosis) and differentiate into diverse specialized cell types and can self-renew to produce more stem cells. In mammals, there are two broad types of stem cells: embryonic stem cells, which are isolated from the inner cell mass of blastocysts, and adult stem cells, which are found in various tissues. In adult organisms, stem cells and progenitor cells act as a repair system for the body, replenishing adult tissues.
Transfusion reaction	In medicine, a transfusion reaction is any adverse event which occurs because of a blood transfusion. These events can take the form of an allergic reaction, a transfusion-related infection, hemolysis related to an incompatible blood type, or an alteration of the immune system related to the transfusion. The risk of a transfusion reaction must always be balanced against the anticipated benefit of a blood transfusion.

Chapter 8. HEMATOLOGY-ONCOLOGY

1. _____ is overactivity of the parathyroid glands resulting in excess production of parathyroid hormone (PTH). The parathyroid hormone regulates calcium and phosphate levels and helps to maintain these levels. Excessive PTH secretion may be due to problems in the glands themselves, in which case it is referred to as primary _____ and which leads to hypercalcemia (raised calcium levels).

   a. Hypoparathyroidism
   b. Parathyroid disease
   c. Hyperparathyroidism
   d. Parathyroid gland

2. _____ is the flexible tissue found in the interior of bones. In humans, red blood cells are produced in the heads of long bones, in a process known as hematopoesis. On average, _____ constitutes 4% of the total body mass of humans; in an adult weighing 65 kilograms (140 lb), _____ accounts for approximately 2.6 kilograms (5.7 lb).

   a. Bone marrow
   b. Microcirculation
   c. Precapillary sphincter
   d. Transport maximum

3. In epidemiology, a _____ is a variable associated with an increased risk of disease or infection. Sometimes, determinant is also used, being a variable associated with either increased or decreased risk.

   _____s or determinants are correlational and not necessarily causal, because correlation does not prove causation.

   a. Risk factor
   b. Sensitivity and specificity
   c. Standardized mortality ratio
   d. Surrogate endpoint

4. _____s are a group of drugs used primarily for the treatment of hypertension (high blood pressure) and congestive heart failure. Originally synthesized from compounds found in pit viper venom, they inhibit angiotensin-converting enzyme (ACE), a component of the blood pressure-regulating renin-angiotensin system.

   a. Enalaprilat
   b. ACE inhibitor
   c. abdominal exam
   d. Plantar fasciitis

5. . _____ is an area of healthcare that focuses on relieving and preventing the suffering of patients. Unlike hospice care, palliative medicine is appropriate for patients in all disease stages, including those undergoing treatment for curable illnesses and those living with chronic diseases, as well as patients who are nearing the end of life. Palliative medicine utilizes a multidisciplinary approach to patient care, relying on input from physicians, pharmacists, nurses, chaplains, social workers, psychologists, and other allied health professionals in formulating a plan of care to relieve suffering in all areas of a patient's life.

a. Palliative sedation
b. Patient safety
c. Palliative care
d. Symptomatic treatment

1. c
2. a
3. a
4. b
5. c

You can take the complete Chapter Practice Test

for Chapter 8. HEMATOLOGY-ONCOLOGY
on all key terms, persons, places, and concepts.

Online 99 Cents

http://www.epub219.49.13357.8.cram101.com/

Use www.Cram101.com for all your study needs

including Cram101's online interactive problem solving labs in

chemistry, statistics, mathematics, and more.

CHAPTER OUTLINE: KEY TERMS, PEOPLE, PLACES, CONCEPTS

Renal failure

Renal tubular acidosis

Protease inhibitor

Parenteral nutrition

Glomerular filtration

Hydronephrosis

Acute inflammatory demyelinating polyneuropathy

Differential diagnosis

Intrinsic

Hemolytic-uremic syndrome

Anorexia nervosa

Hyperkalemia

Hemolytic anemia

Cystic fibrosis

Epidemiology

Etiological myth

Pathogenesis

Prognosis

Pathophysiology

_____ | Proximal renal tubular acidosis

_____ | Distal renal tubular acidosis

_____ | Metabolic acidosis

_____ | Urine anion gap

_____ | Anion gap

_____ | Diabetes insipidus

_____ | Gastrointestinal bleeding

_____ | Hypoadrenocorticism

_____ | Minimal change disease

_____ | Nephrotic syndrome

_____ | Hypertensive crisis

_____ | Palliative care

_____ | Blood pressure

_____ | Hypertension

_____ | Prevalence

_____ | Primary

_____ | ACE inhibitor

_____ | Angiotensin I-converting enzyme

_____ | Beta-adrenergic agonist

Chapter 9. RENAL

CHAPTER OUTLINE: KEY TERMS, PEOPLE, PLACES, CONCEPTS

	Enzyme inhibitor
	Terminal sedation
	Renal vein
	Ischaemic
	Crisis management
	Hypertensive emergency
	Cardiogenic shock
	Vomiting

CHAPTER HIGHLIGHTS & NOTES: KEY TERMS, PEOPLE, PLACES, CONCEPTS

Renal failure	Renal failure or kidney failure (formerly called renal insufficiency) describes a medical condition in which the kidneys fail to adequately filter toxins and waste products from the blood. The two forms are acute (acute kidney injury) and chronic (chronic kidney disease); a number of other diseases or health problems may cause either form of renal failure to occur. Renal failure is described as a decrease in glomerular filtration rate.
Renal tubular acidosis	Renal tubular acidosis is a medical condition that involves an accumulation of acid in the body due to a failure of the kidneys to appropriately acidify the urine. When blood is filtered by the kidney, the filtrate passes through the tubules of the nephron, allowing for exchange of salts, acid equivalents, and other solutes before it drains into the bladder as urine. The metabolic acidosis that results from RTA may be caused either by failure to recover sufficient (alkaline) bicarbonate ions from the filtrate in the early portion of the nephron (proximal tubule) or by insufficient secretion of (acid) hydrogen ions into the latter portions of the nephron (distal tubule).

Chapter 9. RENAL

Protease inhibitor	Protease inhibitors are a class of drugs used to treat or prevent infection by viruses, including HIV and Hepatitis C. Protease inhibitors prevent viral replication by inhibiting the activity of proteases, e.g.HIV-1 protease, enzymes used by the viruses to cleave nascent proteins for final assembly of new virons. Protease inhibitors have been developed or are presently undergoing testing for treating various viruses:•HIV/AIDS: antiretroviral protease inhibitors (saquinavir, ritonavir, indinavir, nelfinavir, amprenavir etc).•Hepatitis C: experimental agents: BILN 2061 (All clinical trials of BILN 2061 have been suspended due to cardiac issues), VX 950 (trade name Telaprevir), or SCH 503034 Given the specificity of the target of these drugs there is the risk, as in antibiotics, of the development of drug-resistant mutated viruses. To reduce this risk it is common to use several different drugs together that are each aimed at different targets.
Parenteral nutrition	Parenteral nutrition is feeding a person intravenously, bypassing the usual process of eating and digestion. The person receives nutritional formulae that contain nutrients such as glucose, amino acids, lipids and added vitamins and dietary minerals. It is called total parenteral nutrition or total nutrient admixture (TNA) when no food is given by other routes.
Glomerular filtration	Renal function, in nephrology, is an indication of the state of the kidney and its role in renal physiology. glomerular filtration rate (glomerular filtration R) describes the flow rate of filtered fluid through the kidney. Creatinine clearance rate (C_{Cr}) is the volume of blood plasma that is cleared of creatinine per unit time and is a useful measure for approximating the glomerular filtration R. Both glomerular filtration R and C_{Cr} may be accurately calculated by comparative measurements of substances in the blood and urine, or estimated by formulas using just a blood test result (e glomerular filtration R and eC_{Cr}.)
Hydronephrosis	Hydronephrosis - literally 'water inside the kidney' - refers to distension and dilation of the renal pelvis and calyces, usually caused by obstruction of the free flow of urine from the kidney. Untreated, it leads to progressive atrophy of the kidney. In cases of hydroureteronephrosis, there is distention of both the ureter and the renal pelvis and calices.
Acute inflammatory demyelinating polyneuropathy	Guillain-Barré syndrome (GBS) is an Acute inflammatory demyelinating polyneuropathy , an autoimmune disorder affecting the peripheral nervous system, usually triggered by an acute infectious process.The syndrome was named after the French physicians Guillain, Barré and Strohl, who were the first to describe it in 1916. It is sometimes called Landry's paralysis, after the French physician who first described a variant of it in 1859. It is included in the wider group of peripheral neuropathies. There are several types of GBS, but unless otherwise stated, GBS refers to the most common form, Acute inflammatory demyelinating polyneuropathy . GBS is rare and has an incidence of 1 or 2 people per 100,000.

It is frequently severe and usually exhibits as an ascending paralysis noted by weakness in the legs that spreads to the upper limbs and the face along with complete loss of deep tendon reflexes. With prompt treatment by plasmapheresis or intravenous immunoglobulins and supportive care, the majority of patients will regain full functional capacity.

Differential diagnosis

A differential diagnosis is a systematic diagnostic method used to identify the presence of an entity where multiple alternatives are possible (and the process may be termed differential diagnostic procedure), and may also refer to any of the included candidate alternatives (which may also be termed candidate condition). This method is essentially a process of elimination, or at least, rendering of the probabilities of candidate conditions to negligible levels. In this sense, probabilities are, in fact, imaginative parameters in the mind or hardware of the diagnostician or system, while in reality the target (such as a patient) either has a condition or not with an actual probability of either 0 or 100%.

Intrinsic

The term Intrinsic denotes a property of some thing or action which is essential and specific to that thing or action, and which is wholly independent of any other object, action or consequence. A characteristic which is not essential or inherent is extrinsic.

For example in biology, Intrinsic effects originate from 'inside' an organism or cell, such as an autoimmune disease immunity.

More specific uses of the concepts can be found:

· in philosophy; Intrinsic and extrinsic properties · in physics; intensive and extensive properties · in psychology; Intrinsic and extrinsic motivation · in computing; Intrinsic function. · in mathematics; Intrinsic equations.

Hemolytic-uremic syndrome

Hemolytic-uremic syndrome , abbreviated HUS, is a disease characterized by hemolytic anemia (anemia caused by destruction of red blood cells), acute kidney failure (uremia) and a low platelet count (thrombocytopenia). It predominantly, but not exclusively, affects children. Most cases are preceded by an episode of infectious, sometimes bloody, diarrhea caused by E. coli O157:H7, which is acquired as a foodborne illness or from a contaminated water supply.

Anorexia nervosa

The differential diagnoses of anorexia nervosa (AN) include various medical and psychological conditions which may be misdiagnosed as (AN), in some cases these conditions may be comorbid with anorexia nervosa (AN). The misdiagnosis of AN is not uncommon. In one instance a case of achalasia was misdiagnosed as AN and the patient spent two months confined to a psychiatric hospital.

Hyperkalemia

Hyperkalemia refers to the condition in which the concentration of the electrolyte potassium (K^+) in the blood is elevated.

Extreme hyperkalemia is a medical emergency due to the risk of potentially fatal abnormal heart rhythms (arrhythmia).

Normal serum potassium levels are between 3.5 and 5.0 mEq/L; at least 95% of the body's potassium is found inside cells, with the remainder in the blood.

Hemolytic anemia	Hemolytic anemia is a form of anemia due to hemolysis, the abnormal breakdown of red blood cells (RBCs), either in the blood vessels (intravascular hemolysis) or elsewhere in the human body (extravascular). It has numerous possible causes, ranging from relatively harmless to life-threatening. The general classification of hemolytic anemia is either inherited or acquired.
Cystic fibrosis	Cystic fibrosis is an autosomal recessive genetic disorder affecting most critically the lungs, and also the pancreas, liver, and intestine. It is characterized by abnormal transport of chloride and sodium across an epithelium, leading to thick, viscous secretions.
	The name cystic fibrosis refers to the characteristic scarring (fibrosis) and cyst formation within the pancreas, first recognized in the 1930s.
Epidemiology	Epidemiology is the study of the distribution and patterns of health-events, health-characteristics and their causes or influences in well-defined populations. It is the cornerstone method of public health research and practice, and helps inform policy decisions and evidence-based medicine by identifying risk factors for disease and targets for preventive medicine and public policies. Epidemiologists are involved in the design of studies, collection and statistical analysis of data, and interpretation and dissemination of results (including peer review and occasional systematic review).
Etiological myth	Etiology is the study of causation, or origination.
	The word is most commonly used in medical and philosophical theories, where it is used to refer to the study of why things occur, or even the reasons behind the way that things act, and is used in philosophy, physics, psychology, government, medicine, theology and biology in reference to the causes of various phenomena. An etiological myth is a myth intended to explain a name or create a mythic history for a place or family.
Pathogenesis	The pathogenesis of a disease is the mechanism by which the disease is caused. The term can also be used to describe the origin and development of the disease and whether it is acute, chronic or recurrent. The word comes from the Greek pathos, 'disease', and genesis, 'creation'.
Prognosis	Prognosis is a medical term to describe the likely outcome of an illness.

When applied to large populations, prognostic estimates can be very accurate: for example the statement '45% of patients with severe septic shock will die within 28 days' can be made with some confidence, because previous research found that this proportion of patients died. However, it is much harder to translate this into a prognosis for an individual patient: additional information is needed to determine whether a patient belongs to the 45% who will succumb, or to the 55% who survive.

Pathophysiology	Pathophysiology sample values Pathophysiology is the study of the changes of normal mechanical, physical, and biochemical functions, either caused by a disease, or resulting from an abnormal syndrome. More formally, it is the branch of medicine which deals with any disturbances of body functions, caused by disease or prodromal symptoms. An alternative definition is 'the study of the biological and physical manifestations of disease as they correlate with the underlying abnormalities and physiological disturbances.' The study of pathology and the study of pathophysiology often involves substantial overlap in diseases and processes, but pathology emphasizes direct observations, while pathophysiology emphasizes quantifiable measurements.
Proximal renal tubular acidosis	Proximal renal tubular acidosis is a type of renal tubular acidosis caused by a failure of the proximal tubular cells to reabsorb filtered bicarbonate from the urine, leading to urinary bicarbonate wasting and subsequent acidemia. The distal intercalated cells function normally, so the acidemia is less severe than dRTA and the urine can acidify to a pH of less than 5.3. pRTA also has several causes, and may occasionally be present as a solitary defect, but is usually associated with a more generalised dysfunction of the proximal tubular cells called Fanconi's syndrome where there is also phosphaturia, glycosuria, aminoaciduria, uricosuria and tubular proteinuria. The principal feature of Fanconi's syndrome is bone demineralization (osteomalacia or rickets) due to phosphate wasting.
Distal renal tubular acidosis	Distal renal tubular acidosis is the classical form of RTA, being the first described. Distal RTA is characterized by a failure of acid secretion by the alpha intercalated cells of the cortical collecting duct of the distal nephron. This failure of acid secretion may be due to a number of causes, and it leads to an inability to acidify the urine to a pH of less than 5.3.
Metabolic acidosis	In medicine, metabolic acidosis is a condition that occurs when the body produces too much acid or when the kidneys are not removing enough acid from the body. If unchecked, metabolic acidosis leads to acidemia, i.e., blood pH is low (less than 7.35) due to increased production of hydrogen by the body or the inability of the body to form bicarbonate (HCO_3^-) in the kidney.

Chapter 9. RENAL

Urine anion gap	The urine anion gap is calculated using measured ions found in the urine. It is used to aid in the differential diagnosis of metabolic acidosis. The term 'anion gap' without qualification usually implies serum anion gap.
Anion gap	Pathophysiology sample values The anion gap is the difference in the measured cations and the measured anions in serum, plasma, or urine. The magnitude of this difference (i.e. 'gap') in the serum is often calculated in medicine when attempting to identify the cause of metabolic acidosis. If the gap is greater than normal, then high anion gap metabolic acidosis is diagnosed.
Diabetes insipidus	Diabetes insipidus is a condition characterized by excessive thirst and excretion of large amounts of severely diluted urine, with reduction of fluid intake having no effect on the concentration of the urine. There are several different types of DI, each with a different cause. The most common type in humans is central DI, caused by a deficiency of arginine vasopressin (AVP), also known as antidiuretic hormone (ADH).
Gastrointestinal bleeding	Gastrointestinal bleeding, from the pharynx to the rectum. It has diverse causes, and a medical history, as well as physical examination, generally distinguishes between the main forms. The degree of bleeding can range from nearly undetectable to acute, massive, life-threatening bleeding.
Hypoadrenocorticism	Hypoadrenocorticism is a medical term describing a condition of decreased secretion of adrenocorticotropic hormone. It should not be confused with Addison's disease, which is a primary adrenocortical insufficiency.
Minimal change disease	Minimal Change Disease (also known as Nil Lesions or Nil Disease (lipoid nephrosis)) is a disease of the kidney that causes nephrotic syndrome and usually affects children (peak incidence at 2-3 years of age). Minimal Change Disease is most common in very young children but can occur in older children and adults. It is by far the most common cause of nephrotic syndrome (NS) in children between the ages of 1 and 7, accounting for the majority (about 90%) of these diagnoses.
Nephrotic syndrome	Nephrotic syndrome is a nonspecific disorder in which the kidneys are damaged, causing them to leak large amounts of protein (proteinuria at least 3.5 grams per day per 1.73m^2 body surface area) from the blood into the urine.

Kidneys affected by nephrotic syndrome have small pores in the podocytes, large enough to permit proteinuria (and subsequently hypoalbuminemia, because some of the protein albumin has gone from the blood to the urine) but not large enough to allow cells through (hence no hematuria). By contrast, in nephritic syndrome, RBCs pass through the pores, causing hematuria.

Hypertensive crisis

A hypertensive emergency is severe hypertension (high blood pressure) with acute impairment of an organ system (especially the central nervous system, cardiovascular system and/or the renal system) and the possibility of irreversible organ-damage. In case of a hypertensive emergency, the blood pressure should be lowered aggressively over minutes to hours with an antihypertensive agent.

Several classes of antihypertensive agents are recommended and the choice for the antihypertensive agent depends on the cause for the Hypertensive crisis, the severity of elevated blood pressure and the patient's usual blood pressure before the Hypertensive crisis.

Palliative care

Palliative care is an area of healthcare that focuses on relieving and preventing the suffering of patients. Unlike hospice care, palliative medicine is appropriate for patients in all disease stages, including those undergoing treatment for curable illnesses and those living with chronic diseases, as well as patients who are nearing the end of life. Palliative medicine utilizes a multidisciplinary approach to patient care, relying on input from physicians, pharmacists, nurses, chaplains, social workers, psychologists, and other allied health professionals in formulating a plan of care to relieve suffering in all areas of a patient's life.

Blood pressure

Blood pressure is the pressure exerted by circulating blood upon the walls of blood vessels, and is one of the principal vital signs. When used without further specification, 'blood pressure' usually refers to the arterial pressure of the systemic circulation. During each heartbeat, blood pressure varies between a maximum (systolic) and a minimum (diastolic) pressure.

Hypertension

Hypertension or high blood pressure, sometimes called arterial hypertension, is a chronic medical condition in which the blood pressure in the arteries is elevated. This requires the heart to work harder than normal to circulate blood through the blood vessels. Blood pressure involves two measurements, systolic and diastolic, which depend on whether the heart muscle is contracting (systole) or relaxed between beats (diastole).

Prevalence

In epidemiology, the prevalence of a health-related state (typically disease, but also other things like smoking or seatbelt use) in a statistical population is defined as the total number of cases of the risk factor in the population at a given time, or the total number of cases in the population, divided by the number of individuals in the population. It is used as an estimate of how common a disease is within a population over a certain period of time.

Primary	The Primary (formerly the Primary Association) is a children's organization and an official auxiliary within The Church of Jesus Christ of Latter-day Saints (LDS Church). It acts as a Sunday school organization for the church's children under the age of 12.
	The official purpose of Primary is to help parents in teaching their children to learn and live the gospel of Jesus Christ.
ACE inhibitor	ACE inhibitors are a group of drugs used primarily for the treatment of hypertension (high blood pressure) and congestive heart failure. Originally synthesized from compounds found in pit viper venom, they inhibit angiotensin-converting enzyme (ACE), a component of the blood pressure-regulating renin-angiotensin system.
Angiotensin I-converting enzyme	Angiotensin I-converting enzyme an exopeptidase, is a circulating enzyme that participates in the body's renin-angiotensin system , which mediates extracellular volume (i.e. that of the blood plasma, lymph and interstitial fluid), and arterial vasoconstriction. It is secreted by pulmonary and renal endothelial cells and catalyzes the conversion of decapeptide angiotensin I to octapeptide angiotensin II.
	It has two primary functions:
	· ACE catalyses the conversion of angiotensin I to angiotensin II, a potent vasoconstrictor in a substrate concentration dependent manner. · ACE degrades bradykinin, a potent vasodilator, and other vasoactive peptides,
	These two actions make ACE inhibition a goal in the treatment of conditions such as high blood pressure, heart failure, diabetic nephropathy, and type 2 diabetes mellitus. Inhibition of ACE (by ACE inhibitors) results in the decreased formation of angiotensin II and decreased metabolism of bradykinin, leading to systematic dilation of the arteries and veins and a decrease in arterial blood pressure. In addition, inhibiting angiotension II formation diminishes angiotensin II-mediated aldosterone secretion from the adrenal cortex, leading to a decrease in water and sodium reabsorption and a reduction in extracellular volume.
Beta-adrenergic agonist	Beta-adrenergic agonists are adrenergic agonists which act upon the beta receptors.
	β_1 agonists
	β_1 agonists: stimulates adenylyl cyclase activity; opening of calcium channel. (cardiac stimulants; used to treat cardiogenic shock, acute heart failure, bradyarrhythmias).
Enzyme inhibitor	An enzyme inhibitor is a molecule that binds to enzymes and decreases their activity.

Since blocking an enzyme's activity can kill a pathogen or correct a metabolic imbalance, many drugs are enzyme inhibitors. They are also used as herbicides and pesticides.

Terminal sedation	In medicine, specifically in end-of-life care, terminal sedation is the palliative practice of relieving distress in a terminally ill person in the last hours or days of a dying patient's life, usually by means of a continuous intravenous or subcutaneous infusion of a sedative drug. This is a option of last resort for patients whose symptoms cannot be controlled by any other means. This should be differentiated from euthanasia as the goal of palliative sedation is to control symptoms through sedation but not shorten the patient's life, while in euthanasia the goal is to shorten life to relieve symptoms.
Renal vein	The renal veins are veins that drain the kidney. They connect the kidney to the inferior vena cava. They carry the blood purified by the kidney.
Ischaemic	Ischaemic or ischemic heart disease (IHD), or myocardial ischaemia, is a disease characterized by reduced blood supply to the heart muscle, usually due to coronary artery disease (atherosclerosis of the coronary arteries). Its risk increases with age, smoking, hypercholesterolaemia (high cholesterol levels), diabetes, hypertension (high blood pressure) and is more common in men and those who have close relatives with Ischaemic heart disease. Symptoms of stable Ischaemic heart disease include angina (characteristic chest pain on exertion) and decreased exercise tolerance.
Crisis management	Crisis management is the process by which an organization deals with a major event that threatens to harm the organization, its stakeholders, or the general public. The study of crisis management originated with the large scale industrial and environmental disasters in the 1980s. Three elements are common to most definitions of crisis: (a) a threat to the organization, (b) the element of surprise, and (c) a short decision time.
Hypertensive emergency	A hypertensive emergency is severe hypertension (high blood pressure) with acute impairment of one or more organ systems (especially the central nervous system, cardiovascular system and/or the renal system) that can result in irreversible organ damage. In a hypertensive emergency, the blood pressure should be substantially lowered over a period of minutes to hours with an antihypertensive agent. The eyes may show retinal hemorrhage or an exudate.
Cardiogenic shock	Cardiogenic shock is based upon an inadequate circulation of blood due to primary failure of the ventricles of the heart to function effectively. Since this is a type of shock there is insufficient perfusion of tissue (i.e.

	the heart) to meet the required demands for oxygen and nutrients. Cardiogenic shock is a largely irreversible condition and as such is more often fatal than not.
Vomiting	Vomiting is the forceful expulsion of the contents of one's stomach through the mouth and sometimes the nose. Vomiting can be caused by a wide variety of conditions; it may present as a specific response to ailments like gastritis or poisoning, or as a non-specific sequela of disorders ranging from brain tumors and elevated intracranial pressure to overexposure to ionizing radiation. The feeling that one is about to vomit is called nausea, which usually precedes, but does not always lead to, vomiting.

1. _____s are adrenergic agonists which act upon the beta receptors.

   β_1 agonists

   β_1 agonists: stimulates adenylyl cyclase activity; opening of calcium channel. (cardiac stimulants; used to treat cardiogenic shock, acute heart failure, bradyarrhythmias).

   a. Bambuterol
   b. Bitolterol
   c. Bromoacetylalprenololmenthane
   d. Beta-adrenergic agonist

2. _____ (also known as Nil Lesions or Nil Disease (lipoid nephrosis)) is a disease of the kidney that causes nephrotic syndrome and usually affects children (peak incidence at 2-3 years of age).

   _____ is most common in very young children but can occur in older children and adults. It is by far the most common cause of nephrotic syndrome (NS) in children between the ages of 1 and 7, accounting for the majority (about 90%) of these diagnoses.

   a. Nephritic syndrome
   b. Lipoid congenital adrenal hyperplasia
   c. Minimal change disease
   d. Primary aldosteronism

3. . _____, from the pharynx to the rectum. It has diverse causes, and a medical history, as well as physical examination, generally distinguishes between the main forms. The degree of bleeding can range from nearly undetectable to acute, massive, life-threatening bleeding.

   a. Gastrojejunocolic fistula

Chapter 9. RENAL

b. Gastrointestinal bleeding

c. High altitude flatus expulsion

d. Hyperchlorhydria

4. _____ is the forceful expulsion of the contents of one's stomach through the mouth and sometimes the nose. _____ can be caused by a wide variety of conditions; it may present as a specific response to ailments like gastritis or poisoning, or as a non-specific sequela of disorders ranging from brain tumors and elevated intracranial pressure to overexposure to ionizing radiation. The feeling that one is about to vomit is called nausea, which usually precedes, but does not always lead to, _____.

a. Bacteriophage

b. Catamenial pneumothorax

c. Vomiting

d. Cervical pregnancy

5. An _____ is a molecule that binds to enzymes and decreases their activity. Since blocking an enzyme's activity can kill a pathogen or correct a metabolic imbalance, many drugs are _____s. They are also used as herbicides and pesticides.

a. Epoxide hydrolase

b. Ethyl glucuronide

c. Excretion

d. Enzyme inhibitor

1. d
2. c
3. b
4. c
5. d

You can take the complete Chapter Practice Test

for Chapter 9. RENAL
on all key terms, persons, places, and concepts.

Online 99 Cents

http://www.epub219.49.13357.9.cram101.com/

Use www.Cram101.com for all your study needs

including Cram101's online interactive problem solving labs in

chemistry, statistics, mathematics, and more.

Chapter 10. VASCULITIS/ RHEUMATOLOGIC

CHAPTER OUTLINE: KEY TERMS, PEOPLE, PLACES, CONCEPTS

Epidemiology

Pathogenesis

Acute hemorrhagic edema of infancy

Differential diagnosis

ACE inhibitor

Angiotensin I-converting enzyme

Enzyme inhibitor

Prognosis

Terminal sedation

Basic life support

Kawasaki disease

Etiological myth

Life support

Coronary arteries

Juvenile idiopathic arthritis

Hemophagocytic lymphohistiocytosis

Ohtahara syndrome

Activation syndrome

Oligoarthritis

CHAPTER OUTLINE: KEY TERMS, PEOPLE, PLACES, CONCEPTS

Polyarthritis

Rheumatic fever

Systemics

Pain assessment

Psoriatic arthritis

Methylmalonic acidemia

Stem cell

Anti-nuclear antibodies

Lupus erythematosus

Pathophysiology

Musculoskeletal

Systemic lupus erythematosus

Lupus nephritis

Gastrointestinal

Pulmonary

Renal failure

Serositis

Gastrointestinal bleeding

Cerebrospinal fluid

Griscelli syndrome

Virulence factor

Erythema marginatum

Acute rheumatic fever

Carditis

Chorea

Dermatomyositis

Polyethylene glycol

Scleroderma

Sicca syndrome

Connective tissue

Takayasu's arteritis

Vasculitis

Polyarteritis nodosa

Sarcoidosis

Goodpasture's syndrome

Microscopic polyangiitis

Vancomycin-resistant

Epidemiology	Epidemiology is the study of the distribution and patterns of health-events, health-characteristics and their causes or influences in well-defined populations. It is the cornerstone method of public health research and practice, and helps inform policy decisions and evidence-based medicine by identifying risk factors for disease and targets for preventive medicine and public policies. Epidemiologists are involved in the design of studies, collection and statistical analysis of data, and interpretation and dissemination of results (including peer review and occasional systematic review).
Pathogenesis	The pathogenesis of a disease is the mechanism by which the disease is caused. The term can also be used to describe the origin and development of the disease and whether it is acute, chronic or recurrent. The word comes from the Greek pathos, 'disease', and genesis, 'creation'.
Acute hemorrhagic edema of infancy	Acute hemorrhagic edema of infancy is a skin condition that affects children under the age of two with a recent history of upper respiratory illness, a course of antibiotics, or both.
Differential diagnosis	A differential diagnosis is a systematic diagnostic method used to identify the presence of an entity where multiple alternatives are possible (and the process may be termed differential diagnostic procedure), and may also refer to any of the included candidate alternatives (which may also be termed candidate condition). This method is essentially a process of elimination, or at least, rendering of the probabilities of candidate conditions to negligible levels. In this sense, probabilities are, in fact, imaginative parameters in the mind or hardware of the diagnostician or system, while in reality the target (such as a patient) either has a condition or not with an actual probability of either 0 or 100%.
ACE inhibitor	ACE inhibitors are a group of drugs used primarily for the treatment of hypertension (high blood pressure) and congestive heart failure. Originally synthesized from compounds found in pit viper venom, they inhibit angiotensin-converting enzyme (ACE), a component of the blood pressure-regulating renin-angiotensin system.
Angiotensin I-converting enzyme	Angiotensin I-converting enzyme an exopeptidase, is a circulating enzyme that participates in the body's renin-angiotensin system , which mediates extracellular volume (i.e. that of the blood plasma, lymph and interstitial fluid), and arterial vasoconstriction. It is secreted by pulmonary and renal endothelial cells and catalyzes the conversion of decapeptide angiotensin I to octapeptide angiotensin II. It has two primary functions: · ACE catalyses the conversion of angiotensin I to angiotensin II, a potent vasoconstrictor in a substrate concentration dependent manner. · ACE degrades bradykinin, a potent vasodilator, and other vasoactive peptides,

These two actions make ACE inhibition a goal in the treatment of conditions such as high blood pressure, heart failure, diabetic nephropathy, and type 2 diabetes mellitus. Inhibition of ACE (by ACE inhibitors) results in the decreased formation of angiotensin II and decreased metabolism of bradykinin, leading to systematic dilation of the arteries and veins and a decrease in arterial blood pressure. In addition, inhibiting angiotension II formation diminishes angiotensin II-mediated aldosterone secretion from the adrenal cortex, leading to a decrease in water and sodium reabsorption and a reduction in extracellular volume.

Enzyme inhibitor	An enzyme inhibitor is a molecule that binds to enzymes and decreases their activity. Since blocking an enzyme's activity can kill a pathogen or correct a metabolic imbalance, many drugs are enzyme inhibitors. They are also used as herbicides and pesticides.
Prognosis	Prognosis is a medical term to describe the likely outcome of an illness. When applied to large populations, prognostic estimates can be very accurate: for example the statement '45% of patients with severe septic shock will die within 28 days' can be made with some confidence, because previous research found that this proportion of patients died. However, it is much harder to translate this into a prognosis for an individual patient: additional information is needed to determine whether a patient belongs to the 45% who will succumb, or to the 55% who survive.
Terminal sedation	In medicine, specifically in end-of-life care, terminal sedation is the palliative practice of relieving distress in a terminally ill person in the last hours or days of a dying patient's life, usually by means of a continuous intravenous or subcutaneous infusion of a sedative drug. This is a option of last resort for patients whose symptoms cannot be controlled by any other means. This should be differentiated from euthanasia as the goal of palliative sedation is to control symptoms through sedation but not shorten the patient's life, while in euthanasia the goal is to shorten life to relieve symptoms.
Basic life support	Basic life support is the level of medical care which is used for patients with life-threatening illnesses or injuries until the patient can be given full medical care at a hospital. It can be provided by trained medical personnel, including emergency medical technicians, paramedics, and by laypersons who have received BLS training. BLS is generally used in the pre-hospital setting, and can be provided without medical equipment.
Kawasaki disease	Kawasaki disease also known as Kawasaki syndrome, lymph node syndrome and mucocutaneous lymph node syndrome, is an autoimmune disease in which the medium-sized blood vessels throughout the body become inflamed. It is largely seen in children under five years of age.

Etiological myth	Etiology is the study of causation, or origination. The word is most commonly used in medical and philosophical theories, where it is used to refer to the study of why things occur, or even the reasons behind the way that things act, and is used in philosophy, physics, psychology, government, medicine, theology and biology in reference to the causes of various phenomena. An etiological myth is a myth intended to explain a name or create a mythic history for a place or family.
Life support	Life support in medicine is a broad term that applies to any therapy used to sustain a patient's life while they are critically ill or injured, as part of intensive-care medicine. There are many therapies and techniques that may be used by clinicians to achieve the goal of sustaining life. Some examples include:•Feeding tube•Total parenteral nutrition•Mechanical ventilation•Heart/Lung bypass•Urinary catheterization•Dialysis•Cardiopulmonary resuscitation•Defibrillation•Artificial pacemaker These techniques are applied most commonly in the Emergency Department, Intensive Care Unit and, Operating Rooms.
Coronary arteries	Coronary circulation is the circulation of blood in the blood vessels of the heart muscle. Although blood fills the chambers of the heart, the muscle tissue of the heart (the myocardium) is so thick that it requires coronary blood vessels to deliver blood deep into it. The vessels that deliver oxygen-rich blood to the myocardium are known as Coronary arteries.
Juvenile idiopathic arthritis	Juvenile idiopathic arthritis (aka Juvenile Rheumatoid Arthritis JRA) is the most common form of persistent arthritis in children. (Juvenile in this context refers to an onset before age 16, idiopathic refers to a condition with no defined cause, and arthritis is the inflammation of the synovium of a joint). JIA is a subset of arthritis seen in childhood, which may be transient and self-limited or chronic.
Hemophagocytic lymphohistiocytosis	Hemophagocytic lymphohistiocytosis also known as hemophagocytic syndrome, is an uncommon hematologic disorder that, typically, clinically manifests as fever, hepatosplenomegaly, lymphadenopathy, jaundice and rash, with laboratory findings of lymphocytosis and histiocytosis, and the pathologic finding of hemophagocytosis. Pancytopenia (anemia, neutropenia, and thrombocytopenia), markely elevated serum ferritin levels, and abnormal liver enzymes are frequently present. Primary HLH, also known as familial hemophagocytic lymphohistioctosis (FHL) or familial erythrophagocytic lymphohistiocytosis, is a heterogeneous autosomal recessive disorder found to be more prevalent with parental consanguinity.

Chapter 10. VASCULITIS/ RHEUMATOLOGIC

Ohtahara syndrome	Ohtahara syndrome also known as Early Infantile Epileptic Encephalopathy with Burst-Suppression (EIEE), is a progressive epileptic encephalopathy. The syndrome is outwardly characterized by tonic spasms and partial seizures, and receives its more elaborate name from the pattern of burst activity on an electroencephalogram (EEG). It is an extremely debilitating progressive neurological disorder, involving intractable seizures and severe mental retardation.
Activation syndrome	Activation syndrome is a form of sometimes suicidal or homicidal stimulation or agitation that can occur in response to some psychoactive drugs. A study of paroxetine found that 21 out of 93 (23 percent) of youth taking Paxil reported manic-like symptoms which included hostility, emotional lability and nervousness. Pfizer has denied that sertraline can cause such effects.
Oligoarthritis	Oligoarthritis is defined as arthritis affecting one to four joints during the first six months of disease.
Polyarthritis	Polyarthritis is any type of arthritis which involves 5 or more joints simultaneously. It is usually associated with autoimmune conditions. Polyarthritis may be experienced at any age and is not gender specific.
Rheumatic fever	Rheumatic fever is an inflammatory disease that occurs following a Streptococcus pyogenes infection, such as streptococcal pharyngitis or scarlet fever. Believed to be caused by antibody cross-reactivity that can involve the heart, joints, skin, and brain, the illness typically develops two to three weeks after a streptococcal infection. Acute rheumatic fever commonly appears in children between the ages of 6 and 15, with only 20% of first-time attacks occurring in adults.
Systemics	In the context of systems science and systems philosophy, the term systemics refers to an initiative to study systems from a holistic point of view. It is an attempt at developing logical, mathematical, engineering and philosophical paradigms and frameworks in which physical, technological, biological, social, cognitive, and metaphysical systems can be studied and modeled. The term 'systemics' was coined in the 1970s by Mario Bunge and others, as an alternative paradigm for research related to general systems theory and systems science.
Pain assessment	Pain is often regarded as the fifth vital sign in regard to healthcare because it is accepted now in healthcare that pain, like other vital signs, is an objective sensation rather than subjective. As a result nurses are trained and expected to assess pain. Pain assessment and re-assessment after administration of analgesics or pain management is regulated in healthcare facilities by accreditation bodies, like the Joint Commission.

Psoriatic arthritis	Psoriatic arthritis is a type of inflammatory arthritis that, according to the National Psoriasis Foundation, will develop in up to 30 percent of people who have the chronic skin condition psoriasis. Psoriatic arthritis is said to be a seronegative spondyloarthropathy and therefore occurs more commonly in patients with tissue type HLA-B27.

Common symptoms of psoriatic arthritis include:•Pain, swelling, or stiffness in one or more joints.•Joints that are red or warm to the touch.•Sausage-like swelling in the fingers or toes, known as dactylitis.•Pain in and around the feet and ankles, especially tendinitis in the Achilles tendon or Plantar fasciitis in the sole of the foot.•Changes to the nails, such as pitting or separation from the nail bed.•Pain in the area of the Sacrum (the lower back, above the tailbone).

Along with the above noted pain and inflammation, there is extreme exhaustion that does not go away with adequate rest. |
| Methylmalonic acidemia | Methylmalonic acidemia also called methylmalonic aciduria, is an autosomal recessive metabolic disorder. It is a classical type of organic acidemia.

Methylmalonic acidemia stems from several genotypes, all forms of the disorder usually diagnosed in the early neonatal period, presenting progressive encephalopathy, and secondary hyperammonemia. |
Stem cell	Stem cells are biological cells found in all multicellular organisms, that can divide (through mitosis) and differentiate into diverse specialized cell types and can self-renew to produce more stem cells. In mammals, there are two broad types of stem cells: embryonic stem cells, which are isolated from the inner cell mass of blastocysts, and adult stem cells, which are found in various tissues. In adult organisms, stem cells and progenitor cells act as a repair system for the body, replenishing adult tissues.
Anti-nuclear antibodies	Anti-nuclear antibodies are antibodies directed against the cell nucleus. They are raised in several conditions, usually in an auto-immune condition where the immune system makes antibodies to fight its own body. Normally a test is administered in people with many arthritic type symptoms or skin rashes to exclude systemic lupus erythematosus(SLE).
Lupus erythematosus	Lupus erythematosus is a category for a collection of diseases with similar underlying problems with immunity (autoimmune disease). Symptoms of these diseases can affect many different body systems, including joints, skin, kidneys, blood cells, heart, and lungs. Four main types of lupus exist: systemic lupus erythematosus, discoid lupus erythematosus, drug-induced lupus erythematosus, and neonatal lupus erythematosus.
Pathophysiology	Pathophysiology sample values

Pathophysiology is the study of the changes of normal mechanical, physical, and biochemical functions, either caused by a disease, or resulting from an abnormal syndrome. More formally, it is the branch of medicine which deals with any disturbances of body functions, caused by disease or prodromal symptoms.

An alternative definition is 'the study of the biological and physical manifestations of disease as they correlate with the underlying abnormalities and physiological disturbances.'

The study of pathology and the study of pathophysiology often involves substantial overlap in diseases and processes, but pathology emphasizes direct observations, while pathophysiology emphasizes quantifiable measurements.

Musculoskeletal	A musculoskeletal system (also known as the locomotor system) is an organ system that gives animals (including humans) the ability to move using the muscular and skeletal systems. The musculoskeletal system provides form, stability, and movement to the body. It is made up of the body's bones (the skeleton), muscles, cartilage, tendons, ligaments, joints, and other connective tissue (the tissue that supports and binds tissues and organs together).
Systemic lupus erythematosus	Systemic lupus erythematosus often abbreviated to SLE or lupus, is a systemic autoimmune disease that can affect any part of the body. As occurs in other autoimmune diseases, the immune system attacks the body's cells and tissue, resulting in inflammation and tissue damage. It is a Type III hypersensitivity reaction caused by antibody-immune complex formation.
Lupus nephritis	Lupus nephritis is an inflammation of the kidney caused by systemic lupus erythematosus (SLE), a disease of the immune system. Apart from the kidneys, SLE can also damage the skin, joints, nervous system and virtually any organ or system in the body. General Symptoms of Lupus include: Malar Rash, Discoid rash, photosensitivity, oral ulcers, nonerosive arthritis, pleuropericarditis, renal disease, neurologic manifestaions, and hematologic disorders.
Gastrointestinal	The digestive tract is the system of organs within multicellular animals that takes in food, digests it to extract energy and nutrients, and expels the remaining matter. The major function of the gastrointestinal tract are ingestion, digestion, absorption, and defecation. The GI tract differs substantially from animal to animal.
Pulmonary	The lung or pulmonary system is the essential respiration organ in air-breathing animals, including most tetrapods, a few fish and a few snails. In mammals and the more complex life forms, the two lungs are located in the chest on either side of the heart.

Renal failure	Renal failure or kidney failure (formerly called renal insufficiency) describes a medical condition in which the kidneys fail to adequately filter toxins and waste products from the blood. The two forms are acute (acute kidney injury) and chronic (chronic kidney disease); a number of other diseases or health problems may cause either form of renal failure to occur. Renal failure is described as a decrease in glomerular filtration rate.
Serositis	Serositis refers to inflammation of the serous tissues of the body, the tissues lining the lungs (pleura), heart (pericardium), and the inner lining of the abdomen (peritoneum) and organs within. It is commonly found with fat wrapping or creeping fat. Serositis is seen in numerous conditions:•Lupus erythematosus (SLE), for which it is one of the criteria,•Rheumatoid arthritis•Familial Mediterranean fever (FMF),•Chronic renal failure•Juvenile idiopathic arthritis•Inflammatory bowel disease (especially Crohn's disease)•Acute appendicitis.
Gastrointestinal bleeding	Gastrointestinal bleeding, from the pharynx to the rectum. It has diverse causes, and a medical history, as well as physical examination, generally distinguishes between the main forms. The degree of bleeding can range from nearly undetectable to acute, massive, life-threatening bleeding.
Cerebrospinal fluid	Cerebrospinal fluid Liquor cerebrospinalis, is a clear, colorless, bodily fluid, that occupies the subarachnoid space and the ventricular system around and inside the brain and spinal cord. The CSF occupies the space between the arachnoid mater (the middle layer of the brain cover, meninges) and the pia mater (the layer of the meninges closest to the brain). It constitutes the content of all intra-cerebral (inside the brain, cerebrum) ventricles, cisterns, and sulci, as well as the central canal of the spinal cord.
Griscelli syndrome	Griscelli syndrome is a rare autosomal recessive disorder characterized by albinism (hypopigmentation) with immunodeficiency, that usually causes death by early childhood. Griscelli syndrome is a disorder of melanosome transport, and divided into several types:Presentation Griscelli syndrome is defined by the characteristic hypopigmentation, with frequent pyogenic infection, hepatosplenomegaly, neutropenia, thrombocytopenia, and immunodeficiency. Very often there is also impaired natural killer cell activity, absent delayed-type hypersensitivity and a poor cell proliferation response to antigenic challenge.

Chapter 10. VASCULITIS/ RHEUMATOLOGIC

Virulence factor	Virulence factors are molecules expressed and secreted by pathogens (bacteria, viruses, fungi and protozoa) that enable them to achieve the following:•colonization of a niche in the host (this includes adhesion to cells)•Immunoevasion, evasion of the host's immune response•Immunosuppression, inhibition of the host's immune response•entry into and exit out of cells (if the pathogen is an intracellular one)•obtain nutrition from the host. Virulence factors are very often responsible for causing disease in the host as they inhibit certain host functions. Pathogens possess a wide array of virulence factors. Some are intrinsic to the bacteria (e.g. capsules and endotoxin) whereas others are obtained from plasmids (e.g. some toxins).
Erythema marginatum	Erythema marginatum is described as the presence of pink rings on the trunk and inner surfaces of the limbs which come and go for as long as several months. It is found primarily on extensor surfaces. An association with bradykinin has been proposed in the case of hereditary angioedema.
Acute rheumatic fever	Rheumatic fever is an inflammatory disease that may develop two to three weeks after a Group A streptococcal infection (such as strep throat or scarlet fever). It is believed to be caused by antibody cross-reactivity and can involve the heart, joints, skin, and brain. Acute rheumatic fever commonly appears in children between ages 5 and 15, with only 20% of first time attacks occurring in adults.
Carditis	Carditis is the inflammation of the heart or its surroundings. It is usually studied and treated by specifying it as: · PeriCarditis is the inflammation of the pericardium · MyoCarditis is the inflammation of the heart muscle · EndoCarditis is the inflammation of the endocardium, is a bacterial infection of the endocardium that causes symptoms such as night sweats, fevers, weight loss, and other symptoms. It is treated with intravenus antibiotics. Reflux Carditis refers to a possible outcome of esophageal reflux (also known as GERD)
Chorea	Chorea is an abnormal involuntary movement disorder, one of a group of neurological disorders called dyskinesias. The term chorea is derived from the Greek word χορε?α , as the quick movements of the feet or hands are comparable to dancing.

Dermatomyositis	Dermatomyositis is a connective-tissue disease related to polymyositis (PM) that is characterized by inflammation of the muscles and the skin. While DM most frequently affects the skin and muscles, it is a systemic disorder that may also affect the joints, the esophagus, the lungs, and, less commonly, the heart. The cause is unknown, but it may result from either a viral infection or an autoimmune reaction.
Polyethylene glycol	Polyethylene glycol is a polyether compound with many applications from industrial manufacturing to medicine. The structure of PEG is (note the repeated element in parentheses):HO-CH$_2$-(CH$_2$-O-CH$_2$-)$_n$-CH$_2$-OH PEG is also known as polyethylene oxide (PEO) or polyoxyethylene (POE), depending on its molecular weight, and under the tradename Carbowax. Available forms and nomenclature PEG, PEO, or POE refers to an oligomer or polymer of ethylene oxide.
Scleroderma	Scleroderma is a chronic systemic autoimmune disease (primarily of the skin) characterized by fibrosis , vascular alterations, and autoantibodies. There are two major forms: Limited systemic sclerosis/scleroderma involves cutaneous manifestations that mainly affect the hands, arms, and face. It was previously called CREST syndrome in reference to the following complications: Calcinosis, Raynaud's phenomenon, Esophageal dysfunction, Sclerodactyly, and Telangiectasias.
Sicca syndrome	Sjögren's syndrome, also known as 'Mikulicz disease' and 'Sicca syndrome', is a systemic autoimmune disease in which immune cells attack and destroy the exocrine glands that produce tears and saliva. Nine out of ten Sjögren's patients are women and the average age of onset is late 40s, although Sjögren's occurs in all age groups in both women and men. It is estimated to affect as many as 4 million people in the United States alone, making it the second most common autoimmune rheumatic disease.
Connective tissue	Connective tissue is a form of fibrous tissue.. It is one of the four types of tissue in traditional classifications (the others being epithelial, muscle, and nervous tissue). Collagen is the main protein of Connective tissue in animals and the most abundant protein in mammals, making up about 25% of the total protein content. It is largely a category of exclusion rather than one with a precise defintion, but all or most tissues in this category are similarly:

	· Involved in structure and support. · Derived from mesoderm, usually. · Characterized largely by the traits of non-living tissue.
Takayasu's arteritis	Takayasu's arteritis is a form of large vessel granulomatous vasculitis with massive intimal fibrosis and vascular narrowing affecting often young or middle-aged women of Asian decent. It mainly affects the aorta (the main blood vessel leaving the heart) and its branches, as well as the pulmonary arteries. Females are about 8-9 times more likely to be affected than males.
Vasculitis	Vasculitis refers to a heterogeneous group of disorders that are characterized by inflammatory destruction of blood vessels. Both arteries and veins are affected. Lymphangitis is sometimes considered a type of vasculitis.
Polyarteritis nodosa	Polyarteritis nodosa is a vasculitis of medium & small-sized arteries, which become swollen and damaged from attack by rogue immune cells. Polyarteritis nodosa is also called Kussmaul disease or Kussmaul-Maier disease. Infantile polyarteritis nodosa is a type of PAN restricted to infants.
Sarcoidosis	Sarcoidosis also called sarcoid, Besnier-Boeck disease or Besnier-Boeck-Schaumann disease, is a disease in which abnormal collections of chronic inflammatory cells (granulomas) form as nodules in multiple organs. The cause of sarcoidosis is unknown. The granulomas that appear are usually of the non-necrotizing variety and are most often located in the lungs or the lymph nodes, but virtually any organ can be affected.
Goodpasture's syndrome	Goodpasture's syndrome is a rare condition characterized by glomerulonephritis and hemorrhaging of the lungs. Although many diseases can present with these symptoms, the name Goodpasture's syndrome is usually reserved for the autoimmune disease triggered when the patient's immune system attacks Goodpasture antigen (a type II hypersensitivity reaction), which is found in the kidney and lung, and in time, causing damage to these organs. The disease bears the name of the American pathologist Dr. Ernest Goodpasture of Vanderbilt University, whose 1919 description is regarded as the first report on the existence of the condition.
Microscopic polyangiitis	Microscopic polyangiitis is an ill-defined autoimmune disease characterized by a systemic, pauci-immune, necrotizing, small-vessel vasculitis without clinical or pathological evidence of necrotizing granulomatous inflammation. Clinical features may include constitutional symptoms like fever, anorexia, weight loss, fatigue, and renal failure. A majority of patients may have hematuria and proteinuria.

Vancomycin-resistant	Vancomycin-resistant enterococcus (VRE) is the name given to a group of bacterial species of the genus Enterococcus that is resistant to the antibiotic vancomycin.
	Enterococci are enteric gram-positive coccoid shaped bacteria that can be found in the digestive and urinary tracts of some humans. VRE was discovered in 1985 and is particularly dangerous to immunocompromised individuals.

CHAPTER QUIZ: KEY TERMS, PEOPLE, PLACES, CONCEPTS

1. _____ is a vasculitis of medium & small-sized arteries, which become swollen and damaged from attack by rogue immune cells. _____ is also called Kussmaul disease or Kussmaul-Maier disease. Infantile _____ is a type of PAN restricted to infants.

   a. Primary lymphedema associated with yellow nails and pleural effusion
   b. Venous ulcer
   c. Polyarteritis nodosa
   d. Bacteriophage

2. _____ (aka Juvenile Rheumatoid Arthritis JRA) is the most common form of persistent arthritis in children. (Juvenile in this context refers to an onset before age 16, idiopathic refers to a condition with no defined cause, and arthritis is the inflammation of the synovium of a joint).

   JIA is a subset of arthritis seen in childhood, which may be transient and self-limited or chronic.

   a. Juvenile idiopathic arthritis
   b. Great vessels
   c. Hot aches
   d. High endothelial venules

3. An _____ is a molecule that binds to enzymes and decreases their activity. Since blocking an enzyme's activity can kill a pathogen or correct a metabolic imbalance, many drugs are _____s. They are also used as herbicides and pesticides.

   a. Epoxide hydrolase
   b. Enzyme inhibitor
   c. Excretion
   d. IdMOC

4. . _____ is a chronic systemic autoimmune disease (primarily of the skin) characterized by fibrosis , vascular alterations, and autoantibodies. There are two major forms:

Limited systemic sclerosis/_____ involves cutaneous manifestations that mainly affect the hands, arms, and face. It was previously called CREST syndrome in reference to the following complications: Calcinosis, Raynaud's phenomenon, Esophageal dysfunction, Sclerodactyly, and Telangiectasias.

a. Scleroderma
b. Systemic scleroderma
c. Thrombotic thrombocytopenic purpura
d. Vitiligo

5. _____ in medicine is a broad term that applies to any therapy used to sustain a patient's life while they are critically ill or injured, as part of intensive-care medicine. There are many therapies and techniques that may be used by clinicians to achieve the goal of sustaining life. Some examples include:•Feeding tube•Total parenteral nutrition•Mechanical ventilation•Heart/Lung bypass•Urinary catheterization•Dialysis•Cardiopulmonary resuscitation•Defibrillation•Artificial pacemaker

These techniques are applied most commonly in the Emergency Department, Intensive Care Unit and, Operating Rooms.

a. Medical biology
b. Monitoring
c. Pediatric ependymoma
d. Life support

1. c
2. a
3. b
4. a
5. d

You can take the complete Chapter Practice Test

for Chapter 10. VASCULITIS/ RHEUMATOLOGIC
on all key terms, persons, places, and concepts.

Online 99 Cents

http://www.epub219.49.13357.10.cram101.com/

Use www.Cram101.com for all your study needs

including Cram101's online interactive problem solving labs in

chemistry, statistics, mathematics, and more.

CHAPTER OUTLINE: KEY TERMS, PEOPLE, PLACES, CONCEPTS

| | Outbreak |

| | Meningitis |

| | Epidemiology |

| | Pathogenesis |

| | Pathogen |

| | Intracranial pressure |

| | Genital herpes |

| | Lyme disease |

| | Valproic acid |

| | Community-acquired pneumonia |

| | Prognosis |

| | Herpes simplex |

| | Differential diagnosis |

| | Etiological myth |

| | Physical examination |

| | Computed tomography |

| | Abdominal mass |

| | Encephalitis |

| | Naegleria fowleri |

Aspiration

Aspiration pneumonia

Parapneumonic effusion

Hospital-acquired pneumonia

Bronchiolitis

Risk factor

Beta-adrenergic agonist

Chest radiograph

Bronchiolitis obliterans

Palivizumab

Prevention

Orbital cellulitis

Periorbital cellulitis

Pathophysiology

Cystic fibrosis

Imaging

Rheumatic fever

Fungus

Cystitis

CHAPTER OUTLINE: KEY TERMS, PEOPLE, PLACES, CONCEPTS

Pyelonephritis

Urethritis

Urinary tract infection

Prevalence

Septic arthritis

Vesicoureteral reflux

Renal failure

Blood culture

Cellulitis

Ecthyma

Erysipelas

Erysipeloid

Pasteurella multocida

Staphylococcus aureus

Necrotizing fasciitis

Mantoux test

Mycobacterium tuberculosis

Tuberculosis

Pleural effusion

Chapter 11. INFECTIOUS DISEASES
CHAPTER OUTLINE: KEY TERMS, PEOPLE, PLACES, CONCEPTS

_____ Scrofula

_____ Lymphadenopathy

_____ Nervous system

_____ Tuberculous meningitis

_____ Human immunodeficiency virus

_____ Subtyping

_____ Retrovir

_____ Monitoring

_____ Herpes simplex virus

_____ Transmission

_____ Herpes labialis

_____ Herpes gladiatorum

_____ Herpetic whitlow

_____ Substance abuse

_____ Skin infection

_____ Common variable immunodeficiency

_____ X-linked hypogammaglobulinemia

_____ Primary

_____ Primary immunodeficiency

CHAPTER OUTLINE: KEY TERMS, PEOPLE, PLACES, CONCEPTS

_____ Bone marrow

_____ 22q11.2 deletion syndrome

_____ Howell-Jolly bodies

_____ Aplastic anemia

_____ Osteomyelitis

_____ Bone scan

_____ Osteoarthritis

_____ Vertebral osteomyelitis

_____ Pelvic

_____ Sneakers

_____ Vertebral

_____ Croup

_____ Thumbprint sign

_____ Epiglottitis

_____ Entry inhibitor

_____ Mechanical ventilation

_____ Retropharyngeal abscess

_____ Chlamydia trachomatis

_____ Neisseria gonorrhoeae

Abdominal pain

Gastroesophageal reflux

Pelvic inflammatory disease

Fitz-Hugh-Curtis syndrome

Perihepatitis

Neisseria meningitidis

Purpura fulminans

Immunization

Meningococcal vaccine

Ehlers-Danlos syndrome

Tick-borne disease

Babesiosis

Ehrlichiosis

Borrelia burgdorferi

Erythema migrans

Rickettsia rickettsii

Rocky Mountains

Rocky Mountain spotted fever

Staphylococcal scalded skin syndrome

Toxic shock syndrome

Streptococcal toxic shock syndrome

Genetics

Coccidioides immitis

Isovaleric acidemia

Endocarditis

Histoplasmosis

Aspergillus

Central venous catheter

Trade name

Urine

Amphetamine

Formulation

Cartilage-hair hypoplasia

Adverse effect

Resistance

Cerebrospinal fluid

Polymyxin B

Influenza

Chapter 11. INFECTIOUS DISEASES

Avian influenza

Influenza pandemic

Influenza prevention

Pandemic

Infection control

Personal protective equipment

Transmission-based precautions

Protective equipment

Terminal sedation

Nosocomial infection

Infectious disease

Outbreak	Outbreak is a term used in epidemiology to describe an occurrence of disease greater than would otherwise be expected at a particular time and place. It may affect a small and localized group or impact upon thousands of people across an entire continent. Two linked cases of a rare infectious disease may be sufficient to constitute an outbreak.
Meningitis	Meningitis is inflammation of the protective membranes covering the brain and spinal cord, known collectively as the meninges. The inflammation may be caused by infection with viruses, bacteria, or other microorganisms, and less commonly by certain drugs. Meningitis can be life-threatening because of the inflammation's proximity to the brain and spinal cord; therefore the condition is classified as a medical emergency.
Epidemiology	Epidemiology is the study of the distribution and patterns of health-events, health-characteristics and their causes or influences in well-defined populations. It is the cornerstone method of public health research and practice, and helps inform policy decisions and evidence-based medicine by identifying risk factors for disease and targets for preventive medicine and public policies. Epidemiologists are involved in the design of studies, collection and statistical analysis of data, and interpretation and dissemination of results (including peer review and occasional systematic review).
Pathogenesis	The pathogenesis of a disease is the mechanism by which the disease is caused. The term can also be used to describe the origin and development of the disease and whether it is acute, chronic or recurrent. The word comes from the Greek pathos, 'disease', and genesis, 'creation'.
Pathogen	A pathogen (Greek: π?θος pathos, 'suffering, passion' and γεν?ς genes (-gen) 'producer of') or infectious agent -- in colloquial terms, a germ -- is a microorganism such as a virus, bacterium, prion, or fungus, that causes disease in its animal or plant host. There are several substrates including pathways wherein pathogens can invade a host; the principal pathways have different episodic time frames, but soil contamination has the longest or most persistent potential for harboring a pathogen. Not all pathogens are negative.
Intracranial pressure	Intracranial pressure is the pressure inside the skull and thus in the brain tissue and cerebrospinal fluid (CSF). The body has various mechanisms by which it keeps the ICP stable, with CSF pressures varying by about 1 mmHg in normal adults through shifts in production and absorption of CSF. CSF pressure has been shown to be influenced by abrupt changes in intrathoracic pressure during coughing (intraabdominal pressure), valsalva (Queckenstedt's maneuver), and communication with the vasculature (venous and arterial systems). ICP is measured in millimeters of mercury (mmHg) and, at rest, is normally 7-15 mmHg for a supine adult, and becomes negative (averaging −10 mmHg) in the vertical position.

Chapter 11. INFECTIOUS DISEASES

Genital herpes	Herpes genitalis (or genital herpes) refers to a genital infection by Herpes simplex virus. Following the classification HSV into two distinct categories of HSV-1 and HSV-2 in the 1960s, it was established that 'HSV-2 was below the waist, HSV-1 was above the waist'. Although genital herpes is largely believed to be caused by HSV-2, genital HSV-1 infections are increasing and now exceed 50% in certain populations, and that rule of thumb no longer applies.
Lyme disease	Lyme disease, is an emerging infectious disease caused by at least three species of bacteria belonging to the genus Borrelia. Borrelia burgdorferi sensu stricto is the main cause of Lyme disease in the United States, whereas Borrelia afzelii and Borrelia garinii cause most European cases. he town of Lyme, Connecticut, USA, where a number of cases were identified in 1975. Although Allen Steere realized that Lyme disease was a tick-borne disease in 1978, the cause of the disease remained a mystery until 1981, when B. burgdorferi was identified by Willy Burgdorfer.
Valproic acid	Valproic acid is a chemical compound and an acid that has found clinical use as an anticonvulsant and mood-stabilizing drug, primarily in the treatment of epilepsy, bipolar disorder, and, less commonly, major depression. It is also used to treat migraine headaches and schizophrenia. VPA is a liquid at room temperature, but it can be reacted with a base such as sodium hydroxide to form the salt sodium valproate, which is a solid.
Community-acquired pneumonia	Community-acquired pneumonia is a term used to describe one of several diseases in which individuals who have not recently been hospitalized develop an infection of the lungs (pneumonia). Community acquired pneumonia is a common illness and can affect people of all ages. Community acquired pneumonia often causes problems like difficulty in breathing, fever, chest pains, and a cough.
Prognosis	Prognosis is a medical term to describe the likely outcome of an illness. When applied to large populations, prognostic estimates can be very accurate: for example the statement '45% of patients with severe septic shock will die within 28 days' can be made with some confidence, because previous research found that this proportion of patients died. However, it is much harder to translate this into a prognosis for an individual patient: additional information is needed to determine whether a patient belongs to the 45% who will succumb, or to the 55% who survive.
Herpes simplex	Herpes simplex is a viral disease from the herpesviridae family caused by both Herpes simplex virus type 1 (HSV-1) and type 2 (HSV-2). Infection with the herpes virus is categorized into one of several distinct disorders based on the site of infection. Oral herpes, the visible symptoms of which are colloquially called cold sores or fever blisters, is an infection of the face or mouth.

Differential diagnosis	A differential diagnosis is a systematic diagnostic method used to identify the presence of an entity where multiple alternatives are possible (and the process may be termed differential diagnostic procedure), and may also refer to any of the included candidate alternatives (which may also be termed candidate condition). This method is essentially a process of elimination, or at least, rendering of the probabilities of candidate conditions to negligible levels. In this sense, probabilities are, in fact, imaginative parameters in the mind or hardware of the diagnostician or system, while in reality the target (such as a patient) either has a condition or not with an actual probability of either 0 or 100%.
Etiological myth	Etiology is the study of causation, or origination.
	The word is most commonly used in medical and philosophical theories, where it is used to refer to the study of why things occur, or even the reasons behind the way that things act, and is used in philosophy, physics, psychology, government, medicine, theology and biology in reference to the causes of various phenomena. An etiological myth is a myth intended to explain a name or create a mythic history for a place or family.
Physical examination	A physical examination, medical examination, or clinical examination (more popularly known as a check-up or medical) is the process by which a doctor investigates the body of a patient for signs of disease. It generally follows the taking of the medical history -- an account of the symptoms as experienced by the patient. Together with the medical history, the physical examination aids in determining the correct diagnosis and devising the treatment plan.
Computed tomography	Computed tomography is a medical imaging method employing tomography created by computer processing. Digital geometry processing is used to generate a three-dimensional image of the inside of an object from a large series of two-dimensional X-ray images taken around a single axis of rotation.
	Computed tomography produces a volume of data which can be manipulated, through a process known as 'windowing', in order to demonstrate various bodily structures based on their ability to block the X-ray/Röntgen beam.
Abdominal mass	An abdominal mass is any localized enlargement or swelling in the human abdomen. Depending on its location, the abdominal mass may be caused by an enlarged liver (hepatomegaly), enlarged spleen (splenomegaly), protruding kidney, a pancreatic mass, a retroperitoneal mass (a mass in the posterior of the peritoneum), an abdominal aortic aneurysm, or various tumours, such as those caused by abdominal carcinomatosis and omental metastasis. The treatments depend on the cause, and may range from watchful waiting to radical surgery.
Encephalitis	Encephalitis is an acute inflammation of the brain.

Encephalitis with meningitis is known as meningoencephalitis. Symptoms include headache, fever, confusion, drowsiness, and fatigue.

Naegleria fowleri	Naegleria fowleri is a free-living excavate form of protist typically found in warm bodies of fresh water, such as ponds, lakes, rivers, and hot springs. It is also found in soil, near warm-water discharges of industrial plants, and unchlorinated swimming pools in an amoeboid or temporary flagellate stage. There is no evidence of this organism living in ocean water.
Aspiration	In phonetics, aspiration is the strong burst of air that accompanies either the release or, in the case of preaspiration, the closure of some obstruents. To feel or see the difference between aspirated and unaspirated sounds, one can put a hand or a lit candle in front of one's mouth, and say pin and then bin . One should either feel a puff of air or see a flicker of the candle flame with pin that one does not get with bin.
Aspiration pneumonia	Aspiration pneumonia is bronchopneumonia that develops due to the entrance of foreign materials that enter the bronchial tree, usually oral or gastric contents (including food, saliva, or nasal secretions). Depending on the acidity of the aspirate, a chemical pneumonitis can develop, and bacterial pathogens (particularly anaerobic bacteria) may add to the inflammation. Aspiration pneumonia is often caused by an incompetent swallowing mechanism, such as occurs in some forms of neurological disease (a common cause being strokes) or while a person is intoxicated.
Parapneumonic effusion	A Parapneumonic effusion is a type of pleural effusion that arises as a result of a pneumonia. There are three types of Parapneumonic effusions: uncomplicated effusions, complicated effusions, and empyema. Uncomplicated effusions generally respond well to appropriate antibiotic treatment.
Hospital-acquired pneumonia	Hospital-acquired pneumonia or nosocomial pneumonia refers to any pneumonia contracted by a patient in a hospital at least 48-72 hours after being admitted. It is usually caused by a bacterial infection, rather than a virus. HAP is the second most common nosocomial infection (urinary tract infection is the most common) and accounts for 15-20% of the total.
Bronchiolitis	Bronchiolitis is inflammation of the bronchioles, the smallest air passages of the lungs. It usually occurs in children less than two years of age and presents with coughing, wheezing, and shortness of breath. This inflammation is usually caused by respiratory syncytial virus.
Risk factor	In epidemiology, a risk factor is a variable associated with an increased risk of disease or infection.

Sometimes, determinant is also used, being a variable associated with either increased or decreased risk.

Risk factors or determinants are correlational and not necessarily causal, because correlation does not prove causation.

Beta-adrenergic agonist	Beta-adrenergic agonists are adrenergic agonists which act upon the beta receptors.

β_1 agonists

β_1 agonists: stimulates adenylyl cyclase activity; opening of calcium channel. (cardiac stimulants; used to treat cardiogenic shock, acute heart failure, bradyarrhythmias).

Chest radiograph	In medicine, a chest radiograph, commonly called a chest X-ray (CXR), is a projection radiograph of the chest used to diagnose conditions affecting the chest, its contents, and nearby structures. Chest radiographs are among the most common films taken, being diagnostic of many conditions.

Like all methods of radiography, chest radiography employs ionizing radiation in the form of X-rays to generate images of the chest.

Bronchiolitis obliterans	Bronchiolitis obliterans also called obliterative bronchiolitis (OB) and constrictive bronchiolitis (CB), is a rare and life-threatening form of non-reversible obstructive lung disease in which the bronchioles (small airway branches) are compressed and narrowed by fibrosis (scar tissue) and/or inflammation. Bronchiolitis obliterans is also sometimes used to refer to a particularly severe form of pediatric bronchiolitis caused by adenovirus.

Bronchiolitis means inflammation of the bronchioles and obliterans refers to the fact that the inflammation or fibrosis of the bronchioles partially or completely obliterates the airways.

Palivizumab	Palivizumab is a monoclonal antibody produced by recombinant DNA technology. It is used in the prevention of respiratory syncytial virus (RSV) infections. It is recommended for infants that are high-risk because of prematurity or other medical problems such as congenital heart disease.
Prevention	Prevention refers to:

· Preventive medicine · Hazard Prevention, the process of risk study and elimination and mitigation in emergency management · Risk Prevention · Risk management · Preventive maintenance · Crime Prevention

Chapter 11. INFECTIOUS DISEASES

	· Prevention, an album by Scottish band De Rosa · Prevention a magazine about health in the United States · Prevent (company), a textile company from Slovenia
Orbital cellulitis	Orbital cellulitis is an infection of eye tissues posterior to the orbital septum. It most commonly refers to an acute spread of infection into the eye socket from either the adjacent sinuses or through the blood. When it affects the rear of the eye, it is known as retro-orbital cellulitis.
Periorbital cellulitis	Periorbital cellulitis, which is behind the septum), is an inflammation and infection of the eyelid and portions of skin around the eye, anterior to the orbital septum. It may be caused by breaks in the skin around the eye, and subsequent spread to the eyelid; infection of the sinuses around the nose (sinusitis); or from spread of an infection elsewhere through the blood. Periorbital cellulitis must be differentiated from orbital cellulitis, which is an emergency and requires intravenous (IV) antibiotics.
Pathophysiology	Pathophysiology sample values Pathophysiology is the study of the changes of normal mechanical, physical, and biochemical functions, either caused by a disease, or resulting from an abnormal syndrome. More formally, it is the branch of medicine which deals with any disturbances of body functions, caused by disease or prodromal symptoms. An alternative definition is 'the study of the biological and physical manifestations of disease as they correlate with the underlying abnormalities and physiological disturbances.' The study of pathology and the study of pathophysiology often involves substantial overlap in diseases and processes, but pathology emphasizes direct observations, while pathophysiology emphasizes quantifiable measurements.
Cystic fibrosis	Cystic fibrosis is an autosomal recessive genetic disorder affecting most critically the lungs, and also the pancreas, liver, and intestine. It is characterized by abnormal transport of chloride and sodium across an epithelium, leading to thick, viscous secretions. The name cystic fibrosis refers to the characteristic scarring (fibrosis) and cyst formation within the pancreas, first recognized in the 1930s.
Imaging	Imaging is the representation or reproduction of an object's outward form; especially a visual representation (i.e., the formation of an image). · Chemical Imaging, the simultaneous measurement of spectra and pictures

Rheumatic fever	Rheumatic fever is an inflammatory disease that occurs following a Streptococcus pyogenes infection, such as streptococcal pharyngitis or scarlet fever. Believed to be caused by antibody cross-reactivity that can involve the heart, joints, skin, and brain, the illness typically develops two to three weeks after a streptococcal infection. Acute rheumatic fever commonly appears in children between the ages of 6 and 15, with only 20% of first-time attacks occurring in adults.
Fungus	A fungus is a member of a large group of eukaryotic organisms that includes microorganisms such as yeasts and molds, as well as the more familiar mushrooms. These organisms are classified as a kingdom, Fungi, which is separate from plants, animals, and bacteria. One major difference is that fungal cells have cell walls that contain chitin, unlike the cell walls of plants, which contain cellulose.
Cystitis	Cystitis is a term that refers to urinary bladder inflammation that results from any one of a number of distinct syndromes. It is most commonly caused by a bacterial infection in which case it is referred to as a urinary tract infection. •Pressure in the lower pelvis•Painful urination (dysuria)•Frequent urination (polyuria) or urgent need to urinate (urinary urgency)•Need to urinate at night (nocturia)•Urine that contains traces of blood (haematuria)•Dark, cloudy or strong-smelling urine•Pain above the pubic bone, or in the lower back or abdomen•Feeling unwell, weak or feverishSubtypes

There are several medically distinct types of cystitis, each having a unique etiology and therapeutic approach:•Traumatic cystitis is probably the most common form of cystitis in the female, and is due to bruising of the bladder, usually by abnormally forceful sexual intercourse. |
| Pyelonephritis | Pyelonephritis is an ascending urinary tract infection that has reached the pyelum or pelvis of the kidney. It is a form of nephritis that is also referred to as pyelitis. Severe cases of pyelonephritis can lead to pyonephrosis (pus accumulation around the kidney), urosepsis (a systemic inflammatory response of the body to infection), kidney failure and even death. |
| Urethritis | Urethritis is inflammation of the urethra. The most common symptom is painful or difficult urination.

The disease is classified as either gonococcal urethritis, caused by Neisseria gonorrhoeae, or non-gonococcal urethritis most commonly caused by Chlamydia trachomatis. |
| Urinary tract infection | A urinary tract infection is a bacterial infection that affects part of the urinary tract. When it affects the lower urinary tract it is known as a simple cystitis (a bladder infection) and when it affects the upper urinary tract it is known as pyelonephritis (a kidney infection). Symptoms from a lower urinary tract include painful urination and either frequent urination or urge to urinate , while those of pyelonephritis include fever and flank pain in addition to the symptoms of a lower UTI. |

Chapter 11. INFECTIOUS DISEASES

Prevalence	In epidemiology, the prevalence of a health-related state (typically disease, but also other things like smoking or seatbelt use) in a statistical population is defined as the total number of cases of the risk factor in the population at a given time, or the total number of cases in the population, divided by the number of individuals in the population. It is used as an estimate of how common a disease is within a population over a certain period of time. It helps physicians or other health professionals understand the probability of certain diagnoses and is routinely used by epidemiologists, health care providers, government agencies and insurers.
Septic arthritis	Septic arthritis is the purulent invasion of a joint by an infectious agent which produces arthritis. People with artificial joints are more at risk than the general population but have slightly different symptoms, are infected with different organisms and require different treatment. Septic arthritis is considered a medical emergency.
Vesicoureteral reflux	Vesicoureteral reflux is an abnormal movement of urine from the bladder into ureters or kidneys. Urine normally travels from the kidneys via the ureters to the bladder. In vesicoureteral reflux the direction of urine flow is reversed (retrograde).
Renal failure	Renal failure or kidney failure (formerly called renal insufficiency) describes a medical condition in which the kidneys fail to adequately filter toxins and waste products from the blood. The two forms are acute (acute kidney injury) and chronic (chronic kidney disease); a number of other diseases or health problems may cause either form of renal failure to occur. Renal failure is described as a decrease in glomerular filtration rate.
Blood culture	Blood culture is a microbiological culture of blood. It is employed to detect infections that are spreading through the bloodstream (such as bacteremia, septicemia amongst others). This is possible because the bloodstream is usually a sterile environment.
Cellulitis	Cellulitis is a localized or diffuse inflammation of connective tissue with severe inflammation of dermal and subcutaneous layers of the skin. Cellulitis can be caused by normal skin flora or by exogenous bacteria, and often occurs where the skin has previously been broken: cracks in the skin, cuts, blisters, burns, insect bites, surgical wounds, intravenous drug injection or sites of intravenous catheter insertion. Skin on the face or lower legs is most commonly affected by this infection, though cellulitis can occur on any part of the body.
Ecthyma	Ecthyma is an ulcerative pyoderma of the skin caused by bacteria such as Streptococcus pyogenes, Pseudomonas and Staphylococcus aureus. Because ecthyma extends into the dermis, it is often referred to as a deeper form of impetigo. Causes include Insect bites and an ignored minor trauma.

Chapter 11. INFECTIOUS DISEASES

Erysipelas	Erysipelas is an acute streptococcus bacterial infection of the upper dermis and superficial lymphatics. This disease is most common among the elderly, infants, and children. People with immune deficiency, diabetes, alcoholism, skin ulceration, fungal infections and impaired lymphatic drainage (e.g., after mastectomy, pelvic surgery, bypass grafting) are also at increased risk.
Erysipeloid	In humans, Erysipelothrix rhusiopathiae infections most commonly present in a mild cutaneous form known as erysipeloid. E. rhusiopathiae can cause an indolent cellulitis, more commonly in individuals who handle fish and raw meat. It gains entry typically by abrasions in the hand.
Pasteurella multocida	Pasteurella multocida is a Gram-negative, nonmotile, penicillin-sensitive coccobacillus belonging to the Pasteurellaceae family. It can cause avian cholera in birds and a zoonotic infection in humans, which typically is a result of bites or scratches from domestic pets. Many mammals and fowl harbor it as part of their normal respiratory microbiota, displaying asymptomatic colonization.
Staphylococcus aureus	Staphylococcus aureus is a bacterial species named from Greek σταφυλ?κοκκος meaning the 'golden grape-cluster berry'. Also known as 'golden staph' and Oro staphira, it is a facultative anaerobic Gram-positive coccal bacterium. It is frequently found as part of the normal skin flora on the skin and nasal passages.
Necrotizing fasciitis	Necrotizing fasciitis commonly known as flesh-eating disease or Flesh-eating bacteria syndrome, is a rare infection of the deeper layers of skin and subcutaneous tissues, easily spreading across the fascial plane within the subcutaneous tissue. Necrotizing fasciitis is a quickly progressing and severe disease of sudden onset and is usually treated immediately with high doses of intravenous antibiotics. Type I describes a polymicrobial infection, whereas Type II describes a monomicrobial infection.
Mantoux test	The Mantoux test (also known as the Mantoux screening test, tuberculin sensitivity test, Pirquet test, or PPD test for (purified protein derivative) is a diagnostic tool for tuberculosis. It is one of the two major tuberculin skin tests around the world, largely replacing multiple-puncture tests such as the Tine test. Until 2005, the Heaf test was used in the United Kingdom, but the Mantoux test is now used.
Mycobacterium tuberculosis	Mycobacterium tuberculosis is a pathogenic bacterial species in the genus Mycobacterium and the causative agent of most cases of tuberculosis (TB). First discovered in 1882 by Robert Koch, M.

Chapter 11. INFECTIOUS DISEASES

tuberculosis has an unusual, waxy coating on its cell surface (primarily mycolic acid), which makes the cells impervious to Gram staining, so acid-fast detection techniques are used, instead. The physiology of M. tuberculosis is highly aerobic and requires high levels of oxygen.

Tuberculosis	Tuberculosis, MTB or TB (short for tubercles bacillus) is a common and in some cases deadly infectious disease caused by various strains of mycobacteria, usually Mycobacterium tuberculosis in humans. Tuberculosis usually attacks the lungs but can also affect other parts of the body. It is spread through the air when people who have an active MTB infection cough, sneeze, or otherwise transmit their saliva through the air.
Pleural effusion	Pleural effusion is excess fluid that accumulates between the two pleural layers, the fluid-filled space that surrounds the lungs. Excessive amounts of such fluid can impair breathing by limiting the expansion of the lungs during ventilation.
	Pleural fluid is secreted by the parietal layer of the pleura and reabsorbed by the visceral layer of the pleura.
Scrofula	Tuberculous cervical lymphadenitis, also known as scrofula, refers to a lymphadenitis of the cervical lymph nodes associated with tuberculosis.
	Scrofula is the term used for tuberculosis of the neck, or, more precisely, a cervical tuberculous lymphadenopathy. Scrofula is usually a result of an infection in the lymph nodes, known as lymphadenitis and is most often observed in immunocompromised patients (about 50% of cervical tuberculous lymphadenopathy).
Lymphadenopathy	Lymphadenopathy is a term meaning 'disease of the lymph nodes.' It is, however, almost synonymously used with 'swollen/enlarged lymph nodes'. It could be due to infection, auto-immune disease, or malignancy.
	Inflammation of a lymph node is called lymphadenitis.
Nervous system	The nervous system is an organ system containing a network of specialized cells called neurons that coordinate the actions of an animal and transmit signals between different parts of its body. In most animals the nervous system consists of two parts, central and peripheral. The central nervous system of vertebrates (such as humans) contains the brain, spinal cord, and retina.
Tuberculous meningitis	Tuberculous meningitis is also known as TB meningitis or tubercular meningitis.
	Tuberculous meningitis is Mycobacterium tuberculosis infection of the meninges--the system of membranes which envelops the central nervous system.

Human immunodeficiency virus	Human immunodeficiency virus is a lentivirus (a member of the retrovirus family) that can lead to acquired immunodeficiency syndrome (AIDS), a condition in humans in which the immune system begins to fail, leading to life-threatening opportunistic infections. Previous names for the virus include human T-lymphotropic virus-III (HTLV-III), lymphadenopathy-associated virus (LAV), and AIDS-associated retrovirus (ARV.)

Infection with Human immunodeficiency virus occurs by the transfer of blood, semen, vaginal fluid, pre-ejaculate, or breast milk. |
| Subtyping | In programming language theory, subtyping or subtype polymorphism is a form of type polymorphism in which a subtype is a datatype that is related to another datatype (the supertype) by some notion of substitutability, meaning that program constructs, typically subroutines or functions, written to operate on elements of the supertype can also operate on elements of the subtype. If S is a subtype of T, the subtyping relation is often written S <: T, to mean that any term of type S can be safely used in a context where a term of type T is expected. The precise semantics of subtyping crucially depends on the particulars of what 'safely used in a context where' means in a given programming language. |
| Retrovir | Zidovudine or azidothymidine (AZT) (also called ZDV) is a nucleoside analog reverse transcriptase inhibitor (NRTI), a type of antiRetroviral drug. It is an analog of thymidine.

AZT was the first approved treatment for HIV, sold under the names Retrovir and Retrovis. |
| Monitoring | In medicine, monitoring is the evaluation of a disease or condition over time.

It can be performed by continuously measuring certain parameters (for example, by continuously measuring vital signs by a bedside monitor), and/or by repeatedly performing medical tests (such as blood glucose monitoring in people with diabetes mellitus).

Transmitting data from a monitor to a distant monitoring station is known as telemetry or biotelemetry. |
| Herpes simplex virus | Herpes simplex virus 1 and 2 (Herpes simplex virus-1 and Herpes simplex virus-2), also known as Human herpes virus 1 and 2 (HHV-1 and -2), are two members of the herpes virus family, Herpesviridae, that infect humans. Both Herpes simplex virus-1 (which produces cold sores) and Herpes simplex virus-2 (which produces genital herpes) are ubiquitous and contagious. They can be spread when an infected person is producing and shedding the virus. |
| Transmission | A machine consists of a power source and a power transmission system, which provides controlled application of the power. |

	Merriam-Webster defines transmission as: an assembly of parts including the speed-changing gears and the propeller shaft by which the power is transmitted from an engine to a live axle. Often transmission refers simply to the gearbox that uses gears and gear trains to provide speed and torque conversions from a rotating power source to another device.
Herpes labialis	Herpes labialis is an infection of the lip by herpes simplex virus (HSV-1). An outbreak typically causes small blisters or sores on or around the mouth commonly known as cold sores or fever blisters. The sores typically heal within 2-3 weeks, but the herpes virus remains dormant in the facial nerves, following orofacial infection, periodically reactivating (in symptomatic people) to create sores in the same area of the mouth or face at the site of the original infection.
Herpes gladiatorum	Herpes Gladiatorum is one of the most infectious of herpes-caused diseases, and is transmissible by skin-to-skin contact. The disease was first described in the 1960s in the New England Journal of Medicine. It is caused by cutaneous infection with Human Herpes Simplex Virus type 1 (HSV-1), which more commonly causes cold sores.
Herpetic whitlow	A herpetic whitlow is a lesion (whitlow) on a finger or thumb caused by the herpes simplex virus. It is a painful infection that typically affects the fingers or thumbs. Occasionally infection occurs on the toes or on the nail cuticle.
Substance abuse	Substance abuse, refers to a maladaptive patterned use of a substance (drug) in which the user consumes the substance in amounts or with methods not condoned by medical professionals. Substance abuse/drug abuse is not limited to mood-altering or psycho-active drugs. Activity is also considered substance abuse when inappropriately used (as in steroids for performance enhancement in sports).
Skin infection	A skin infection is an infection of the skin. Infection of the skin is distinguished from dermatitis, which is inflammation of the skin, but a skin infection can result in skin inflammation. Skin inflammation due to skin infection is called infective dermatitis.
Common variable immunodeficiency	Common variable immunodeficiency (also known as Acquired hypogammaglobulinemia) is a group of approximately 150 primary immunodeficiencies (PIDs), which have a common set of features (including hypogammaglobulinemia) but which have different underlying causes. Common variable immunodeficiency is the most commonly encountered primary immunodeficiency. Causes and types CVID is shown to be a genetically determined primary immune defect; however, the underlying causes are different.

X-linked hypogammaglobuline mia	X-linked agammaglobulinemia (also called X-linked hypogammaglobulinemia, XLA, Bruton type agammaglobulinemia, Bruton syndrome, or Sex-linked agammaglobulinemia) is a rare X-linked genetic disorder discovered in 1952 that affects the body's ability to fight infection. XLA is an X-linked disorder, and therefore is more common in males. XLA patients do not generate mature B cells, which manifests as a complete lack of antibodies in their bloodstream.
Primary	The Primary (formerly the Primary Association) is a children's organization and an official auxiliary within The Church of Jesus Christ of Latter-day Saints (LDS Church). It acts as a Sunday school organization for the church's children under the age of 12. The official purpose of Primary is to help parents in teaching their children to learn and live the gospel of Jesus Christ.
Primary immunodeficiency	Primary immunodeficiencies are disorders in which part of the body's immune system is missing or does not function properly. To be considered a primary immunodeficiency, the cause of the immune deficiency must not be secondary in nature (i.e., caused by other disease, drug treatment, or environmental exposure to toxins). Most primary immunodeficiencies are genetic disorders; the majority are diagnosed in children under the age of one, although milder forms may not be recognized until adulthood.
Bone marrow	Bone marrow is the flexible tissue found in the interior of bones. In humans, red blood cells are produced in the heads of long bones, in a process known as hematopoesis. On average, bone marrow constitutes 4% of the total body mass of humans; in an adult weighing 65 kilograms (140 lb), bone marrow accounts for approximately 2.6 kilograms (5.7 lb).
22q11.2 deletion syndrome	22q11.2 deletion syndrome, also known as DiGeorge syndrome, DiGeorge anomaly, velo-cardio-facial syndrome, Shprintzen syndrome, conotruncal anomaly face syndrome, Strong syndrome, congenital thymic aplasia, and thymic hypoplasia is a syndrome caused by the deletion of a small piece of chromosome 22. The deletion occurs near the middle of the chromosome at a location designated q11.2 i.e., on the long arm of one of the pair of chromosomes 22. It has a prevalence estimated at 1:4000. The syndrome was described in 1968 by the pediatric endocrinologist Angelo DiGeorge. The features of this syndrome vary widely, even among members of the same family, and affect many parts of the body. Characteristic signs and symptoms may include birth defects such as congenital heart disease, defects in the palate, most commonly related to neuromuscular problems with closure (velo-pharyngeal insufficiency), learning disabilities, mild differences in facial features, and recurrent infections.
Howell-Jolly bodies	Howell-Jolly bodies are histopathological findings of basophilic nuclear remnants (clusters of DNA) in circulating erythrocytes.

During maturation in the bone marrow erythrocytes normally expel their nuclei, but in some cases a small portion of DNA remains.

It is named for William Henry Howell and Justin Marie Jolly.

Aplastic anemia	Aplastic anemia is a condition where bone marrow does not produce sufficient new cells to replenish blood cells. The condition, as the name indicates, involves both aplasia and anemia. Typically, anemia refers to low red blood cell counts, but aplastic anemia patients have lower counts of all three blood cell types: red blood cells, white blood cells, and platelets, termed pancytopenia.
Osteomyelitis	Osteomyelitis simply means an infection of the bone or bone marrow. It can be usefully subclassified on the basis of the causative organism (pyogenic bacteria or mycobacteria), the route, duration and anatomic location of the infection. In general, microorganisms may infect bone through one or more of three basic methods: via the bloodstream, contiguously from local areas of infection (as in cellulitis), or penetrating trauma, including iatrogenic causes such as joint replacements or internal fixation of fractures or root-canaled teeth.
Bone scan	A Bone scan are triggering the bone's attempts to heal. It is primarily used to help diagnose a number of conditions relating to bones, including: cancer of the bone or cancers that have spread (metastasized) to the bone, locating some sources of bone inflammation (e.g. bone pain such as lower back pain due to a fracture), the diagnosis of fractures that may not be visible in traditional X-ray images, and the detection of damage to bones due to certain infections and other problems. Nuclear medicine bone scans are one of a number of methods of bone imaging, all of which are used to visually detect bone abnormalities.
Osteoarthritis	Osteoarthritis also known as degenerative arthritis or degenerative joint disease or osteoarthrosis, is a group of mechanical abnormalities involving degradation of joints, including articular cartilage and subchondral bone. Symptoms may include joint pain, tenderness, stiffness, locking, and sometimes an effusion. A variety of causes--hereditary, developmental, metabolic, and mechanical--may initiate processes leading to loss of cartilage.
Vertebral osteomyelitis	The term osteomyelitis describes any new infection in the bone and bone marrow. Vertebral osteomyelitis is a specific type of this disease; the term describes a rare bone infection concentrated in the spinal region. Cases of vertebral osteomyelitis are so rare that only 2-4% of all bone infections are attributed to the disease.

Pelvic	In human anatomy, the pelvis is the part of the trunk inferioposterior to the abdomen in the transition area between the trunk and the lower limbs. The term is used to denote several structures: · the Pelvic girdle or bony pelvis, the irregular ring-shaped bony structure connecting the spine to the femurs, · the Pelvic cavity, the space enclosed by the Pelvic girdle, subdivided into · the greater or false pelvis (inferior part of the abdominal cavity) and · the lesser or true pelvis which provides the skeletal framework for the perineum and the Pelvic cavity (which are separated by the Pelvic diaphragm), · the Pelvic region. 'Pelvis' is the Latin word for a 'basin' and the pelvis thus got its name from its shape. It is also known as hip girdle or coxa girdle.
Sneakers	Sneakers are footwear of flexible material, typically featuring a sole made of rubber. The upper part is made of leather or canvas. Sneakers were originally sporting apparel, but are today worn much more widely as casual footwear.
Vertebral	A vertebra (plural: vertebrae) is an individual bone in the flexible column that defines vertebrate animals, via humans. The vertebral column encases and protects the spinal cord, which runs from the base of the cranium down the dorsal side of the animal until reaching the pelvis. From there, vertebra continue into the tail.
Croup	Croup is a respiratory condition that is usually triggered by an acute viral infection of the upper airway. The infection leads to swelling inside the throat, which interferes with normal breathing and produces the classical symptoms of a 'barking' cough, stridor, and hoarseness. It may produce mild, moderate, or severe symptoms, which often worsen at night.
Thumbprint sign	In radiology, the thumbprint sign, is a radiologic sign found on a lateral C-spine radiograph that suggests the diagnosis of epiglottitis. The sign is caused by a thickened free edge of the epiglottis, which causes it to appear more radiopaque than normal, resembling the distal thumb. In an abdominal X-ray, thumbprinting has the similar appearance of thumbs protruding into the intestinal lumen, but are caused by thickened edematous mucosal folds.
Epiglottitis	Epiglottitis is an inflammation of the epiglottis -- the flap at the base of the tongue that keeps food from going into the trachea (windpipe). Due to its place in the airway, swelling of this structure can interfere with breathing, and constitutes a medical emergency. Infection can cause the epiglottis to obstruct or completely close off the windpipe.

Chapter 11. INFECTIOUS DISEASES

Entry inhibitor	Entry inhibitors, also known as fusion inhibitors, are a class of antiretroviral drugs, used in combination therapy for the treatment of HIV infection. This class of drugs interferes with the binding, fusion and entry of an HIV virion to a human cell. By blocking this step in HIV's replication cycle, such agents slow the progression from HIV infection to AIDS.
Mechanical ventilation	In medicine, mechanical ventilation is a method to mechanically assist or replace spontaneous breathing. This may involve a machine called a ventilator or the breathing may be assisted by a physician, respiratory therapist or other suitable person compressing a bag or set of bellows. Traditionally divided into negative-pressure ventilation, where air is essentially sucked into the lungs, or positive pressure ventilation, where air is pushed into the trachea.
Retropharyngeal abscess	Most commonly seen in infants and young children, retropharyngeal abscess is an abscess located in the tissues in the back of the throat behind the posterior pharyngeal wall (the retropharyngeal space). Because RPA's typically occur in deep tissue, they are difficult to diagnose by physical examination alone. RPA is a relatively uncommon illness, and therefore may not receive early diagnosis in children presenting with stiff neck, malaise, difficulty swallowing, or other symptoms listed below.
Chlamydia trachomatis	Chlamydia trachomatis, an obligate intracellular human pathogen, is one of three bacterial species in the genus Chlamydia. C. trachomatis is a Gram-negative bacteria, therefore its cell wall components retain the counter-stain safranin and appear pink under a light microscope. The inclusion bodies of Chlamydia trachomatis were first described in 1907, the Chlamydia trachomatis agent was first cultured in the yolk sacs of eggs by Feifan Tang et al in 1957.
Neisseria gonorrhoeae	Neisseria gonorrhoeae, or gonococcus, is a species of Gram-negative coffee bean-shaped diplococci bacteria responsible for the sexually transmitted infection gonorrhea. N. gonorrhoea was first described by Albert Neisser in 1879. Microbiology Neisseria are fastidious Gram-negative cocci that require nutrient supplementation to grow in laboratory cultures.
Abdominal pain	Abdominal pain can be one of the symptoms associated with transient disorders or serious disease. Making a definitive diagnosis of the cause of abdominal pain can be difficult, because many diseases can result in this symptom. Abdominal pain is a common problem.
Gastroesophageal reflux	Gastroesophageal reflux disease (GERD), gastro-oesophageal reflux disease (GORD), gastric reflux disease, or acid reflux disease is defined as chronic symptoms or mucosal damage produced by the abnormal reflux in the oesophagus.

	This is commonly due to transient or permanent changes in the barrier between the oesophagus and the stomach. This can be due to incompetence of the lower esophageal sphincter, transient lower oesophageal sphincter relaxation, impaired expulsion of gastric reflux from the oesophagus, or a hiatal hernia.
Pelvic inflammatory disease	Pelvic inflammatory disease (PID) is a term for inflammation of the uterus, fallopian tubes, and/or ovaries as it progresses to scar formation with adhesions to nearby tissues and organs. This can lead to infertility. PID is a vague term and can refer to viral, fungal, parasitic, though most often bacterial infections.
Fitz-Hugh-Curtis syndrome	Fitz-Hugh-Curtis syndrome is a rare complication of pelvic inflammatory disease (PID) named after the two physicians, Fitz-Hugh and Curtis who first reported this condition in 1934 and 1930 respectively. Fitz-Hugh-Curtis syndrome occurs almost exclusively in women. It is usually caused by gonorrhoea (acute gonococcal perihepatitis) or chlamydia bacteria, which cause a thinning of cervical mucous and allow bacteria from the vagina into the uterus and oviducts, causing infection and inflammation.
Perihepatitis	Perihepatitis is inflammation of the serous or peritoneal coating of the liver. Perihepatitis is often caused by one of the inflammatory disorders of the female upper genital tract, known collectively as Pelvic inflammatory disease. Some patients have sharp right upper abdominal quadrant pain.
Neisseria meningitidis	Neisseria meningitidis, often referred to as meningococcus, is a bacterium that can cause meningitis and other forms of meningococcal disease such as meningococcemia, a life threatening sepsis. N. meningitidis is a major cause of morbidity and mortality during childhood in industrialized countries and has been responsible for epidemics in Africa and in Asia. Upon Gram staining, it appears as a Gram-negative diplococcus and cultures of the bacteria test positive for the enzyme oxidase.
Purpura fulminans	Purpura fulminans is a haemorrhagic condition usually associated with sepsis or previous infection. It occurs mainly in babies and small children. It was first described by Guelliot in 1884.
Immunization	Immunization, is the process by which an individual's immune system becomes fortified against an agent (known as the immunogen).

Chapter 11. INFECTIOUS DISEASES

When this system is exposed to molecules that are foreign to the body, called non-self, it will orchestrate an immune response, and it will also develop the ability to quickly respond to a subsequent encounter because of immunological memory. This is a function of the adaptive immune system.

Meningococcal vaccine	Meningococcal vaccine is a vaccine used against Meningococcus, a bacterium that causes meningitis, meningococcemia, septicemia, and rarely carditis, septic arthritis, or pneumonia.
	Neisseria meningitidis has 13 clinically significant serogroups. These are classified according to the antigenic structure of their polysaccharide capsule.
Ehlers-Danlos syndrome	Ehlers-Danlos syndrome is a group of inherited connective tissue disorders, caused by a defect in the synthesis of collagen. The collagen in connective tissue helps tissues to resist deformation. In the skin, muscles, ligaments, blood vessels, and visceral organs collagen plays a very significant role and with reduced elasticity, secondary to abnormal collagen, pathology results.
Tick-borne disease	Tick-borne diseases are diseases or illnesses transmitted by ticks. As the incidence of tick-borne illnesses increases and the geographic areas in which they are found expand, it becomes increasingly important that health professionals be able to distinguish the diverse, and often overlapping, clinical presentations of these diseases.
	Tick-borne illnesses are caused by infection with a variety of pathogens, including rickettsia and other types of bacteria, viruses, and protozoa.
Babesiosis	Babesiosis is a malaria-like parasitic disease caused by infection with Babesia, a genus of protozoal piroplasms. After trypanosomes, Babesia are thought to be the second most common blood parasites of mammals and they can have a major impact on health of domestic animals in areas without severe winters. Human babesiosis is uncommon, but reported cases have risen recently because of expanded medical awareness.
Ehrlichiosis	Ehrlichiosis (; also known as canine rickettsiosis, canine hemorrhagic fever, canine typhus, tracker dog disease, and tropical canine pancytopenia) is a tick-borne disease of dogs usually caused by the organism Ehrlichia canis. Ehrlichia canis is the pathogen of animals. Humans can become infected by E. canis and other species after tick exposure.
Borrelia burgdorferi	Borrelia burgdorferi is a species of Gram negative bacteria of the spirochete class of the genus Borrelia. B. burgdorferi is predominant in North America, but also exists in Europe, and is the agent of Lyme disease.

Lyme disease is a zoonotic, vector-borne disease transmitted by ticks; the causative agent is named after the researcher Willy Burgdorfer, who first isolated the bacterium in 1982. B. burgdorferi is one of the few pathogenic bacteria that can survive without iron, having replaced all of its iron-sulfur cluster enzymes with enzymes that use manganese, thus avoiding the problem many pathogenic bacteria face in acquiring iron.

Erythema migrans

Erythema chronicum migrans refers to the rash often (though not always) seen in the early stage of Lyme disease. It can appear anywhere from one day to one month after a tick bite. This rash does not represent an allergic reaction to the bite, but rather an actual skin infection with the Lyme bacteria, Borrelia burgdorferi sensu lato. 'Erythema migrans is the only manifestation of Lyme disease in the United States that is sufficiently distinctive to allow clinical diagnosis in the absence of laboratory confirmation.'.

Rickettsia rickettsii

Rickettsia rickettsii is a unicellular, gram-negative coccobacillus that is native to the New World. It belongs to the spotted fever group (SFG) of Rickettsia and is most commonly known as the causative agent of Rocky Mountain spotted fever (RMSF). By nature, R. rickettsii is an obligate intracellular parasite that survive by an endosymbiotic relationship with other cells.

Rocky Mountains

The Rocky Mountains are a major mountain range in western North America. The North American Rocky Mountains stretch more than 4,800 kilometres (2,980 mi) from the northernmost part of British Columbia, in western Canada, to New Mexico, in the southwestern United States. The range's highest peak is Mount Elbert located in Colorado at 14,440 feet (4,401 m) above sea level. Though part of North America's Pacific Cordillera, the Rockies are distinct from the Pacific Coast Ranges or the Pacific Mountain System (as it is known in the United States), which are located directly adjacent to the Pacific coast.

Rocky Mountain spotted fever

Rocky Mountain spotted fever is the most lethal and most frequently reported rickettsial illness in the United States. It has been diagnosed throughout the Americas. Some synonyms for Rocky Mountain spotted fever in other countries include 'tick typhus,' 'Tobia fever' (Colombia), 'São Paulo fever' or 'febre maculosa' (Brazil), and 'fiebre manchada' (Mexico).

Staphylococcal scalded skin syndrome

Staphylococcal scalded skin syndrome, SSSS, also known as Pemphigus neonatorum or Ritter's disease, or Localized bullous impetigo is a dermatological condition caused by Staphylococcus aureus.

The syndrome is induced by epidermolytic exotoxins (exfoliatin) A and B, which are released by S. aureus and cause detachment within the epidermal layer. One of the exotoxins is produced by the bacterial chromosome, while the other is produced by a plasmid.

Chapter 11. INFECTIOUS DISEASES

Toxic shock syndrome	Toxic shock syndrome is a potentially fatal illness caused by a bacterial toxin. Different bacterial toxins may cause toxic shock syndrome, depending on the situation. The causative bacteria include Staphylococcus aureus and Streptococcus pyogenes.
Streptococcal toxic shock syndrome	Toxic shock syndrome (TSS) is a potentially fatal illness caused by a bacterial toxin. Different bacterial toxins may cause toxic shock syndrome, depending on the situation. The causative bacteria include Staphylococcus aureus and Streptococcus pyogenes. Streptococcal TSS is sometimes referred to as toxic shock-like syndrome (TSLS) or streptococcal toxic shock syndrome.
Genetics	Genetics, a discipline of biology, is the science of genes, heredity, and variation in living organisms.
	Genetics deals with the molecular structure and function of genes, gene behavior in context of a cell or organism (e.g. dominance and epigenetics), patterns of inheritance from parent to offspring, and gene distribution, variation and change in populations,such as through Genome-Wide Association Studies. Given that genes are universal to living organisms, genetics can be applied to the study of all living systems, from viruses and bacteria, through plants and domestic animals, to humans (as in medical genetics).
Coccidioides immitis	Coccidioides immitis is a pathogenic fungus that resides in the soil in certain parts of the southwestern United States, northern Mexico, and a few other areas in the Western Hemisphere.
	It, along with its relative Coccidioides posadasii, can cause a disease called coccidioidomycosis (Valley Fever), and it is a rare cause of meningitis, mostly in immunocompromised persons. It has been declared a select agent by both the U.S. Department of Health and Human Services and the U.S. Department of Agriculture, and is considered a biosafety level 3 pathogen.
Isovaleric acidemia	Isovaleric acidemia, is a rare autosomal recessive metabolic disorder which disrupts or prevents normal metabolism of the branched-chain amino acid leucine. It is a classical type of organic acidemia.
	A characteristic feature of isovaleric acidemia is a distinctive odor of sweaty feet.
Endocarditis	Endocarditis is an inflammation of the inner layer of the heart, the endocardium. It usually involves the heart valves (native or prosthetic valves). Other structures that may be involved include the interventricular septum, the chordae tendineae, the mural endocardium, or even on intracardiac devices.

Histoplasmosis	Histoplasmosis is a disease caused by the fungus Histoplasma capsulatum. Symptoms of this infection vary greatly, but the disease primarily affects the lungs. Occasionally, other organs are affected; this is called disseminated histoplasmosis, and it can be fatal if left untreated.
Aspergillus	Aspergillus is a genus consisting of several hundred mold species found in various climates worldwide. Aspergillus was first catalogued in 1729 by the Italian priest and biologist Pier Antonio Micheli. Viewing the fungi under a microscope, Micheli was reminded of the shape of an aspergillum (holy water sprinkler), and named the genus accordingly.
Central venous catheter	In medicine, a central venous catheter is a catheter placed into a large vein in the neck (internal jugular vein), chest (subclavian vein or axillary vein) or groin (femoral vein). It is used to administer medication or fluids, obtain blood tests (specifically the 'mixed venous oxygen saturation'), and directly obtain cardiovascular measurements such as the central venous pressure. There are several types of central venous catheters:Non-tunneled vs. tunneled catheters Non-tunneled catheters are fixed in place at the site of insertion, with the catheter and attachments protruding directly.
Trade name	Meaning 1 A trade name, is the name which a business trades under for commercial purposes, although its registered, legal name, used for contracts and other formal situations, may be another. As an example, the company Panda Chemical Manufacturers, Inc. may use the more friendly name Panda Pharmaceuticals when it holds itself out to the public.
Urine	Urine is a typically sterile liquid by-product of the body secreted by the kidneys through a process called urination and excreted through the urethra. Cellular metabolism generates numerous by-products, many rich in nitrogen, that require elimination from the bloodstream. These by-products are eventually expelled from the body in a process known as micturition, the primary method for excreting water-soluble chemicals from the body.
Amphetamine	Amphetamine or amfetamine (INN) is a psychostimulant drug of the phenethylamine class that produces increased wakefulness and focus in association with decreased fatigue and appetite. Brand names of medications that contain, or metabolize into, amphetamine include Adderall, Dexedrine, Dextrostat, Desoxyn, Didrex, ProCentra, and Vyvanse, as well as Benzedrine in the past.

Chapter 11. INFECTIOUS DISEASES

Formulation	Formulation is a term used in various senses in various applications, both the material and the abstract or formal. Its fundamental meaning is the putting together of components in appropriate relationships or structures, according to a formula. It might help to reflect that etymologically Formula is the diminutive of the Latin Forma, meaning shape.
Cartilage-hair hypoplasia	Cartilage-hair hypoplasia (Cartilage-hair hypoplasiaH), also known as McKusick type metaphyseal chondrodysplasia,[578] is a rare form of short-limbed dwarfism due to skeletal dysplasia. It was first reported in 1965 by McKusick et al. Cartilage-hair hypoplasiaH is an autosomal recessive inherited disorder.
Adverse effect	In medicine, an adverse effect is a harmful and undesired effect resulting from a medication or other intervention such as surgery. An adverse effect may be termed a 'side effect', when judged to be secondary to a main or therapeutic effect. If it results from an unsuitable or incorrect dosage or procedure, this is called a medical error and not a complication.
Resistance	'Resistance' as initially used by Sigmund Freud, referred to patients blocking memories from conscious memory. This was a key concept, since the primary treatment method of Freud's talk therapy required making these memories available to the patient's consciousness. 'Resistance' expanded Later, Freud described five different forms of resistance.
Cerebrospinal fluid	Cerebrospinal fluid Liquor cerebrospinalis, is a clear, colorless, bodily fluid, that occupies the subarachnoid space and the ventricular system around and inside the brain and spinal cord. The CSF occupies the space between the arachnoid mater (the middle layer of the brain cover, meninges) and the pia mater (the layer of the meninges closest to the brain). It constitutes the content of all intra-cerebral (inside the brain, cerebrum) ventricles, cisterns, and sulci, as well as the central canal of the spinal cord.
Polymyxin B	Polymyxin B is an antibiotic primarily used for resistant Gram-negative infections. It is derived from the bacterium Bacillus polymyxa. Polymyxin B is a mixture of two closely related compounds, polymyxin B1 and polymyxin B2. It has a bactericidal action against almost all Gram-negative bacilli except the Proteus group.
Influenza	Influenza, commonly referred to as the flu, is an infectious disease caused by RNA viruses of the family Orthomyxoviridae (the influenza viruses), that affects birds and mammals.

The most common symptoms of the disease are chills, fever, sore throat, muscle pains, severe headache, coughing, weakness/fatigue and general discomfort. Although it is often confused with other influenza-like illnesses, especially the common cold, influenza is a more severe disease than the common cold and is caused by a different type of virus.

Avian influenza	Avian influenza -- known informally as avian flu or bird flu -- refers to 'influenza caused by viruses adapted to birds.' Of the greatest concern is highly pathogenic avian influenza. 'Bird flu' is a phrase similar to 'swine flu,' 'dog flu,' 'horse flu,' or 'human flu' in that it refers to an illness caused by any of many different strains of influenza viruses that have adapted to a specific host. All known viruses that cause influenza in birds belong to the species influenza A virus.
Influenza pandemic	An influenza pandemic is an epidemic of an influenza virus that spreads on a worldwide scale and infects a large proportion of the human population. In contrast to the regular seasonal epidemics of influenza, these pandemics occur irregularly, with the 1918 Spanish flu the most serious pandemic in recent history. Pandemics can cause high levels of mortality, with the Spanish influenza estimated as being responsible for the deaths of over 50 million people.
Influenza prevention	Influenza prevention involves taking steps that one can use to decrease their chances of contracting flu viruses, such as the Pandemic H1N1/09 virus, responsible for the 2009 flu pandemic. People who contract influenza are most infective between the second and third days after infection, and infectivity lasts for around ten days. Children are much more infectious than adults and shed virus from just before they develop symptoms until two weeks after infection.
Pandemic	A pandemic is an epidemic of infectious disease that has spread through human populations across a large region; for instance multiple continents, or even worldwide. A widespread endemic disease that is stable in terms of how many people are getting sick from it is not a pandemic. Further, flu pandemics generally exclude recurrences of seasonal flu.
Infection control	Infection control is the discipline concerned with preventing nosocomial or healthcare-associated infection, a practical (rather than academic) sub-discipline of epidemiology. It is an essential, though often under-recognized and under-supported, part of the infrastructure of health care. Infection control and hospital epidemiology are akin to public health practice, practiced within the confines of a particular health-care delivery system rather than directed at society as a whole.

Chapter 11. INFECTIOUS DISEASES

Personal protective equipment	Personal protective equipment refers to protective clothing, helmets, goggles, or other garment or equipment designed to protect the wearer's body from injury by blunt impacts, electrical hazards, heat, chemicals, and infection, for job-related occupational safety and health purposes, and in sports, martial arts, combat, etc. Personal armor is combat-specialized protective gear. In British legislation the term PPE does not cover items such as armour.
Transmission-based precautions	'Transmission-Based Precautions', also known as additional infection control precautions in health care, are the latest routine infection prevention and control practices applied for patients who are known or suspected to be infected or colonized with infectious agents, including certain epidemiologically important pathogens. The latter require additional control measures to effectively prevent transmission. Transmission-Based Precautions in history of guidelines for isolation precautions in hospitals Rationale behind Transmission-Based Precautions in healthcare setting

Communicable diseases occur as a result of the interaction between:•a source of infectious agents,•a mode of transmission for the agent,•a susceptible host with a portal of entry receptive to the agent,•the environment.

The control of communicable diseases may involve changing one or more of these components, the first three of which are influenced by the environment. |
Protective equipment	Personal protective equipment refers to protective clothing, helmets, goggles, or other garment designed to protect the wearer's body from injury by blunt impacts, electrical hazards, heat, chemicals, and infection, for job-related occupational safety and health purposes, and in sports, martial arts, combat, etc. Personal armor is combat-specialized protective gear. In British legislation the term PPE does not cover items such as armour.
Terminal sedation	In medicine, specifically in end-of-life care, terminal sedation is the palliative practice of relieving distress in a terminally ill person in the last hours or days of a dying patient's life, usually by means of a continuous intravenous or subcutaneous infusion of a sedative drug. This is a option of last resort for patients whose symptoms cannot be controlled by any other means. This should be differentiated from euthanasia as the goal of palliative sedation is to control symptoms through sedation but not shorten the patient's life, while in euthanasia the goal is to shorten life to relieve symptoms.
Nosocomial infection	A nosocomial infection also known as a hospital-acquired infection or HAI, is an infection whose development is favoured by a hospital environment, such as one acquired by a patient during a hospital visit or one developing among hospital staff. Such infections include fungal and bacterial infections and are aggravated by the reduced resistance of individual patients.

Infectious disease	Infectious diseases, also known as transmissible diseases or communicable diseases comprise clinically evident illness (i.e., characteristic medical signs and/or symptoms of disease) resulting from the infection, presence and growth of pathogenic biological agents in an individual host organism. In certain cases, infectious diseases may be asymptomatic for much or even all of their course in a given host. In the latter case, the disease may only be defined as a 'disease' (which by definition means an illness) in hosts who secondarily become ill after contact with an asymptomatic carrier.

CHAPTER QUIZ: KEY TERMS, PEOPLE, PLACES, CONCEPTS

1. _____ is a lentivirus (a member of the retrovirus family) that can lead to acquired immunodeficiency syndrome (AIDS), a condition in humans in which the immune system begins to fail, leading to life-threatening opportunistic infections. Previous names for the virus include human T-lymphotropic virus-III (HTLV-III), lymphadenopathy-associated virus (LAV), and AIDS-associated retrovirus (ARV.)

   Infection with _____ occurs by the transfer of blood, semen, vaginal fluid, pre-ejaculate, or breast milk.

   a. Blown pupil
   b. Nervous tissue
   c. Human immunodeficiency virus
   d. Neuroanatomy

2. _____ is a pathogenic bacterial species in the genus Mycobacterium and the causative agent of most cases of tuberculosis (TB). First discovered in 1882 by Robert Koch, M. tuberculosis has an unusual, waxy coating on its cell surface (primarily mycolic acid), which makes the cells impervious to Gram staining, so acid-fast detection techniques are used, instead. The physiology of M. tuberculosis is highly aerobic and requires high levels of oxygen.

   a. Accessory breasts
   b. Skin window technique
   c. Mycobacterium tuberculosis
   d. Tattoo removal

3. . _____ is an inflammatory disease that occurs following a Streptococcus pyogenes infection, such as streptococcal pharyngitis or scarlet fever. Believed to be caused by antibody cross-reactivity that can involve the heart, joints, skin, and brain, the illness typically develops two to three weeks after a streptococcal infection. Acute _____ commonly appears in children between the ages of 6 and 15, with only 20% of first-time attacks occurring in adults.

   a. Rheumatic fever
   b. Ophthalmoscopy
   c. Insurance policy

Chapter 11. INFECTIOUS DISEASES

4. A _____ is a lesion (whitlow) on a finger or thumb caused by the herpes simplex virus. It is a painful infection that typically affects the fingers or thumbs. Occasionally infection occurs on the toes or on the nail cuticle.

    a. Herpetic whitlow
    b. HSUR
    c. Human herpesvirus 6
    d. Human herpesvirus 7

5. _____ are histopathological findings of basophilic nuclear remnants (clusters of DNA) in circulating erythrocytes. During maturation in the bone marrow erythrocytes normally expel their nuclei, but in some cases a small portion of DNA remains.

It is named for William Henry Howell and Justin Marie Jolly.

    a. Lardacein
    b. Mallory body
    c. Howell-Jolly bodies
    d. Psammoma body

ANSWER KEY
Chapter 11. INFECTIOUS DISEASES

1. c
2. c
3. a
4. a
5. c

You can take the complete Chapter Practice Test

for Chapter 11. INFECTIOUS DISEASES
on all key terms, persons, places, and concepts.

Online 99 Cents

http://www.epub219.49.13357.11.cram101.com/

Use www.Cram101.com for all your study needs

including Cram101's online interactive problem solving labs in

chemistry, statistics, mathematics, and more.

Chapter 12. ENDOCRINE

CHAPTER OUTLINE: KEY TERMS, PEOPLE, PLACES, CONCEPTS

Diabetes mellitus

Etiological myth

Insulin resistance

Glucose transporter

Hypoglycemia

Diabetic ketoacidosis

Pathogenesis

Monitoring

Venous thrombosis

Intracranial pressure

Chapter 12. ENDOCRINE

Diabetes mellitus	Diabetes mellitus, often simply referred to as diabetes, is a group of metabolic diseases in which a person has high blood sugar, either because the body does not produce enough insulin, or because cells do not respond to the insulin that is produced. This high blood sugar produces the classical symptoms of polyuria (frequent urination), polydipsia (increased thirst) and polyphagia (increased hunger).
	The three main types of diabetes mellitus are:•Type 1 DM results from the body's failure to produce insulin, and presently requires the person to inject insulin.
Etiological myth	Etiology is the study of causation, or origination.
	The word is most commonly used in medical and philosophical theories, where it is used to refer to the study of why things occur, or even the reasons behind the way that things act, and is used in philosophy, physics, psychology, government, medicine, theology and biology in reference to the causes of various phenomena. An etiological myth is a myth intended to explain a name or create a mythic history for a place or family.
Insulin resistance	Insulin resistance is the condition in which normal amounts of insulin are inadequate to produce a normal insulin response from fat, muscle and liver cells. Insulin resistance in fat cells reduces the effects of insulin and results in elevated hydrolysis of stored triglycerides in the absence of measures which either increase insulin sensitivity or which provide additional insulin. Increased mobilization of stored lipids in these cells elevates free fatty acids in the blood plasma.
Glucose transporter	Glucose transporters (GLUT or SLC2A family) are a family of membrane proteins found in most mammalian cells.
	Structure
	Glucose transporters are integral membrane proteins that contain 12 membrane-spanning helices with both the amino and carboxyl termini exposed on the cytoplasmic side of the plasma membrane. Glucose transporter proteins transport glucose and related hexoses according to a model of alternate conformation, which predicts that the transporter exposes a single substrate binding site toward either the outside or the inside of the cell.
Hypoglycemia	Hypoglycemia, hypoglycæmia or low blood sugar (not to be confused with hyperglycemia) is an abnormally diminished content of glucose in the blood. The term literally means 'low sugar blood' . It can produce a variety of symptoms and effects but the principal problems arise from an inadequate supply of glucose to the brain, resulting in impairment of function (neuroglycopenia).

Diabetic ketoacidosis	Diabetic ketoacidosis is a potentially life-threatening complication in patients with diabetes mellitus. It happens predominantly in those with type 1 diabetes, but it can occur in those with type 2 diabetes under certain circumstances. DKA results from a shortage of insulin; in response the body switches to burning fatty acids and producing acidic ketone bodies that cause most of the symptoms and complications.
Pathogenesis	The pathogenesis of a disease is the mechanism by which the disease is caused. The term can also be used to describe the origin and development of the disease and whether it is acute, chronic or recurrent. The word comes from the Greek pathos, 'disease', and genesis, 'creation'.
Monitoring	In medicine, monitoring is the evaluation of a disease or condition over time. It can be performed by continuously measuring certain parameters (for example, by continuously measuring vital signs by a bedside monitor), and/or by repeatedly performing medical tests (such as blood glucose monitoring in people with diabetes mellitus). Transmitting data from a monitor to a distant monitoring station is known as telemetry or biotelemetry.
Venous thrombosis	A venous thrombosis is a blood clot (thrombus) that forms within a vein. Thrombosis is a medical term for a blood clot occurring inside a blood vessel. A classical venous thrombosis is deep vein thrombosis (DVT), which can break off (embolize), and become a life-threatening pulmonary embolism (PE).
Intracranial pressure	Intracranial pressure is the pressure inside the skull and thus in the brain tissue and cerebrospinal fluid (CSF). The body has various mechanisms by which it keeps the ICP stable, with CSF pressures varying by about 1 mmHg in normal adults through shifts in production and absorption of CSF. CSF pressure has been shown to be influenced by abrupt changes in intrathoracic pressure during coughing (intraabdominal pressure), valsalva (Queckenstedt's maneuver), and communication with the vasculature (venous and arterial systems). ICP is measured in millimeters of mercury (mmHg) and, at rest, is normally 7-15 mmHg for a supine adult, and becomes negative (averaging −10 mmHg) in the vertical position.

Chapter 12. ENDOCRINE

1. _____ is the condition in which normal amounts of insulin are inadequate to produce a normal insulin response from fat, muscle and liver cells. _____ in fat cells reduces the effects of insulin and results in elevated hydrolysis of stored triglycerides in the absence of measures which either increase insulin sensitivity or which provide additional insulin. Increased mobilization of stored lipids in these cells elevates free fatty acids in the blood plasma.

   a. Oral glucose gel
   b. United Kingdom Prospective Diabetes Study
   c. Insulin resistance
   d. Accu-chek

2. Etiology is the study of causation, or origination.

   The word is most commonly used in medical and philosophical theories, where it is used to refer to the study of why things occur, or even the reasons behind the way that things act, and is used in philosophy, physics, psychology, government, medicine, theology and biology in reference to the causes of various phenomena. An _____ is a myth intended to explain a name or create a mythic history for a place or family.

   a. Etiology
   b. abdominal exam
   c. Acquired vision
   d. Etiological myth

3. _____, often simply referred to as diabetes, is a group of metabolic diseases in which a person has high blood sugar, either because the body does not produce enough insulin, or because cells do not respond to the insulin that is produced. This high blood sugar produces the classical symptoms of polyuria (frequent urination), polydipsia (increased thirst) and polyphagia (increased hunger).

   The three main types of _____ are:•Type 1 DM results from the body's failure to produce insulin, and presently requires the person to inject insulin.

   a. Dietary Reference Values
   b. Diabetes mellitus
   c. Health Management Resources
   d. History of USDA nutrition guides

4. . _____s (GLUT or SLC2A family) are a family of membrane proteins found in most mammalian cells.

   Structure

   _____s are integral membrane proteins that contain 12 membrane-spanning helices with both the amino and carboxyl termini exposed on the cytoplasmic side of the plasma membrane. _____ proteins transport glucose and related hexoses according to a model of alternate conformation, which predicts that the transporter exposes a single substrate binding site toward either the outside or the inside of the cell.

   a. Voltage-gated ion channel

b. United Kingdom Prospective Diabetes Study

c. Untethered regimen

d. Glucose transporter

5. _____, hypoglycæmia or low blood sugar (not to be confused with hyperglycemia) is an abnormally diminished content of glucose in the blood. The term literally means 'low sugar blood' . It can produce a variety of symptoms and effects but the principal problems arise from an inadequate supply of glucose to the brain, resulting in impairment of function (neuroglycopenia).

a. Ketotic hypoglycemia

b. Reactive hypoglycemia

c. Hypoglycemia

d. Stress hyperglycemia

1. c
2. d
3. b
4. d
5. c

You can take the complete Chapter Practice Test

for Chapter 12. ENDOCRINE
on all key terms, persons, places, and concepts.

Online 99 Cents

http://www.epub219.49.13357.12.cram101.com/

Use www.Cram101.com for all your study needs

including Cram101's online interactive problem solving labs in

chemistry, statistics, mathematics, and more.

CHAPTER OUTLINE: KEY TERMS, PEOPLE, PLACES, CONCEPTS

	Diabetes insipidus
	Primary polydipsia
	Bronchopulmonary dysplasia
	Etiological myth
	Regulation
	Fluid deprivation test
	Pathogenesis
	Amiloride
	Abdominal mass
	Heart failure
	Terminal sedation
	Venous thrombosis
	Adrenal gland
	Androgen
	Glucocorticoid
	Adrenal hyperplasia
	Organogenesis
	Pathophysiology
	Primary

Secretion

Thyrotropin-releasing hormone

Congenital hypothyroidism

Pendred syndrome

Ethylene glycol

Hyperthermia

Thyroxine-binding globulin

Euthyroid sick syndrome

Beta-adrenergic agonist

Methimazole

Propylthiouracil

Hyperthyroidism

Methylmalonic acidemia

Thyroid hormone

Thyroid cancer

Thyroidectomy

Prognosis

Parathyroid gland

Hypocalcemia

CHAPTER OUTLINE: KEY TERMS, PEOPLE, PLACES, CONCEPTS

Barakat syndrome

22q11.2 deletion syndrome

Vitamin B6

Hypoparathyroidism

Parenteral nutrition

Vitamin D

Calcium gluconate

Chvostek sign

Blue diaper syndrome

Fat necrosis

Hypophosphatasia

Osteitis fibrosa cystica

Williams syndrome

Computed tomography

Hyperparathyroidism

Growth hormone

Pituitary adenomas

Septo-optic dysplasia

Panhypopituitarism

Ballard score

Gestational age

Caput succedaneum

Cephalhematoma

Eyes

Hypertensive crisis

Mucous retention cyst

Poland anomaly

Umbilical cord

Chest

Genitalia

Musculoskeletal

Chordee

Epispadias

Hypopituitarism

Inguinal hernia

Polydactyly

Syndactyly

Physical examination

Heart disease

Pulse oximetry

Chest radiograph

Hyperoxia test

Cyanosis

Glucose transporter

Hyperinsulinemia

Hypoglycemia

Sepsis

Differential diagnosis

Glucose-6-phosphate dehydrogenase

Hyperbilirubinemia

Kernicterus

Cardiopulmonary resuscitation

Physiology

Exchange transfusion

Home care

Phototherapy

Annular pancreas

Chapter 13. COMMON AND UNCOMMON PROBLEMS OF THE TERM NEWBORN
CHAPTER OUTLINE: KEY TERMS, PEOPLE, PLACES, CONCEPTS

_____ | Duodenal atresia

_____ | Esophageal atresia

_____ | Gastroesophageal reflux

_____ | Intestinal malrotation

_____ | Muscular dystrophies

_____ | Tracheoesophageal fistula

_____ | Vomiting

_____ | Cerebral palsy

_____ | Supraventricular tachycardia

_____ | Necrotizing enterocolitis

_____ | Imaging

_____ | Nasogastric tube

_____ | Hemostasis

_____ | Thrombocytopenia

_____ | Thrombocytopenic purpura

_____ | Disseminated intravascular coagulation

_____ | Vitamin K

_____ | Genetics

_____ | Hemorrhagic disease of the newborn

CHAPTER OUTLINE: KEY TERMS, PEOPLE, PLACES, CONCEPTS

Liver disease

Hyperekplexia

Sandifer syndrome

Seizure

Status epilepticus

Febrile seizure

Palliative care

Pyridoxine deficiency

Kyphoscoliosis

Subgaleal hemorrhage

Risk factor

Intracranial hemorrhage

Skull fracture

Subconjunctival hemorrhage

Brachial plexus

Clavicle fracture

Humerus fracture

Phrenic nerve

Spinal cord

Nerve injury

Respiratory distress

Neonatal sepsis

Prevention

Blood culture

C-reactive protein

Genital herpes

Weight gain

Aplastic anemia

Thermoregulation

Immunization

Substance abuse

Drug use

Pain management

Regional analgesia

Koplik spots

Syphilis

Toxoplasmosis

Tuberculosis

Community-acquired pneumonia

Congenital syphilis

Leydig cell

Sertoli cell

Sex determination

Y chromosome

High-mobility group

Androgen insensitivity syndrome

Gonadal dysgenesis

Congenital adrenal hyperplasia

Mixed gonadal dysgenesis

True hermaphroditism

Turner syndrome

Sex assignment

Surgery

Genetic disorder

CHARGE syndrome

Dysmorphic feature

Goldenhar syndrome

Tetralogy of Fallot

Deletion

Hypotonia

Urea cycle

Fatty acid

Oxidative phosphorylation

Pyruvate dehydrogenase

Process

Sickle-cell disease

Hemoglobinopathies

Newborn screening

Cystic fibrosis

Immunoreactive trypsinogen

Binge eating

Biotinidase deficiency

Eating disorder

Galactosemia

Hypothyroidism

Mass spectrometry

CHAPTER OUTLINE: KEY TERMS, PEOPLE, PLACES, CONCEPTS

Phenylketonuria

Tandem mass spectrometry

Homocystinuria

Maple syrup urine disease

Organic acid

Tyrosinemia

Urea cycle disorder

Propionic acidemia

Continuous positive airway pressure

Mechanical ventilation

Oxygen

Respiratory failure

Arnold-Chiari malformation

Neural tube

Neural tube defect

Chapter 13. COMMON AND UNCOMMON PROBLEMS OF THE TERM NEWBORN

Diabetes insipidus	Diabetes insipidus is a condition characterized by excessive thirst and excretion of large amounts of severely diluted urine, with reduction of fluid intake having no effect on the concentration of the urine. There are several different types of DI, each with a different cause. The most common type in humans is central DI, caused by a deficiency of arginine vasopressin (AVP), also known as antidiuretic hormone (ADH).
Primary polydipsia	Primary polydipsia is a special form of polydipsia. It is usually associated with a patient's increasing fluid intake due to the sensation of having a dry mouth.
	When the term 'psychogenic polydipsia' is used, it implies that the condition is caused by mental disorders.
Bronchopulmonary dysplasia	Bronchopulmonary dysplasia is a chronic lung disorder that is most common among children who were born prematurely, with low birthweights and who received prolonged mechanical ventilation to treat respiratory distress syndrome. The classic diagnosis of BPD may be assigned at 28 days of life if the following criteria are met (Bureau of Maternal and Child Health, 1989): (1) Positive pressure ventilation during the first 2 weeks of life for a minimum of 3 days.(2) Clinical signs of abnormal respiratory function.(3) Requirements for supplemental oxygen for longer than 28 days of age to maintain PaO2 above 50 mm Hg.(4) Chest radiograph with diffuse abnormal findings characteristic of BPD.
Etiological myth	Etiology is the study of causation, or origination.
	The word is most commonly used in medical and philosophical theories, where it is used to refer to the study of why things occur, or even the reasons behind the way that things act, and is used in philosophy, physics, psychology, government, medicine, theology and biology in reference to the causes of various phenomena. An etiological myth is a myth intended to explain a name or create a mythic history for a place or family.
Regulation	Regulation is 'controlling human or societal behavior by rules or restrictions.' Regulation can take many forms: legal restrictions promulgated by a government authority, self-regulation by an industry such as through a trade association, social regulation co-regulation and market regulation. One can consider regulation as actions of conduct imposing sanctions (such as a fine). This action of administrative law, or implementing regulatory law, may be contrasted with statutory or case law.
Fluid deprivation test	A fluid deprivation test or water deprivation test is a medical test which can be used to determine whether the patient has diabetes insipidus as opposed to other causes of polydipsia (a condition of excessive thirst that causes an excessive intake of water). The patient is required, for a prolonged period, to forgo intake of water completely, to determine the cause of the thirst.

Pathogenesis	The pathogenesis of a disease is the mechanism by which the disease is caused. The term can also be used to describe the origin and development of the disease and whether it is acute, chronic or recurrent. The word comes from the Greek pathos, 'disease', and genesis, 'creation'.
Amiloride	Amiloride is a potassium-sparing diuretic, first approved for use in 1967 (then known as MK 870), used in the management of hypertension and congestive heart failure. Amiloride was also tested as treatment of cystic fibrosis, but it was revealed inefficient in vivo due to its short time of action, therefore longer-acting ENaC inhibitors may prove more effective, e.g. Benzamil. Amiloride is a guanidinium group containing pyrazine derivative.
Abdominal mass	An abdominal mass is any localized enlargement or swelling in the human abdomen. Depending on its location, the abdominal mass may be caused by an enlarged liver (hepatomegaly), enlarged spleen (splenomegaly), protruding kidney, a pancreatic mass, a retroperitoneal mass (a mass in the posterior of the peritoneum), an abdominal aortic aneurysm, or various tumours, such as those caused by abdominal carcinomatosis and omental metastasis. The treatments depend on the cause, and may range from watchful waiting to radical surgery.
Heart failure	Heart failure often called congestive heart failure or congestive cardiac failure (CCF) is the inability of the heart to provide sufficient pump action to distribute blood flow to meet the needs of the body. Heart failure can cause a number of symptoms including shortness of breath, leg swelling, and exercise intolerance. The condition is diagnosed with echocardiography and blood tests.
Terminal sedation	In medicine, specifically in end-of-life care, terminal sedation is the palliative practice of relieving distress in a terminally ill person in the last hours or days of a dying patient's life, usually by means of a continuous intravenous or subcutaneous infusion of a sedative drug. This is a option of last resort for patients whose symptoms cannot be controlled by any other means. This should be differentiated from euthanasia as the goal of palliative sedation is to control symptoms through sedation but not shorten the patient's life, while in euthanasia the goal is to shorten life to relieve symptoms.
Venous thrombosis	A venous thrombosis is a blood clot (thrombus) that forms within a vein. Thrombosis is a medical term for a blood clot occurring inside a blood vessel. A classical venous thrombosis is deep vein thrombosis (DVT), which can break off (embolize), and become a life-threatening pulmonary embolism (PE).
Adrenal gland	In mammals, the adrenal glands (also known as suprarenal glands) are endocrine glands that sit atop the kidneys; in humans, the right adrenal gland is triangular shaped, while the left adrenal gland is semilunar shaped.

They are chiefly responsible for releasing hormones in response to stress through the synthesis of corticosteroids such as cortisol and catecholamines such as epinephrine (adrenaline) and norepinephrine. They also produce androgens.

Androgen

Androgen, is the generic term for any natural or synthetic compound, usually a steroid hormone, that stimulates or controls the development and maintenance of male characteristics in vertebrates by binding to androgen receptors. This includes the activity of the accessory male sex organs and development of male secondary sex characteristics. Androgens were first discovered in 1936. Androgens are also the original anabolic steroids and the precursor of all estrogens, the female sex hormones.

Glucocorticoid

Glucocorticoids (GC) are a class of steroid hormones that bind to the glucocorticoid receptor (GR), which is present in almost every vertebrate animal cell.

Glucocorticoids are part of the feedback mechanism in the immune system that turns immune activity (inflammation) down. They are therefore used in medicine to treat diseases that are caused by an overactive immune system, such as allergies, asthma, autoimmune diseases and sepsis.

Adrenal hyperplasia

Congenital adrenal hyperplasia refers to any of several autosomal recessive diseases resulting from mutations of genes for enzymes mediating the biochemical steps of production of cortisol from cholesterol by the adrenal glands (steroidogenesis).

Most of these conditions involve excessive or deficient production of sex steroids and can alter development of primary or secondary sex characteristics in some affected infants, children, or adults. Associated conditions

The symptoms of CAH vary depending upon the form of CAH and the gender of the patient.

Organogenesis

In animal development, organogenesis is the process by which the ectoderm, endoderm, and mesoderm develop into the internal organs of the organism. Internal organs initiate development in humans within the 3rd to 8th weeks in utero. The germ layers in organogenesis differ by three processes: folds, splits, and condensation.

Pathophysiology

Pathophysiology sample values

Pathophysiology is the study of the changes of normal mechanical, physical, and biochemical functions, either caused by a disease, or resulting from an abnormal syndrome. More formally, it is the branch of medicine which deals with any disturbances of body functions, caused by disease or prodromal symptoms.

	An alternative definition is 'the study of the biological and physical manifestations of disease as they correlate with the underlying abnormalities and physiological disturbances.' The study of pathology and the study of pathophysiology often involves substantial overlap in diseases and processes, but pathology emphasizes direct observations, while pathophysiology emphasizes quantifiable measurements.
Primary	The Primary (formerly the Primary Association) is a children's organization and an official auxiliary within The Church of Jesus Christ of Latter-day Saints (LDS Church). It acts as a Sunday school organization for the church's children under the age of 12. The official purpose of Primary is to help parents in teaching their children to learn and live the gospel of Jesus Christ.
Secretion	Secretion is the process of elaborating, releasing, and oozing chemicals, or a secreted chemical substance from a cell or gland. In contrast to excretion, the substance may have a certain function, rather than being a waste product. Secretion in bacterial species means the transport or translocation of effector molecules for example proteins, enzymes or toxins (such as cholera toxin in pathogenic bacteria for example Vibrio cholerae) from across the interior (cytoplasm or cytosol) of a bacterial cell to its exterior.
Thyrotropin-releasing hormone	Thyrotropin-releasing hormone also called thyrotropin-releasing factor (TRF), thyroliberin or protirelin, is a tropic, tripeptidal hormone that stimulates the release of TSH and prolactin from the anterior pituitary. TRH has been used clinically for the treatment of spinocerebellar degeneration and disturbance of consciousness in humans. TRH is produced by the hypothalamus in medial neurons of the paraventricular nucleus.
Congenital hypothyroidism	Congenital hypothyroidism is a condition of thyroid hormone deficiency present at birth. Approximately 1 in 4000 newborn infants has a severe deficiency of thyroid function, while even more have mild or partial degrees. If untreated for several months after birth, severe congenital hypothyroidism can lead to growth failure and permanent mental retardation.
Pendred syndrome	Pendred syndrome is a genetic disorder leading to congenital bilateral (both sides) sensorineural hearing loss and goitre with occasional hypothyroidism (decreased thyroid gland function). There is no specific treatment, other than supportive measures for the hearing loss and thyroid hormone supplementation in case of hypothyroidism. It is named Dr Vaughan Pendred (1869-1946), the English doctor who first described the condition in an Irish family living in Durham in 1896.

Chapter 13. COMMON AND UNCOMMON PROBLEMS OF THE TERM NEWBORN

Ethylene glycol	Ethylene glycol is an organic compound widely used as an automotive antifreeze and a precursor to polymers. In its pure form, it is an odorless, colorless, syrupy, liquid. Ethylene glycol is toxic, and ingestion can result in death.
Hyperthermia	Hyperthermia is an elevated body temperature due to failed thermoregulation. Hyperthermia occurs when the body produces or absorbs more heat than it can dissipate. When the elevated body temperatures are sufficiently high, hyperthermia is a medical emergency and requires immediate treatment to prevent disability or death.
Thyroxine-binding globulin	Thyroxine-binding globulin binds thyroid hormone in circulation. It is one of three proteins (along with transthyretin and albumin) responsible for carrying the thyroid hormones thyroxine (T4) and 3,5,3'-triiodothyronine (T3) in the bloodstream. Of these three proteins, TBG has the highest affinity for T4 and T3, but is present in the lowest concentration.
Euthyroid sick syndrome	Euthyroid sick syndrome, sick euthyroid syndrome, non-thyroidal illness syndrome or low T_3 low T_4 syndrome is a state of adaptation or dysregulation of thyrotropic feedback control where the levels of T3 and/or T4 are at unusual levels, but the thyroid gland does not appear to be dysfunctional. This condition is often seen in starvation, critical illness or patients in intensive care unit. Causes of euthyroid sick syndrome include a number of acute and chronic conditions, including pneumonia, fasting, starvation, sepsis, trauma, cardiopulmonary bypass, malignancy, stress, heart failure, hypothermia, myocardial infarction, chronic renal failure, cirrhosis, and diabetic ketoacidosis.
Beta-adrenergic agonist	Beta-adrenergic agonists are adrenergic agonists which act upon the beta receptors. β_1 agonists β_1 agonists: stimulates adenylyl cyclase activity; opening of calcium channel. (cardiac stimulants; used to treat cardiogenic shock, acute heart failure, bradyarrhythmias).
Methimazole	Methimazole is an antithyroid drug, and part of the thioamide group. Methimazole is a drug used to treat hyperthyroidism, a condition that usually occurs when the thyroid gland is producing too much thyroid hormone. It may also be taken before thyroid surgery to lower thyroid hormone levels and minimize the effects of thyroid manipulation.
Propylthiouracil	Propylthiouracil or 6-n-propylthiouracil is a thiouracil-derived drug used to treat hyperthyroidism (including Graves' disease) by decreasing the amount of thyroid hormone produced by the thyroid gland. Its notable side effects include a risk of agranulocytosis.

Hyperthyroidism	Hyperthyroidism, often referred to as an 'overactive thyroid', is when the thyroid gland produces and secretes excessive amounts of the free - not protein bound and circulating in the blood - thyroid hormones, triiodothyronine (T3) and/or thyroxine (T4). This is the opposite of hypothyroidism ('sluggish thyroid'), which is the reduced production and secretion of T3 and/or T4.Hyperthyroidism is a type of thyrotoxicosis, a hypermetabolic clinical syndrome which occurs when there are elevated serum levels of T3 and/or T4.Graves disease is the most common form of hyperthyroidism. While hyperthyroidism may cause thyrotoxicosis they are not synonymous medical conditions; some patients may develop thyrotoxicosis as a result of inflammation of the thyroid gland (thyroiditis), which may cause the release of excessive thyroid hormone already stored in the gland but does not cause accelerated hormone production.
Methylmalonic acidemia	Methylmalonic acidemia also called methylmalonic aciduria, is an autosomal recessive metabolic disorder. It is a classical type of organic acidemia. Methylmalonic acidemia stems from several genotypes, all forms of the disorder usually diagnosed in the early neonatal period, presenting progressive encephalopathy, and secondary hyperammonemia.
Thyroid hormone	The thyroid hormones, thyroxine (T_4) and triiodothyronine (T_3), are tyrosine-based hormones produced by the thyroid gland primarily responsible for regulation of metabolism. An important component in the synthesis of thyroid hormones is iodine. The major form of thyroid hormone in the blood is thyroxine (T_4), which has a longer half life than T_3. The ratio of T_4 to T_3 released into the blood is roughly 20 to 1. Thyroxine is converted to the active T_3 (three to four times more potent than T_4) within cells by deiodinases (5'-iodinase). These are further processed by decarboxylation and deiodination to produce iodothyronamine (T_1a) and thyronamine (T_0a).
Thyroid cancer	Thyroid cancer is a thyroid neoplasm that is malignant. It can be treated with radioactive iodine or surgical resection of the thyroid gland. Chemotherapy or radiotherapy may also be used.
Thyroidectomy	A thyroidectomy is an operation that involves the surgical removal of all or part of the thyroid gland. Surgeons often perform a thyroidectomy when a patient has thyroid cancer or some other condition of the thyroid gland (such as hyperthyroidism) or goiter. Other indications for surgery include cosmetic (very enlarged thyroid), or symptomatic obstruction (causing difficulties in swallowing or breathing).
Prognosis	Prognosis is a medical term to describe the likely outcome of an illness. When applied to large populations, prognostic estimates can be very accurate: for example the statement '45% of patients with severe septic shock will die within 28 days' can be made with some confidence, because previous research found that this proportion of patients died.

Chapter 13. COMMON AND UNCOMMON PROBLEMS OF THE TERM NEWBORN

Parathyroid gland	The parathyroid glands are small endocrine glands in the neck that produce parathyroid hormone. Humans usually have four parathyroid glands, which are usually located on the rear surface of the thyroid gland, or, in rare cases, within the thyroid gland itself or in the chest. Parathyroid glands control the amount of calcium in the blood and within the bones.
Hypocalcemia	In medicine, Hypocalcemia is the presence of low serum calcium levels in the blood, usually taken as less than 2.1 mmol/L or 9 mg/dl or an ionized calcium level mm of less than 1.1 mmol/L (4.5 mg/dL). It is a type of electrolyte disturbance. In the blood, about half of all calcium is bound to proteins such as serum albumin, but it is the unbound, or ionized, calcium that the body regulates.
Barakat syndrome	Barakat syndrome, was first described by Amin J. Barakat et al. in 1977.
	The frequency is unknown, but the disease is considered to be very rare. Presentation
	It is a genetic developmental disorder with clinical diversity characterized by hypoparathyroidism, sensorineural deafness and renal disease.
22q11.2 deletion syndrome	22q11.2 deletion syndrome, also known as DiGeorge syndrome, DiGeorge anomaly, velo-cardio-facial syndrome, Shprintzen syndrome, conotruncal anomaly face syndrome, Strong syndrome, congenital thymic aplasia, and thymic hypoplasia is a syndrome caused by the deletion of a small piece of chromosome 22. The deletion occurs near the middle of the chromosome at a location designated q11.2 i.e., on the long arm of one of the pair of chromosomes 22. It has a prevalence estimated at 1:4000. The syndrome was described in 1968 by the pediatric endocrinologist Angelo DiGeorge.
	The features of this syndrome vary widely, even among members of the same family, and affect many parts of the body. Characteristic signs and symptoms may include birth defects such as congenital heart disease, defects in the palate, most commonly related to neuromuscular problems with closure (velo-pharyngeal insufficiency), learning disabilities, mild differences in facial features, and recurrent infections.
Vitamin B6	Vitamin B_6 is a water-soluble vitamin and is part of the vitamin B complex group. Several forms of the vitamin are known, but pyridoxal phosphate (PLP) is the active form and is a cofactor in many reactions of amino acid metabolism, including transamination, deamination, and decarboxylation. PLP also is necessary for the enzymatic reaction governing the release of glucose from glycogen.
	Vitamin B_6 is a water-soluble compound that was discovered in the 1930s during nutrition studies on rats. In 1934, a Hungarian physician, Paul György discovered a substance that was able to cure a skin disease in rats (dermititis acrodynia), this substance he named vitamin B_6.

In 1938, Samuel Lepkovsky isolated vitamin B_6 from rice bran. Harris and Folkers in 1939 determined the structure of pyridoxine, and, in 1945, Snell was able to show that there are two forms of vitamin B_6, pyridoxal and pyridoxamine. Vitamin B_6 was named pyridoxine to indicate its structural homology to pyridine. All three forms of vitamin B_6 are precursors of an activated compound known as pyridoxal 5'-phosphate (PLP), which plays a vital role as the co-factor of a large number of essential enzymes in the human body.

Enzymes dependent on PLP focus a wide variety of chemical reactions mainly involving amino acids. The reactions carried out by the PLP-dependent enzymes that act on amino acids include transfer of the amino group, decarboxylation, racemization, and beta- or gamma-elimination or replacement. Such versatility arises from the ability of PLP to covalently bind the substrate, and then to act as an electrophilic catalyst, thereby stabilizing different types of carbanionic reaction intermediates.

Overall, the Enzyme Commission has catalogued more than 140 PLP-dependent activities, corresponding to ~4% of all classified activities. Forms

Seven forms of this vitamin are known:•Pyridoxine (PN), the form that is most commonly given as vitamin B_6 supplement•Pyridoxine 5'-phosphate (PNP)•Pyridoxal (PL)•Pyridoxal 5'-phosphate (PLP), the metabolically active form (sold as 'P-5-P' vitamin supplement)•Pyridoxamine (PM)•Pyridoxamine 5'-phosphate (PMP)•4-Pyridoxic acid (PA), the catabolite which is excreted in the urine

All forms except PA can be interconverted. Functions

Pyridoxal phosphate, the metabolically active form of vitamin B_6, is involved in many aspects of macronutrient metabolism, neurotransmitter synthesis, histamine synthesis, hemoglobin synthesis and function and gene expression. Pyridoxal phosphate generally serves as a coenzyme for many reactions and can help facilitate decarboxylation, transamination, racemization, elimination, replacement and beta-group interconversion reactions. The liver is the site for vitamin B_6 metabolism. Amino acid metabolism

Pyridoxal phosphate (PLP) is a cofactor in transaminases that can catabolize amino acids. PLP is also an essential component of two enzymes that converts methionine to cysteine via two reactions. Low vitamin B_6 status will result in decreased activity of these enzymes. PLP is also an essential cofactor for enzymes involved in the metabolism of selenomethionine to selenohomocysteine and then from selenohomocysteine to hydrogen selenide. Vitamin B_6 is also required for the conversion of tryptophan to niacin and low vitamin B_6 status will impair this conversion. PLP is also used to create physiologically active amines by decarboxylation of amino acids.

Some notable examples of this include: histidine to histamine, tryptophan to serotonin, glutamate to gamma-aminobutyric acid (GABA), and dihydroxyphenylalanine to dopamine. Gluconeogenesis

Vitamin B_6 also plays a role in gluconeogenesis. Pyridoxal phosphate can catalyze transamination reactions that are essential for the providing amino acids as a substrate for gluconeogenesis. Also, vitamin B_6 is a required coenzyme of glycogen phosphorylase, the enzyme that is necessary for glycogenolysis to occur. Lipid metabolism

Vitamin B_6 is an essential component of enzymes that facilitate the biosynthesis of sphingolipids. Particularly, the synthesis of ceramide requires PLP. In this reaction serine is decarboxylated and combined with palmitoyl-CoA to form sphinganine which is combined with a fatty acyl CoA to form dihydroceramide. Dihydroceramide is then further desaturated to form ceramide. In addition, the breakdown of sphingolipids is also dependent on vitamin B_6 since S1P lyase, the enzyme responsible for breaking down sphingosine-1-phosphate, is also PLP dependent. Metabolic functions

The primary role of vitamin B_6 is to act as a coenzyme to many other enzymes in the body that are involved predominantly in metabolism. This role is performed by the active form, pyridoxal phosphate. This active form is converted from the two other natural forms founds in food: pyridoxal, pyridoxine and pyridoxamine.

Vitamin B_6 is involved in the following metabolic processes:•amino acid, glucose and lipid metabolism•neurotransmitter synthesis•histamine synthesis•hemoglobin synthesis and function•gene expressionAmino acid metabolism

Pyridoxal phosphate is involved in almost all amino acid metabolism, from synthesis to breakdown. •Transamination: transaminase enzymes needed to break down amino acids are dependent on the presence of pyridoxal phosphate. The proper activity of these enzymes are crucial for the process of moving amine groups from one amino acid to another.•Transsulfuration: Pyridoxal phosphate is a coenzyme needed for the proper function of the enzymes cystathionine synthase and cystathionase. These enzymes work to transform methionine into cysteine.•Selenoamino acid metabolism: Selenomethionine is the primary dietary form of selenium. Pyridoxal phosphate is needed as a cofactor for the enzymes that allow selenium to be used from the dietary form. Pyridoxal phosphate also plays a cofactor role in releasing selenium from selenohomocysteine to produce hydrogen selenide. This hydrogen selenide can then be used to incorporate selenium into selenoproteins.•Vitamin B_6 is also required for the conversion of tryptophan to niacin and low vitamin B_6 status will impair this conversion.Neurotransmitter synthesis

Pyridoxal phosphate-dependent enzymes play a role in the biosynthesis of four important neurotransmitters: serotonin, epinephrine, norepinephrine and gamma-aminobutyric acid. Serine racemase, which synthesizes the neuromodulator D-serine, is also a pyridoxal phosphate-dependent enzyme. Histamine synthesis

Pyridoxal phosphate is involved in the metabolism of histamine. Hemoglobin synthesis and function

Pyridoxal phosphate aids in the synthesis of heme, by serving as a coenzyme for the enzyme ALA synthase. It also binds to two sites on hemoglobin to enhance the oxygen binding of hemoglobin. Gene expression

It transforms homocysteine into cistation then into cysteine. Pyridoxal phosphate has been implicated in increasing or decreasing the expression of certain genes. Increased intracellular levels of the vitamin will lead to a decrease in the transcription of glucocorticoid hormones. Also, vitamin B_6 deficiency will lead to the increased expression of albumin mRNA. Also, pyridoxal phosphate will influence gene expression of glycoprotein IIb by interacting with various transcription factors. The result is inhibition of platelet aggregation. Dietary reference intakes

The Institute of Medicine notes that 'No adverse effects associated with vitamin B_6 from food have been reported. This does not mean that there is no potential for adverse effects resulting from high intakes. Because data on the adverse effects of vitamin B_6 are limited, caution may be warranted. Sensory neuropathy has occurred from high intakes of supplemental forms.' Food sources

Vitamin B_6 is widely distributed in foods in both its free and bound forms. Good sources include meats, whole grain products, vegetables, nuts and bananas. Cooking, storage and processing losses of vitamin B_6 vary and in some foods may be more than 50%, depending on the form of vitamin present in the food. Plant foods lose the least during processing as they contain mostly pyridoxine which is far more stable than the pyridoxal or pyridoxamine found in animal foods. For example, milk can lose 30-70% of its vitamin B_6 content when dried. Vitamin B_6 is found in the germ and aleurone layer of grains and milling results to the reduction of this vitamin in white flour. Freezing and canning are other food processing methods that results in the loss of vitamin B_6 in foods. Absorption and excretion

Vitamin B_6 is absorbed in the jejunum and ileum via passive diffusion. With the capacity for absorption being so great, animals are able to absorb quantities much greater than what is needed for physiological demands. The absorption of pyridoxal phosphate and pyridoxamine phosphate involves their dephosphorylation catalyzed by a membrane-bound alkaline phosphatase.

Those products and non-phosphorylated vitamers in the digestive tract are absorbed by diffusion, which is driven by trapping of the vitamin as 5'-phosphates through the action of phosphorylation (by a pyridoxal kinase) in the jejunal mucosa. The trapped pyridoxine and pyridoxamine are oxidized to pyridoxal phosphate in the tissue.

The products of vitamin B_6 metabolism are excreted in the urine; the major product of which is 4-pyridoxic acid. It has been estimated that 40-60% of ingested vitamin B_6 is oxidized to 4-pyridoxic acid. Several studies have shown that 4-pyridoxic acid is undetectable in the urine of vitamin B_6 deficient subjects, making it a useful clinical marker to assess the vitamin B_6 status of an individual. Other products of vitamin B_6 metabolism that are excreted in the urine when high doses of the vitamin have been given include pyridoxal, pyridoxamine, and pyridoxine and their phosphates. A small amount of vitamin B_6 is also excreted in the feces. Deficiencies

The classic clinical syndrome for B_6 deficiency is a seborrhoeic dermatitis-like eruption, atrophic glossitis with ulceration, angular cheilitis, conjunctivitis, intertrigo, and neurologic symptoms of somnolence, confusion, and neuropathy.

While severe vitamin B_6 deficiency results in dermatologic and neurologic changes, less severe cases present with metabolic lesions associated with insufficient activities of the coenzyme pyridoxal phosphate. The most prominent of the lesions is due to impaired tryptophan-niacin conversion. This can be detected based on urinary excretion of xanthurenic acid after an oral tryptophan load. Vitamin B_6 deficiency can also result from impaired transsulfuration of methionine to cysteine. The pyridoxal phosphate-dependent transaminases and glycogen phosphorylase provide the vitamin with its role in gluconeogenesis, so deprivation of vitamin B_6 results in impaired glucose tolerance.

A deficiency of vitamin B_6 alone is relatively uncommon and often occurs in association with other vitamins of the B complex. The elderly and alcoholics have an increased risk of vitamin B_6 deficiency, as well as other micronutrient deficiencies. Renal patients undergoing dialysis may experience vitamin B_6 deficiency. Also, patients with liver disease, rheumatoid arthritis and those infected with HIV also appear to be at risk, despite adequate dietary intakes. The availability of vitamin B_6 to the body can be affected by certain drugs such as anticonvulsants and corticosteroids. The drug isoniazid (used in the treatment of tuberculosis), and cycloserine, penicillamine, and hydrocortisone all interfere with vitamin B_6 metabolism. These drugs may form a complex with vitamin B_6 that is inhibitory for pyridoxal kinase, or they may positively displace PLP from binding sites. Clinical assessment of vitamin B_6

The biochemical assessment of vitamin B_6 status is essential, as the clinical signs and symptoms of vitamin B_6 deficiency are very nonspecific.

The three biochemical tests most widely used are the activation coefficient for the erythrocyte enzyme aspartate aminotransferase, plasma pyridoxal phosphate (PLP) concentrations, and the urinary excretion of vitamin B_6 degradation products, specifically urinary pyridoxic acid. Of these, plasma PLP is probably the best single measure because it reflects tissue stores. When plasma pyridoxal phosphate is less than 10nmol/L, it is indicative of vitamin B_6 deficiency. Urinary 4-pyridoxic acid is also an indicator of vitamin B_6 deficiency. Urinary 4-pyridoxic of less than 3.0 mmol/day is suggestive of vitamin B_6 deficiency. Toxicity

Adverse effects have only been documented from vitamin B_6 supplements and never from food sources Toxicologic animal studies identify specific destruction of the dorsal root ganglia which is documented in human cases of overdosage of pyridoxine. Although vitamin B_6 is a water-soluble vitamin and is excreted in the urine, doses of pyridoxine in excess of the RDI over long periods of time thus result in painful and ultimately irreversible neurological problems.

The primary symptoms are pain and numbness of the extremities, and in severe cases difficulty walking. Sensory neuropathy typically develops at doses of pyridoxine in excess of 1,000 mg per day. However, there have been a few case reports of individuals who developed sensory neuropathies at doses of less than 500 mg daily over a period of months. None of the studies, in which an objective neurological examination was performed, found evidence of sensory nerve damage at intakes of pyridoxine below 200 mg/day. This condition is usually reversible when supplementation is stopped.

Existing authorisations and valuations vary considerably worldwide. In 1993 the European Community Scientific Committee on Food defines intakes of 50 mg vitamin B6 per day as harmful and established tolerable upper intake level of 25 mg/day for adults in 2000.

Hypoparathyroidism	Hypoparathyroidism is decreased function of the parathyroid glands with under production of parathyroid hormone. This can lead to low levels of calcium in the blood, often causing cramping and twitching of muscles or tetany (involuntary muscle contraction), and several other symptoms. The condition can be inherited, but it is also encountered after thyroid or parathyroid gland surgery, and it can be caused by immune system-related damage as well as a number of rarer causes.
Parenteral nutrition	Parenteral nutrition is feeding a person intravenously, bypassing the usual process of eating and digestion. The person receives nutritional formulae that contain nutrients such as glucose, amino acids, lipids and added vitamins and dietary minerals. It is called total parenteral nutrition or total nutrient admixture (TNA) when no food is given by other routes.
Vitamin D	Vitamin D is a group of fat-soluble prohormones, the two major forms of which are Vitamin D_2 (or ergocalciferol) and Vitamin D_3 (or cholecalciferol).

	Vitamin D obtained from sun exposure, food, and supplements, is biologically inert and must undergo two hydroxylation reactions to be activated in the body. Calcitriol (1,25-Dihydroxycholecalciferol) is the active form of Vitamin D found in the body.
Calcium gluconate	Calcium gluconate is a mineral supplement. It is manufactured by the neutralization of gluconic acid with lime or calcium carbonate. Hypocalcemia 10% calcium gluconate solution (given intravenously) is the form of calcium most widely used in the treatment of hypocalcemia.
Chvostek sign	The Chvostek sign is one of the signs of tetany seen in hypocalcemia. It refers to an abnormal reaction to the stimulation of the facial nerve. When the facial nerve is tapped at the angle of the jaw (i.e. masseter muscle), the facial muscles on the same side of the face will contract momentarily (typically a twitch of the nose or lips) because of hypocalcemia (i.e. from hypoparathyroidism, pseudohypoparathyroidism, hypovitaminosis D) with resultant hyperexcitability of nerves.
Blue diaper syndrome	Blue diaper syndrome is a rare, autosomal recessive metabolic disorder characterized in infants by bluish urine-stained diapers. It is caused by a defect in tryptophan absorption. Bacterial degradation of tryptophan in the intestine leads to excessive indole production and thus to indicanuria which, on oxidation to indigo blue, causes a peculiar bluish discoloration of the diaper.
Fat necrosis	Fat necrosis is a form of necrosis characterized by the action upon fat by digestive enzymes. In fat necrosis the enzyme lipase releases fatty acids from triglycerides. The fatty acids then complex with calcium to form soaps.
Hypophosphatasia	Hypophosphatasia is a rare, and sometimes fatal metabolic bone disease. Clinical symptoms are heterogeneous ranging from the rapidly fatal perinatal variant, with profound skeletal hypomineralization and respiratory compromise to a milder, progressive osteomalacia later in life. Tissue non-specific alkaline phosphatase (TNSALP) deficiency in osteoblasts and chondrocytes impairs bone mineralization, leading to rickets or osteomalacia.
Osteitis fibrosa cystica	Osteitis fibrosa cystica abbreviated OFC, and also known as osteitis fibrosa, osteodystrophia fibrosa, Von Recklinghausen's Disease of Bone, not to be confused with Von Recklinghausen's disease (neurofibromatosis type I). Osteitis Fibrosa Cystica is a skeletal disorder caused by a surplus of parathyroid hormone from over-active parathyroid glands.

Williams syndrome	Williams syndrome is a rare neurodevelopmental disorder characterized by a distinctive, 'elfin' facial appearance, along with a low nasal bridge; an unusually cheerful demeanor and ease with strangers; developmental delay coupled with strong language skills; and cardiovascular problems, such as supravalvular aortic stenosis and transient hypercalcaemia.
	It is caused by a deletion of about 26 genes from the long arm of chromosome 7. The syndrome was first identified in 1961 by Dr. J. C. P. Williams of New Zealand and has an estimated prevalence of 1 in 7,500 to 1 in 20,000 births.
	Signs and symptoms
	The most common symptoms of Williams syndrome are mental disability, heart defects, and unusual facial features.
Computed tomography	Computed tomography is a medical imaging method employing tomography created by computer processing. Digital geometry processing is used to generate a three-dimensional image of the inside of an object from a large series of two-dimensional X-ray images taken around a single axis of rotation.
	Computed tomography produces a volume of data which can be manipulated, through a process known as 'windowing', in order to demonstrate various bodily structures based on their ability to block the X-ray/Röntgen beam.
Hyperparathyroidism	Hyperparathyroidism is overactivity of the parathyroid glands resulting in excess production of parathyroid hormone (PTH). The parathyroid hormone regulates calcium and phosphate levels and helps to maintain these levels. Excessive PTH secretion may be due to problems in the glands themselves, in which case it is referred to as primary hyperparathyroidism and which leads to hypercalcemia (raised calcium levels).
Growth hormone	Growth hormone is a peptide hormone that stimulates growth, cell reproduction and regeneration in humans and other animals. Growth hormone is a 191-amino acid, single-chain polypeptide that is synthesized, stored, and secreted by the somatotroph cells within the lateral wings of the anterior pituitary gland. Somatotropin (STH) refers to the growth hormone 1 produced naturally in animals, whereas the term somatropin refers to growth hormone produced by recombinant DNA technology, and is abbreviated 'HGH' in humans.
Pituitary adenomas	Pituitary adenomas are tumors that occur in the pituitary gland, and account for about 10% of intracranial neoplasms. They often remain undiagnosed, and small pituitary tumors have an estimated prevalence of 16.7% (14.4% in autopsy studies and 22.5% in radiologic studies).

Chapter 13. COMMON AND UNCOMMON PROBLEMS OF THE TERM NEWBORN

Septo-optic dysplasia	Septo-optic dysplasia also known as de Morsier syndrome is a congenital malformation syndrome made manifest by hypoplasia (underdevelopment) of the optic nerve and absence of the septum pellucidum (a midline part of the brain). Vision in each eye can be unaffected, partially lost, or in some patients, completely absent. Although not included in the name, hypopituitarism is sometimes included in the definition.
Panhypopituitarism	Hypopituitarism is the decreased (hypo) secretion of one or more of the eight hormones normally produced by the pituitary gland at the base of the brain. If there is decreased secretion of most pituitary hormones, the term Panhypopituitarism is used. The signs and symptoms of hypopituitarism vary, depending on which hormones are undersecreted and on the underlying cause of the abnormality.
Ballard score	The Ballard Maturational Assessment, Ballard score, the sum of all of which is then extrapolated to the gestational age of the baby. These criteria are divided into Physical and Neurological criteria.
Gestational age	Gestational age relates to the age of an embryo or fetus . There is some ambiguity in how it is defined:•In embryology, the term 'gestational age' is seldom used because it lacks precision. The timing of embryonic development starts with fertilization.
Caput succedaneum	Caput succedaneum is a neonatal condition involving a serosanguinous, subcutaneous, extraperiosteal fluid collection with poorly defined margins caused by the pressure of the presenting part of the scalp against the dilating cervix (tourniquet effect of the cervix) during delivery.
Cephalhematoma	A cephalhematoma is a hemorrhage of blood between the skull and the periosteum of a newborn baby secondary to rupture of blood vessels crossing the periosteum. Because the swelling is subperiosteal its boundaries are limited by the individual bones, in contrast to a chignon.
Eyes	eyes are organs that detect light, and send electrical impulses along the optic nerve to the visual and other areas of the brain. Complex optical systems with resolving power have come in ten fundamentally different forms, and 96% of animal species possess a complex optical system. Image-resolving eyes are present in cnidaria, molluscs, chordates, annelids and arthropods.
Hypertensive crisis	A hypertensive emergency is severe hypertension (high blood pressure) with acute impairment of an organ system (especially the central nervous system, cardiovascular system and/or the renal system) and the possibility of irreversible organ-damage.

In case of a hypertensive emergency, the blood pressure should be lowered aggressively over minutes to hours with an antihypertensive agent.

Several classes of antihypertensive agents are recommended and the choice for the antihypertensive agent depends on the cause for the Hypertensive crisis, the severity of elevated blood pressure and the patient's usual blood pressure before the Hypertensive crisis.

Mucous retention cyst	A mucous retention cyst is a cyst caused by an obstruction of a duct, usually belonging to the parotid gland or a minor salivary gland.
Poland anomaly	The Poland anomaly is a human developmental problem, and is a predominantly sporadic developmental field defect in which hypoplasia or absence of the nipple and/or breast is associated with ipsilateral aplasia of the sternal head of the pectoralis major muscle, patchy absence of axillary hair, and symbrachydactyly.
Umbilical cord	In placental mammals, the umbilical cord is the connecting cord from the developing embryo or fetus to the placenta. During prenatal development, the umbilical cord is physiologically and genetically part of the fetus and (in humans) normally contains two arteries (the umbilical arteries) and one vein (the umbilical vein), buried within Wharton's jelly. The umbilical vein supplies the fetus with oxygenated, nutrient-rich blood from the placenta.
Chest	The chest is a part of the anatomy of humans and various other animals. It is sometimes referred to as the thorax or the bosom. Chest anatomy - humans and other hominids

In hominids, the chest is the region of the body between the neck and the abdomen, along with its internal organs and other contents. |
| Genitalia | A sex organ, or primary sexual characteristic, as narrowly defined, is any of the anatomical parts of the body which are involved in sexual reproduction and constitute the reproductive system in a complex organism; flowers are the reproductive organs of flowering plants, cones are the reproductive organs of coniferous plants , whereas mosses, ferns, and other similar plants have gametangia for reproductive organs.

In mammals, sex organs include:

· Female

· Bartholin's glands · cervix · clitoris

· clitoral hood · clitoral glans (glans clitoridis) · Fallopian tubes · labium · ovaries · Skene's gland · uterus · vagina · vulva |

· Male

· bulbourethral glands · epididymis · penis

· foreskin · glans penis · prostate · scrotum · seminal vesicles · testicles

The Latin term genitalia is used to describe the externally visible sex organs, known as primary genitalia or external genitalia:in males the penis in females the clitoris and vulva.

The other, hidden sex organs are referred to as the secondary genitalia or internal genitalia. The most important of these are the gonads, a pair of sex organs, specifically the testes in the male or the ovaries in the female.

Musculoskeletal	A musculoskeletal system (also known as the locomotor system) is an organ system that gives animals (including humans) the ability to move using the muscular and skeletal systems. The musculoskeletal system provides form, stability, and movement to the body. It is made up of the body's bones (the skeleton), muscles, cartilage, tendons, ligaments, joints, and other connective tissue (the tissue that supports and binds tissues and organs together).
Chordee	Chordee is a condition in which the head of the penis curves downward or upward, at the junction of the head and shaft of the penis. The curvature is usually most obvious during erection, but resistance to straightening is often apparent in the flaccid state as well. In many cases but not all, chordee is associated with hypospadias.
Epispadias	An epispadias is a rare type of malformation of the penis in which the urethra ends in an opening on the upper aspect (the dorsum) of the penis. It can also develop in females when the urethra develops too far anteriorly. It occurs in around 1 in 120,000 male and 1 in 500,000 female births.
Hypopituitarism	Hypopituitarism is the decreased (hypo) secretion of one or more of the eight hormones normally produced by the pituitary gland at the base of the brain. If there is decreased secretion of most pituitary hormones, the term panhypopituitarism is used. The signs and symptoms of hypopituitarism vary, depending on which hormones are undersecreted and on the underlying cause of the abnormality.
Inguinal hernia	An inguinal hernia is a protrusion of abdominal-cavity contents through the inguinal canal. They are very common (lifetime risk 27% for men, 3% for women), and their repair is one of the most frequently performed surgical operations.

| Polydactyly | Polydactyly, also known as hyperdactyly, is a congenital physical anomaly in humans, dogs, and cats having supernumerary fingers or toes.

The extra digit is usually a small piece of soft tissue that can be removed. Occasionally it contains bone without joints; rarely it may be a complete, functioning digit. |
| --- | --- |
| Syndactyly | Syndactyly is a condition wherein two or more digits are fused together. It occurs normally in some mammals, such as the siamang and kangaroo, but is an unusual condition in humans.

Syndactyly can be simple or complex. |
| Physical examination | A physical examination, medical examination, or clinical examination (more popularly known as a check-up or medical) is the process by which a doctor investigates the body of a patient for signs of disease. It generally follows the taking of the medical history -- an account of the symptoms as experienced by the patient. Together with the medical history, the physical examination aids in determining the correct diagnosis and devising the treatment plan. |
| Heart disease | Heart disease is an umbrella term for a variety of diseases affecting the heart. As of 2007, it is the leading cause of death in the United States, England, Canada and Wales, accounting for 25.4% of the total deaths in the United States.

Coronary heart disease refers to the failure of the coronary circulation to supply adequate circulation to cardiac muscle and surrounding tissue. Coronary heart disease is most commonly equated with Coronary artery disease although coronary heart disease can be due to other causes, such as coronary vasospasm. |
| Pulse oximetry | Pulse oximetry is a non-invasive method allowing the monitoring of the oxygenation of a patient's hemoglobin.

A sensor is placed on a thin part of the patient's body, usually a fingertip or earlobe, or in the case of an infant, across a foot. Light of two different wavelengths is passed through the patient to a photodetector. |
| Chest radiograph | In medicine, a chest radiograph, commonly called a chest X-ray (CXR), is a projection radiograph of the chest used to diagnose conditions affecting the chest, its contents, and nearby structures. Chest radiographs are among the most common films taken, being diagnostic of many conditions.

Like all methods of radiography, chest radiography employs ionizing radiation in the form of X-rays to generate images of the chest. |

Chapter 13. COMMON AND UNCOMMON PROBLEMS OF THE TERM NEWBORN

Hyperoxia test	A hyperoxia test is a test that is performed--usually on an infant-- to determine whether the patient's cyanosis is due to lung disease or a problem with blood circulation. It is performed by measuring the arterial blood gases of the patient while he breathes room air, then re-measuring the blood gases after the patient has breathed 100% oxygen for 10 minutes. If the cause of the cyanosis is due to poor oxygen saturation by the lungs, allowing the patient to breath 100% O2 will augment the lungs' ability to saturate the blood with oxygen, and the partial pressure of oxygen in the arterial blood will rise (usually above 150 mmHg).
Cyanosis	Cyanosis is the appearance of a blue or purple coloration of the skin or mucous membranes due to the tissues near the skin surface being low on oxygen. The onset of cyanosis is 2.5 g/dL of deoxyhemoglobin. The bluish color is more readily apparent in those with high hemoglobin counts than it is with those with anemia.
Glucose transporter	Glucose transporters (GLUT or SLC2A family) are a family of membrane proteins found in most mammalian cells. Structure Glucose transporters are integral membrane proteins that contain 12 membrane-spanning helices with both the amino and carboxyl termini exposed on the cytoplasmic side of the plasma membrane. Glucose transporter proteins transport glucose and related hexoses according to a model of alternate conformation, which predicts that the transporter exposes a single substrate binding site toward either the outside or the inside of the cell.
Hyperinsulinemia	Hyperinsulinemia are excess levels of insulin circulating in the blood than expected relative to the level of glucose. While it is often mistaken for diabetes or hyperglycaemia, hyperinsulinemia can result from a variety of metabolic diseases and conditions. While hyperinsulinemia is often seen in people with type two diabetes mellitus, it is not the cause of the condition and is only one symptom of the disease.
Hypoglycemia	Hypoglycemia, hypoglycæmia or low blood sugar (not to be confused with hyperglycemia) is an abnormally diminished content of glucose in the blood. The term literally means 'low sugar blood' . It can produce a variety of symptoms and effects but the principal problems arise from an inadequate supply of glucose to the brain, resulting in impairment of function (neuroglycopenia).
Sepsis	Sepsis is a potentially deadly medical condition that is characterized by a whole-body inflammatory state (called a systemic inflammatory response syndrome or SIRS) and the presence of a known or suspected infection. The body may develop this inflammatory response by the immune system to microbes in the blood, urine, lungs, skin, or other tissues.

Differential diagnosis	A differential diagnosis is a systematic diagnostic method used to identify the presence of an entity where multiple alternatives are possible (and the process may be termed differential diagnostic procedure), and may also refer to any of the included candidate alternatives (which may also be termed candidate condition). This method is essentially a process of elimination, or at least, rendering of the probabilities of candidate conditions to negligible levels. In this sense, probabilities are, in fact, imaginative parameters in the mind or hardware of the diagnostician or system, while in reality the target (such as a patient) either has a condition or not with an actual probability of either 0 or 100%.
Glucose-6-phosphate dehydrogenase	Glucose-6-phosphate dehydrogenase is a cytosolic enzyme in the pentose phosphate pathway , a metabolic pathway that supplies reducing energy to cells (such as erythrocytes) by maintaining the level of the co-enzyme nicotinamide adenine dinucleotide phosphate (NADPH). The NADPH in turn maintains the level of glutathione in these cells that helps protect the red blood cells against oxidative damage. Of greater quantitative importance is the production of NADPH for tissues actively engaged in biosynthesis of fatty acids and/or isoprenoids, such as the liver, mammary glands, adipose tissue, and the adrenal glands.
Hyperbilirubinemia	Jaundice, also known as icterus (attributive adjective: icteric), is a yellowish discoloration of the skin, the conjunctival membranes over the sclerae (whites of the eyes), and other mucous membranes caused by hyperbilirubinemia. This hyperbilirubinemia subsequently causes increased levels of bilirubin in the extracellular fluids. Typically, the concentration of bilirubin in the plasma must exceed 1.5 mg/dL, three times the usual value of approximately 0.5 mg/dL, for the coloration to be easily visible.
Kernicterus	Kernicterus is a term used to describe bilirubin-induced brain dysfunction. Bilirubin is a highly neurotoxic substance that may become elevated in the serum, a condition known as hyperbilirubinemia. Hyperbilirubinemia may cause bilirubin to accumulate in the gray matter of the central nervous system, potentially causing irreversible neurological damage.
Cardiopulmonary resuscitation	Cardiopulmonary resuscitation is an emergency procedure which is performed in an effort to manually preserve intact brain function until further measures are taken to restore spontaneous blood circulation and breathing in a person in cardiac arrest. It is indicated in those who are unresponsive with no breathing or abnormal breathing, for example agonal respirations. It may be performed both in and outside of a hospital.
Physiology	Physiology is the science of the function of living systems. This includes how organisms, organ systems, organs, cells, and bio-molecules carry out the chemical or physical functions that exist in a living system. The highest honor awarded in physiology is the Nobel Prize in Physiology or Medicine, awarded since 1901 by the Royal Swedish Academy of Sciences.

Chapter 13. COMMON AND UNCOMMON PROBLEMS OF THE TERM NEWBORN

Exchange transfusion	An exchange transfusion is a medical treatment in which apheresis is used to remove one person's red blood cells or platelets and replace them with transfused blood products. Exchange transfusion is used in the treatment of a number of diseases, including:•Sickle cell disease•Thrombotic thrombocytopenic purpura (TTP)•Hemolytic disease of the newbornDescription An exchange transfusion requires that the patient's blood can be removed and replaced. In most cases, this involves placing one or more thin tubes, called catheters, into a blood vessel.
Home care	Home Care, (also referred to as domiciliary care or social care), is health care or supportive care provided in the patient's home by healthcare professionals (often referred to as home health care or formal care). Often, the term home care is used to distinguish non-medical care or custodial care, which is care that is provided by persons who are not nurses, doctors, or other licensed medical personnel, as opposed to home health care that is provided by licensed personnel. Professionals providing care Professionals providing home care include: Licensed practical nurses, Registered nurses, Home Care Aids, and Social workers.
Phototherapy	Light therapy or Phototherapy consists of exposure to daylight or to specific wavelengths of light using lasers, light-emitting diodes, fluorescent lamps, dichroic lamps or very bright, full-spectrum light, for a prescribed amount of time and, in some cases, at a specific time of day. Light therapy is used to treat Acne vulgaris, seasonal affective disorder, neonatal jaundice, and is part of the standard treatment regimen for delayed sleep phase syndrome with some support for its use with non-seasonal psychiatric disorders. Sunlight was long known to improve acne, and this was thought to be due to antibacterial and other effects of the ultraviolet spectrum; which cannot be used as a treatment due to the likelihood of skin damage in the long term.
Annular pancreas	Annular pancreas is a rare condition in which the second part of the duodenum is surrounded by a ring of pancreatic tissue continuous with the head of the pancreas. This portion of the pancreas can constrict the duodenum and block or impair the flow of food to the rest of the intestines. It is estimated to occur in 1 out of 12,000 to 15,000 newborns.
Duodenal atresia	Duodenal atresia is the congenital absence or complete closure of a portion of the lumen of the duodenum. Approximately 20-40% of all infants with duodenal atresia have Down syndrome.. Approximately 8% all infants with Down syndrome have duodenal atresia.

Esophageal atresia	Esophageal atresia is a congenital medical condition (birth defect) which affects the alimentary tract. It causes the esophagus to end in a blind-ended pouch rather than connecting normally to the stomach. It comprises a variety of congenital anatomic defects that are caused by an abnormal embryological development of the esophagus.
Gastroesophageal reflux	Gastroesophageal reflux disease (GERD), gastro-oesophageal reflux disease (GORD), gastric reflux disease, or acid reflux disease is defined as chronic symptoms or mucosal damage produced by the abnormal reflux in the oesophagus. This is commonly due to transient or permanent changes in the barrier between the oesophagus and the stomach. This can be due to incompetence of the lower esophageal sphincter, transient lower oesophageal sphincter relaxation, impaired expulsion of gastric reflux from the oesophagus, or a hiatal hernia.
Intestinal malrotation	Intestinal malrotation is a congenital anomaly of rotation of the midgut (embryologically, the gut undergoes a complex rotation outside the abdomen). As a result:•the small bowel is found predominantly on the right side of the abdomen•the cecum is displaced (from its usual position in the right lower quadrant) into the epigastrium - right hypochondrium•the ligament of Treitz is displaced inferiorly and rightward•fibrous bands (of Ladd) course over the horizontal part of the duodenum (DII), causing intestinal obstruction.•the small intestine has an unusually narrow base, and therefore the midgut is prone to volvulus (a twisting that can obstruct the mesenteric blood vessels and cause intestinal ischemia).Associated conditions This can lead to a number of disease manifestations such as:•Acute midgut volvulus•Chronic midgut volvulus•Acute duodenal obstruction•Chronic duodenal obstruction•Internal herniation•Superior mesenteric artery syndromeCauses The exact causes are not known. It is not associated with a particular gene, but there is some evidence of recurrence in families.
Muscular dystrophies	Muscular dystrophy refers to a group of hereditary muscle diseases that weaken the muscles that move the human body. muscular dystrophies are characterized by progressive skeletal muscle weakness, defects in muscle proteins, and the death of muscle cells and tissue. Nine diseases including Duchenne, Becker, limb girdle, congenital, facioscapulohumeral, myotonic, oculopharyngeal, distal, and Emery-Dreifuss are always classified as muscular dystrophy but there are more than 100 diseases in total with similarities to muscular dystrophy.
Tracheoesophageal fistula	A tracheoesophageal fistula is an abnormal connection (fistula) between the esophagus and the trachea. TEF is a common congenital abnormality, but when occurring late in life is usually the sequela of surgical procedures such as a laryngectomy.

Chapter 13. COMMON AND UNCOMMON PROBLEMS OF THE TERM NEWBORN

Vomiting	Vomiting is the forceful expulsion of the contents of one's stomach through the mouth and sometimes the nose. Vomiting can be caused by a wide variety of conditions; it may present as a specific response to ailments like gastritis or poisoning, or as a non-specific sequela of disorders ranging from brain tumors and elevated intracranial pressure to overexposure to ionizing radiation. The feeling that one is about to vomit is called nausea, which usually precedes, but does not always lead to, vomiting.
Cerebral palsy	Cerebral palsy is an umbrella term encompassing a group of non-progressive, non-contagious motor conditions that cause physical disability in human development, chiefly in the various areas of body movement. Cerebral refers to the cerebrum, which is the affected area of the brain (although the disorder most likely involves connections between the cortex and other parts of the brain such as the cerebellum), and palsy refers to disorder of movement. Furthermore, 'paralytic disorders' are not cerebral palsy - the condition of quadriplegia, therefore, should not be confused with spastic quadriplegia, nor tardive dyskinesia with dyskinetic cerebral palsy, nor diplegia with spastic diplegia, and so on.
Supraventricular tachycardia	Supraventricular tachycardia is a general term that refers to any rapid heart rhythm originating above the ventricular tissue. Supraventricular tachycardias can be contrasted to the potentially more dangerous ventricular tachycardias - rapid rhythms that originate within the ventricular tissue. Although technically an SVT can be due to any supraventricular cause, the term is often used by clinicians to refer to one specific cause of SVT, namely Paroxysmal supraventricular tachycardia.
Necrotizing enterocolitis	Necrotizing enterocolitis is a medical condition primarily seen in premature infants, where portions of the bowel undergo necrosis (tissue death). The condition is typically seen in premature infants, and the timing of its onset is generally inversely proportional to the gestational age of the baby at birth, i.e. the earlier a baby is born, the later signs of NEC are typically seen. Initial symptoms include feeding intolerance, increased gastric residuals, abdominal distension and bloody stools.
Imaging	Imaging is the representation or reproduction of an object's outward form; especially a visual representation (i.e., the formation of an image). · Chemical Imaging, the simultaneous measurement of spectra and pictures · Creation of a disk image, a file which contains the exact content of a non-volatile computer data storage medium.

Nasogastric tube	Nasogastric intubation is a medical process involving the insertion of a plastic tube (Nasogastric tube, NG tube) through the nose, past the throat, and down into the stomach. The main use of a Nasogastric tube is for feeding and for administering drugs and other oral agents such as activated charcoal. For drugs and for minimal quantities of liquid, a syringe is used for injection into the tube.
Hemostasis	Hemostasis is a process which causes bleeding to stop, meaning to keep blood within a damaged blood vessel (the opposite of hemostasis is hemorrhage). Most of the time this includes blood changing from a liquid to a solid state. All situations that may lead to hemostasis are portrayed by the Virchow's triad.
Thrombocytopenia	Laboratory findings in various platelet and coagulation disordersDiagnosis Laboratory tests might include: full blood count, liver enzymes, renal function, vitamin B_{12} levels, folic acid levels, erythrocyte sedimentation rate, and peripheral blood smear. If the cause for the low platelet count remains unclear, a bone marrow biopsy is usually recommended, to differentiate whether the low platelet count is due to decreased production or peripheral destruction. Thrombocytopenia in hospitalized alcoholics may be caused by splenomegaly, folate deficiency, and, most frequently, a direct toxic effect of alcohol on production, survival time, and function of platelets.
Thrombocytopenic purpura	Thrombocytopenic purpura are purpura associated with a reduction in circulating blood platelets which can result from a variety of causes. By tradition, the term idiopathic thrombocytopenic purpura is used when the cause is idiopathic. However, most cases are now considered to be immune-mediated.
Disseminated intravascular coagulation	Disseminated intravascular coagulation also known as disseminated intravascular coagulopathy or consumptive coagulopathy, is a pathological activation of coagulation (blood clotting) mechanisms that happens in response to a variety of diseases. DIC leads to the formation of small blood clots inside the blood vessels throughout the body. As the small clots consume coagulation proteins and platelets, normal coagulation is disrupted and abnormal bleeding occurs from the skin (e.g. from sites where blood samples were taken), the gastrointestinal tract, the respiratory tract and surgical wounds.

Chapter 13. COMMON AND UNCOMMON PROBLEMS OF THE TERM NEWBORN

Vitamin K	Vitamin K is a group of structurally similar, fat-soluble vitamins that are needed for the posttranslational modification of certain proteins required for blood coagulation and in metabolic pathways in bone and other tissue. They are 2-methyl-1,4-naphthoquinone (3-) derivatives. This group of vitamins includes two natural vitamers: vitamin K_1 and vitamin K_2.
Genetics	Genetics, a discipline of biology, is the science of genes, heredity, and variation in living organisms.
	Genetics deals with the molecular structure and function of genes, gene behavior in context of a cell or organism (e.g. dominance and epigenetics), patterns of inheritance from parent to offspring, and gene distribution, variation and change in populations,such as through Genome-Wide Association Studies. Given that genes are universal to living organisms, genetics can be applied to the study of all living systems, from viruses and bacteria, through plants and domestic animals, to humans (as in medical genetics).
Hemorrhagic disease of the newborn	Hemorrhagic disease of the newborn is a coagulation disturbance in newborns due to vitamin K deficiency. As a consequence of vitamin K deficiency there is an impaired production of coagulation factors II, VII, IX, X, C and S by the liver.
	Newborns are relatively vitamin K deficient for a variety of reasons.
Liver disease	Liver disease is an umbrella term referring to damage to or disease of the liver.
	The symptoms related to liver dysfunction include both physical signs and a variety of symptoms related to digestive problems, blood sugar problems, immune disorders, abnormal absorption of fats, and metabolism problems.
	The malabsorption of fats may lead to symptoms that include indigestion, reflux, deficit of fatsoluble vitamins, hemorrhoids, gall stones, intolerance to fatty foods, intolerance to alcohol, nausea and vomiting attacks, abdominal bloating, and constipation.
Hyperekplexia	Hyperekplexia is a neurologic disorder classically characterised by startle responses to tactile or acoustic stimuli and hypertonia. The hypertonia may be predominantly truncal, attenuated during sleep and less prominent after a year of age. Hyperekplexia has been linked to genetic defects in a number of different gene families, all of which play an important role in glycine neurotransmission.
Sandifer syndrome	Sandifer syndrome is a rare paediatric medical disorder, characterised by gastrointestinal symptoms and associated neurological features There is a significant correlation between the syndrome and gastroesophageal reflux disease (GERD), however it is estimated to occur in less than 1% of children with reflux.

	Onset is usually confined to infancy and early childhood, with peak prevalence at 18-36 months. In rare cases, particularly where the child is severely mentally impaired, onset may extend to adolescence.
Seizure	An epileptic Seizure, occasionally referred to as a fit, is defined as a transient symptom of 'abnormal excessive or synchronous neuronal activity in the brain'. The outward effect can be as dramatic as a wild thrashing movement (tonic-clonic Seizure) or as mild as a brief loss of awareness. It can manifest as an alteration in mental state, tonic or clonic movements, convulsions, and various other psychic symptoms (such as déjà vu or jamais vu).
Status epilepticus	Status epilepticus is a life-threatening condition in which the brain is in a state of persistent seizure. Definitions vary, but traditionally it is defined as one continuous unremitting seizure lasting longer than 30 minutes, or recurrent seizures without regaining consciousness between seizures for greater than 30 minutes. Treatment is, however, generally started after the seizure has lasted 5 minutes.
Febrile seizure	A febrile seizure, is a convulsion associated with a significant rise in body temperature. They most commonly occur in children between the ages of 6 months to 6 years and are twice as common in boys as in girls. The direct cause of a febrile seizure is not known; however, it is normally precipitated by a recent upper respiratory infection or gastroenteritis.
Palliative care	Palliative care is an area of healthcare that focuses on relieving and preventing the suffering of patients. Unlike hospice care, palliative medicine is appropriate for patients in all disease stages, including those undergoing treatment for curable illnesses and those living with chronic diseases, as well as patients who are nearing the end of life. Palliative medicine utilizes a multidisciplinary approach to patient care, relying on input from physicians, pharmacists, nurses, chaplains, social workers, psychologists, and other allied health professionals in formulating a plan of care to relieve suffering in all areas of a patient's life.
Pyridoxine deficiency	Pyridoxine deficiency is a paediatric disease due to a lack of pyridoxine (or vitamin B6). The disease presents with several key symptoms including seizures, irritability, cheilitis (inflammation of the lips), conjunctivitis and neurologic symptoms. It usually becomes noticeable within the first 12 months of life in infants with a lack of pyridoxine, a coenzyme responsible for numerous essential metabolic reactions in humans.
Kyphoscoliosis	Kyphoscoliosis describes an abnormal curvature of the spine in both a coronal and sagittal plane. It is a combination of kyphosis and scoliosis.

Chapter 13. COMMON AND UNCOMMON PROBLEMS OF THE TERM NEWBORN

Subgaleal hemorrhage	Subgaleal hemorrhage is bleeding in the potential space between the skull periosteum and the scalp galea aponeurosis. Majority (90%) result from vacuum applied to the head at delivery (Ventouse assisted delivery). The vacuum assist ruptures the emissary veins (connections between dural sinus and scalp veins) leading to accumulation of blood under the aponeurosis of the scalp muscle and superficial to the periosteum.
Risk factor	In epidemiology, a risk factor is a variable associated with an increased risk of disease or infection. Sometimes, determinant is also used, being a variable associated with either increased or decreased risk. Risk factors or determinants are correlational and not necessarily causal, because correlation does not prove causation.
Intracranial hemorrhage	An intracranial hemorrhage is a hemorrhage, or bleeding, within the skull. Intracranial bleeding occurs when a blood vessel within the skull is ruptured or leaks. It can result from physical trauma (as occurs in head injury) or nontraumatic causes (as occurs in hemorrhagic stroke) such as a ruptured aneurysm.
Skull fracture	Skull fracture is the term used to describe a break in one or more of the eight bones which form the cranial portion of the skull usually occurring as a result of blunt force trauma. If the force of the impact is excessive the bone may fracture at or near the site of the impact and may cause damage to the underlying physical structures contained within the skull such as the membranes, blood vessels, and brain, even in the absence of a fracture. While an uncomplicated skull fracture can occur without associated physical or neurological damage and is in itself usually not clinically significant, a fracture in healthy bone indicates that a substantial amount of force has been applied and increases the possibility of associated injury.
Subconjunctival hemorrhage	A subconjunctival hemorrhage is bleeding underneath the conjunctiva. The conjunctiva contains many small, fragile blood vessels that are easily ruptured or broken. When this happens, blood leaks into the space between the conjunctiva and sclera.
Brachial plexus	The Brachial plexus is an arrangement of nerve fibers, running from the spine, formed by the ventral rami of the lower four cervical and first thoracic nerve roots (C5-T1). It proceeds through the neck, the axilla (armpit region), and into the arm.

Clavicle fracture	A clavicle fracture is a bone fracture in the clavicle, or collarbone. It is often caused by a fall onto an outstretched upper extremity, a fall onto a shoulder, or a direct blow to the clavicle. Many research projects are underway regarding the medical healing process of clavicle fractures.
Humerus fracture	A humerus fracture can be classified by the location of the humerus involved: the upper end, the shaft, or the lower end. Certain lesions are commonly associated with fractures to specific areas of the humerus. At the upper end, the surgical neck of the humerus and anatomical neck of humerus can both be involved, though fractures of the surgical neck are more common.
Phrenic nerve	The phrenic nerve, but also receives contributions from the 5th and 3rd cervical nerves (C3-C5) in humans. The phrenic nerves contain motor, sensory, and sympathetic nerve fibers. These nerves provide the only motor supply to the diaphragm as well as sensation to the central tendon.
Spinal cord	The Spinal cord is a long, thin, tubular bundle of nervous tissue and support cells that extends from the brain. The brain and Spinal cord together make up the central nervous system. The Spinal cord extends down to the space in between the first and second lumbar vertebrae.
Nerve injury	Nerve injury is injury to nervous tissue. There is no single classification system that can describe all the many variations of nerve injury. Most systems attempt to correlate the degree of injury with symptoms, pathology and prognosis.
Respiratory distress	Respiratory distress is a medical term that refers to both difficulty in breathing, and to the psychological experience associated with such difficulty, even if there is no physiological basis for experiencing such distress. The physical presentation of respiratory distress is generally referred to as labored breathing,s while the sensation of respiratory distress is called shortness of breath or dyspnea. Respiratory distress occurs in connection with various physical ailments, such as acute respiratory distress syndrome, a serious reaction to various forms of injuries to the lung, and infant respiratory distress syndrome, a syndrome in premature infants caused by developmental insufficiency of surfactant production and structural immaturity in the lungs.
Neonatal sepsis	In common clinical usage, neonatal sepsis specifically refers to the presence of a bacterial blood stream infection (BSI) (such as meningitis, pneumonia, pyelonephritis, or gastroenteritis) in the setting of fever. Criteria with regards to hemodynamic compromise or respiratory failure are not useful clinically because these symptoms often do not arise in neonates until death is imminent and unpreventable.

Chapter 13. COMMON AND UNCOMMON PROBLEMS OF THE TERM NEWBORN

Prevention	Prevention refers to: · Preventive medicine · Hazard Prevention, the process of risk study and elimination and mitigation in emergency management · Risk Prevention · Risk management · Preventive maintenance · Crime Prevention · Prevention, an album by Scottish band De Rosa · Prevention a magazine about health in the United States · Prevent (company), a textile company from Slovenia
Blood culture	Blood culture is a microbiological culture of blood. It is employed to detect infections that are spreading through the bloodstream (such as bacteremia, septicemia amongst others). This is possible because the bloodstream is usually a sterile environment.
C-reactive protein	C-reactive protein is a protein found in the blood, the levels of which rise in response to inflammation (i.e. C-reactive protein is an acute-phase protein). Its physiological role is to bind to phosphocholine expressed on the surface of dead or dying cells (and some types of bacteria) in order to activate the complement system via the C1Q complex. CRP is synthesized by the liver in response to factors released by fat cells (adipocytes).
Genital herpes	Herpes genitalis (or genital herpes) refers to a genital infection by Herpes simplex virus. Following the classification HSV into two distinct categories of HSV-1 and HSV-2 in the 1960s, it was established that 'HSV-2 was below the waist, HSV-1 was above the waist'. Although genital herpes is largely believed to be caused by HSV-2, genital HSV-1 infections are increasing and now exceed 50% in certain populations, and that rule of thumb no longer applies.
Weight gain	Weight gain is an increase in body weight. This can be either an increase in muscle mass, fat deposits, or excess fluids such as water. Muscle gain or weight gain can occur as a result of exercise or bodybuilding, in which muscle size is increased through strength training.
Aplastic anemia	Aplastic anemia is a condition where bone marrow does not produce sufficient new cells to replenish blood cells. The condition, as the name indicates, involves both aplasia and anemia. Typically, anemia refers to low red blood cell counts, but aplastic anemia patients have lower counts of all three blood cell types: red blood cells, white blood cells, and platelets, termed pancytopenia.
Thermoregulation	Thermoregulation is the ability of an organism to keep its body temperature within certain boundaries, even when the surrounding temperature is very different.

	This process is one aspect of homeostasis: a dynamic state of stability between an animal's internal environment and its external environment (the study of such processes in zoology has been called ecophysiology or physiological ecology). If the body is unable to maintain a normal temperature and it increases significantly above normal, a condition known as hyperthermia occurs.
Immunization	Immunization, is the process by which an individual's immune system becomes fortified against an agent (known as the immunogen).
	When this system is exposed to molecules that are foreign to the body, called non-self, it will orchestrate an immune response, and it will also develop the ability to quickly respond to a subsequent encounter because of immunological memory. This is a function of the adaptive immune system.
Substance abuse	Substance abuse, refers to a maladaptive patterned use of a substance (drug) in which the user consumes the substance in amounts or with methods not condoned by medical professionals. Substance abuse/drug abuse is not limited to mood-altering or psycho-active drugs. Activity is also considered substance abuse when inappropriately used (as in steroids for performance enhancement in sports).
Drug use	
	Drugs can be used in many different ways, as detailed below.
	People can use drugs to relieve pain or discomfort or to cure or prevent disease.
	Recreational drug use is the use of psychoactive drugs for recreational purposes rather than for work, medical or spiritual purposes, although the distinction is not always clear.
Pain management	Pain management is a branch of medicine employing an interdisciplinary approach for easing the suffering and improving the quality of life of those living with pain. The typical pain management team includes medical practitioners, clinical psychologists, physiotherapists, occupational therapists, and nurse practitioners. Pain sometimes resolves promptly once the underlying trauma or pathology has healed, and is treated by one practitioner, with drugs such as analgesics and (occasionally) anxiolytics.
Regional analgesia	Regional analgesia blocks passage of pain impulses through a nerve by depositing an analgesic drug close to the nerve trunk, cutting off sensory innervation to the region it supplies. The drug is normally injected at a site where the nerve is unprotected by bone.
Koplik spots	Koplik spots are a prodromic viral enanthem of measles manifesting on the first day of rash.

	They are characterized as clustered, white lesions on the buccal mucosa near each Stenson's duct and are pathognomonic for measles. The textbook description of Koplik spots is ulcerated mucosal lesions marked by necrosis, neutrophilic exudate, and neovascularization.
Syphilis	Syphilis is a sexually transmitted infection caused by the spirochete bacterium Treponema pallidum subspecies pallidum. The primary route of transmission is through sexual contact; however, it may also be transmitted from mother to fetus during pregnancy or at birth, resulting in congenital syphilis. Other human diseases caused by related Treponema pallidum include yaws (subspecies pertenue), pinta (subspecies carateum) and bejel (subspecies endemicum).
Toxoplasmosis	Toxoplasmosis is a parasitic disease caused by the protozoan Toxoplasma gondii. The parasite infects most genera of warm-blooded animals, including humans, but the primary host is the felid (cat) family. Animals are infected by eating infected meat, by ingestion of feces of a cat that has itself recently been infected, or by transmission from mother to fetus.
Tuberculosis	Tuberculosis, MTB or TB (short for tubercles bacillus) is a common and in some cases deadly infectious disease caused by various strains of mycobacteria, usually Mycobacterium tuberculosis in humans. Tuberculosis usually attacks the lungs but can also affect other parts of the body. It is spread through the air when people who have an active MTB infection cough, sneeze, or otherwise transmit their saliva through the air.
Community-acquired pneumonia	Community-acquired pneumonia is a term used to describe one of several diseases in which individuals who have not recently been hospitalized develop an infection of the lungs (pneumonia). Community acquired pneumonia is a common illness and can affect people of all ages. Community acquired pneumonia often causes problems like difficulty in breathing, fever, chest pains, and a cough.
Congenital syphilis	Congenital syphilis is syphilis present in utero and at birth, and occurs when a child is born to a mother with secondary syphilis. Untreated syphilis results in a high risk of a bad outcome of pregnancy, including mulberry molars in the fetus. Syphilis can cause miscarriages, premature births, stillbirths, or death of newborn babies.
Leydig cell	Leydig cells, also known as interstitial cells of Leydig, are found adjacent to the seminiferous tubules in the testicle. They produce testosterone in the presence of luteinizing hormone (LH). Leydig cells are polyhedral in shape, display a large prominent nucleus, an eosinophilic cytoplasm and numerous lipid-filled vesicles.
Sertoli cell	A Sertoli cell is a 'nurse' cell of the testes that is part of a seminiferous tubule.

	It is activated by follicle-stimulating hormone and has FSH-receptor on its membranes. It is specifically located in the convoluted seminiferous tubules (since this is the only place in the testes where the spermatozoa is produced). Functions

Because its main function is to nourish the developing sperm cells through the stages of spermatogenesis, the Sertoli cell has also been called the 'mother' or 'nurse' cell. |
| Sex determination | A sex-determination system is a biological system that determines the development of sexual characteristics in an organism. Most sexual organisms have two sexes. In many cases, sex determination is genetic: males and females have different alleles or even different genes that specify their sexual morphology. |
| Y chromosome | The Y chromosome is one of the two sex-determining chromosomes in most mammals, including humans. In mammals, it contains the gene SRY, which triggers testis development if present. The human Y chromosome is composed of about 50 million base pairs. |
| High-mobility group | High-Mobility Group is a group of chromosomal proteins that help with transcription, replication, recombination, and DNA repair.

The proteins are subdivided into 3 superfamilies each containing a characteristic functional domain: •A - contains an AT-hook domain •A1•A2•B - contains a -box domain •B1•B2•B3•B4•N - contains a nucleosomal binding domain domain •N1•N2•N3•N4•Sex-Determining Region Y Protein•TCF Transcription Factors •Lymphoid enhancer-binding factor 1•T Cell Transcription Factor 1

Proteins containing any of these embedded in their sequence are known as motif proteins. -box proteins are found in a variety of eukaryotic organisms. |
| Androgen insensitivity syndrome | Androgen insensitivity syndrome is a condition that results in the partial or complete inability of the cell to respond to androgens. The unresponsiveness of the cell to the presence of androgenic hormones can impair or prevent the masculinization of male genitalia in the developing fetus, as well as the development of male secondary sexual characteristics at puberty, but does not significantly impair female genital or sexual development. As such, the insensitivity to androgens is only clinically significant when it occurs in genetic males (i.e. individuals with a Y-chromosome, or more specifically, an SRY gene). |
| Gonadal dysgenesis | Gonadal dysgenesis is a term used to describe multiple reproductive system development disorders. They are conditions of genetic origin. It is characterized by a progressive loss of primordial germ cells on the developing gonads of an embryo. |

Congenital adrenal hyperplasia	Congenital adrenal hyperplasia refers to any of several autosomal recessive diseases resulting from mutations of genes for enzymes mediating the biochemical steps of production of cortisol from cholesterol by the adrenal glands (steroidogenesis). Most of these conditions involve excessive or deficient production of sex steroids and can alter development of primary or secondary sex characteristics in some affected infants, children, or adults. Associated conditions The symptoms of CAH vary depending upon the form of CAH and the gender of the patient.
Mixed gonadal dysgenesis	Mixed gonadal dysgenesis is a condition of unusual and asymmetrical gonadal development leading to an unassigned sex differentiation. A number of differences have been reported in the karyotype, most commonly a mosaicism 45,X/ 46, XY. If Turner syndrome is defined as a condition where one sex chromosome is absent or abnormal, mixed gonadal dysgenesis may be interpreted as a specific variation of Turner's. The phenotypical expression may be ambiguous, intersex, or male, or female pending the extent of the mosaicism.
True hermaphroditism	True hermaphroditism is a medical term for an intersex condition in which an individual is born with ovarian and testicular tissue. There may be an ovary underneath each testicle on the other, but more commonly one or both gonads is an ovotestis containing both types of tissue. It is rare--so far undocumented--for both types of gonadal tissue to function.
Turner syndrome	Turner syndrome, of which monosomy X (absence of an entire sex chromosome, the Barr body) is most common. It is a chromosomal abnormality in which all or part of one of the sex chromosomes is absent (unaffected humans have 46 chromosomes, of which two are sex chromosomes). Typical females have two X chromosomes, but in Turner syndrome, one of those sex chromosomes is missing or has other abnormalities.
Sex assignment	Sex assignment refers to the assigning (naming) of the biological sex at the birth of a baby. In the majority of births, a relative, midwife, or physician inspects the genitalia when the baby is delivered, sees ordinary male or female genitalia, and declares, 'it's a girl' or 'it's a boy' without the expectation of ambiguity. Assignment may also be done prior to birth through prenatal sex discernment.
Surgery	Surgery is an ancient medical specialty that uses operative manual and instrumental techniques on a patient to investigate and/or treat a pathological condition such as disease or injury, or to help improve bodily function or appearance.

	An act of performing surgery may be called a surgical procedure, operation, or simply surgery. In this context, the verb operate means to perform surgery.
enetic disorder	A genetic disorder is an illness caused by abnormalities in genes or chromosomes, especially a condition that is present from before birth. Most genetic disorders are quite rare and affect one person in every several thousands or millions. A genetic disorder may or may not be a heritable disorder.
HARGE syndrome	CHARGE syndrome is a syndrome caused by a genetic disorder. It was first described in 1979. In 1981, the term 'CHARGE' came into use as an acronym for the set of unusual congenital features seen in a number of newborn children.
ysmorphic feature	Dysmorphic feature is a medical term referring to a difference of body structure that is suggestive of a congenital disorder, genetic syndrome, or birth defect. A dysmorphic feature can be a minor and isolated birth defect (e.g., clinodactyly, not accompanied by other features or problems). Alternatively it can be one of a combination of features signaling a serious multi-system syndrome (e.g., the epicanthal folds of Down's syndrome).
oldenhar syndrome	Goldenhar syndrome (also known as Oculo-Auriculo-Vertebral (OAV) syndrome) is a rare congenital defect characterized by incomplete development of the ear, nose, soft palate, lip, and mandible. It is associated with anomalous development of the first branchial arch and second branchial arch. Common clinical manifestations include limbal dermoids, preauricular skin tags, and strabismus.
etralogy of Fallot	Tetralogy of Fallot is a congenital heart defect which is classically understood to involve four anatomical abnormalities (although only three of them are always present). It is the most common cyanotic heart defect, and the most common cause of blue baby syndrome. It was described in 1672 by Niels Stensen, in 1773 by Edward Sandifort, and in 1888 by the French physician Étienne-Louis Arthur Fallot, after whom it is named.
eletion	In genetics, a deletion (also called gene deletion, deficiency, or deletion mutation) (sign: Δ) is a mutation (a genetic aberration) in which a part of a chromosome or a sequence of DNA is missing. Deletion is the loss of genetic material. Any number of nucleotides can be deleted, from a single base to an entire piece of chromosome.
ypotonia	Hypotonia is a state of low muscle tone (the amount of tension or resistance to movement in a muscle), often involving reduced muscle strength.

	Hypotonia is not a specific medical disorder, but a potential manifestation of many different diseases and disorders that affect motor nerve control by the brain or muscle strength. Recognizing hypotonia, even in early infancy, is usually relatively straightforward, but diagnosing the underlying cause can be difficult and often unsuccessful.
Urea cycle	The urea cycle is a cycle of biochemical reactions occurring in many animals that produces urea $((NH_2)_2CO)$ from ammonia (NH_3). This cycle was the first metabolic cycle discovered (Hans Krebs and Kurt Henseleit, 1932), 5 years before the discovery of the TCA cycle. In mammals, the urea cycle takes place primarily in the liver, and to a lesser extent in the kidney.
Fatty acid	In chemistry, especially biochemistry, a fatty acid is a carboxylic acid with a long aliphatic tail (chain), which is either saturated or unsaturated. Most naturally occurring fatty acids have a chain of an even number of carbon atoms, from 4 to 28. Fatty acids are usually derived from triglycerides or phospholipids. When they are not attached to other molecules, they are known as 'free' fatty acids.
Oxidative phosphorylation	Oxidative phosphorylation is a metabolic pathway that uses energy released by the oxidation of nutrients to produce adenosine triphosphate (ATP). Although the many forms of life on earth use a range of different nutrients, almost all aerobic organisms carry out oxidative phosphorylation to produce ATP, the molecule that supplies energy to metabolism. This pathway is probably so pervasive because it is a highly efficient way of releasing energy, compared to alternative fermentation processes such as anaerobic glycolysis.
Pyruvate dehydrogenase	Pyruvate dehydrogenase is the first component enzyme of pyruvate dehydrogenase complex (PDC). The pyruvate dehydrogenase complex contributes to transforming pyruvate into acetyl-CoA by a process called pyruvate decarboxylation. Acetyl-CoA may then be used in the citric acid cycle to carry out cellular respiration, so pyruvate dehydrogenase contributes to linking the glycolysis metabolic pathway to the citric acid cycle and releasing energy via NADH. EC 1.2.4.1.
Process	In anatomy, a process (apophysis) is a projection or outgrowth of tissue from a larger body. The vertebra has several kinds of processes, such as: transverse process, prezygapophysis, postzygapophysis. Examples of processes include:•the mastoid process•the xiphoid process•the acromion process•the spinous process extends from rearward from the centre of each vertebra.•coracoid process•vertebral transverse processes.
Sickle-cell disease	Sickle-cell disease or sickle-cell anaemia or drepanocytosis, is an autosomal recessive genetic blood disorder with overdominance, characterized by red blood cells that assume an abnormal, rigid, sickle shape. Sickling decreases the cells' flexibility and results in a risk of various complications.

Hemoglobinopathies	Hematologic diseases are disorders which primarily affect the blood.
	· Hemoglobinopathies
	· Sickle-cell disease · Thalassemia · Methemoglobinemia · Anemias (lack of red blood cells or hemoglobin)
	· Iron deficiency anemia · Megaloblastic anemia
	· Vitamin B_{12} deficiency
	· Pernicious anemia · Folate deficiency · Hemolytic anemias (destruction of red blood cells)
	· Genetic disorders of RBC membrane
	· Hereditary spherocytosis · Hereditary elliptocytosis · Genetic disorders of RBC metabolism
	· Glucose-6-phosphate dehydrogenase deficiency (G6PD) · Pyruvate kinase deficiency · Immune mediated hemolytic anemia (direct Coombs test is positive)
	· Autoimmune hemolytic anemia
	· Warm antibody autoimmune hemolytic anemia
	· Idiopathic · Systemic lupus erythematosus (SLE) · Evans' syndrome (antiplatelet antibodies and hemolytic antibodies) · Cold antibody autoimmune hemolytic anemia
	· Idiopathic cold hemagglutinin syndrome · Infectious mononucleosis · Paroxysmal cold hemoglobinuria (rare) · Alloimmune hemolytic anemia
	· Hemolytic disease of the newborn (HDN)
	· Rh disease (Rh D) · ABO hemolytic disease of the newborn · Anti-Kell hemolytic disease of the newborn · Rhesus c hemolytic disease of the newborn · Rhesus E hemolytic disease of the newborn · Other blood group incompatibility (RhC, Rhe, Kid, Duffy, MN, P and others) · Drug induced immune mediated hemolytic anemia
	· Penicillin (high dose) · Methyldopa · Hemoglobinopathies · Paroxysmal nocturnal hemoglobinuria (rare acquired clonal disorder of red blood cell surface proteins) · Direct physical damage to RBCs

· Microangiopathic hemolytic anemia · Secondary to artificial heart valve(s) · Aplastic anemia

· Fanconi anemia · Diamond-Blackfan anemia · Acquired pure red cell aplasia · Decreased numbers of cells

· Myelodysplastic syndrome · Myelofibrosis · Neutropenia (decrease in the number of neutrophils) · Agranulocytosis · Glanzmann's thrombasthenia · Thrombocytopenia (decrease in the number of platelets)

· Idiopathic thrombocytopenic purpura (ITP) · Thrombotic thrombocytopenic purpura (TTP) · Heparin-induced thrombocytopenia (HIT)

· Myeloproliferative disorders (Increased numbers of cells)

· Polycythemia vera (increase in the number of cells in general) · Leukocytosis (increase in the number of white blood cells) · Thrombocytosis (increase in the number of platelets) · Myeloproliferative disorder

· Coagulopathies (disorders of bleeding and coagulation)

· Thrombocytosis · Recurrent thrombosis · Disseminated intravascular coagulation · Disorders of clotting proteins

· Hemophilia

· Hemophilia A · Hemophilia B (also known as Christmas disease) · Hemophilia C · Von Willebrand disease · Disseminated intravascular coagulation · Protein S deficiency · Antiphospholipid syndrome · Disorders of platelets

· Thrombocytopenia · Glanzmann's thrombasthenia · Wiskott-Aldrich syndrome

· Hematological malignancies

· Lymphomas

· Hodgkin's disease · Non-Hodgkin's lymphoma{includes the next eight entries} · Burkitt's lymphoma · Anaplastic large cell lymphoma · Splenic marginal zone lymphoma · Hepatosplenic T-cell lymphoma · Angioimmunoblastic T-cell lymphoma (AILT) · Myelomas

· Multiple myeloma · Waldenström macroglobulinemia · Plasmacytoma · Leukemias

	· Acute lymphocytic leukemia (ALL) · Chronic lymphocytic leukemia (CLL){now included in theCLL/SCLL type NHL} · Acute myelogenous leukemia (AML) · Chronic myelogenous leukemia (CML) · T-cell prolymphocytic leukemia (T-PLL) · B-cell prolymphocytic leukemia (B-PLL) · Chronic neutrophilic leukemia (CNL) · Hairy cell leukemia (HCL) · T-cell large granular lymphocyte leukemia (T-LGL) · Aggressive NK-cell leukemia
	· Hemochromatosis · Asplenia · Hypersplenism
	· Gauchers disease · Monoclonal gammopathy of undetermined significance · Hemophagocytic lymphohistiocytosis
	· Anemia of chronic disease · Infectious mononucleosis · AIDS · Malaria · Leishmaniasis .
ewborn screening	Newborn screening is the process by which infants are screened shortly after birth for a list of disorders that are treatable, but difficult or impossible to detect clinically. Screening programs are often run by state or national governing bodies with the goal of screening all infants born in the jurisdiction. Newborn screening originated when Robert Guthrie developed a method to screen for phenylketonuria, a disorder which could be managed by dietary adjustment if diagnosed early.
ystic fibrosis	Cystic fibrosis is an autosomal recessive genetic disorder affecting most critically the lungs, and also the pancreas, liver, and intestine. It is characterized by abnormal transport of chloride and sodium across an epithelium, leading to thick, viscous secretions.
	The name cystic fibrosis refers to the characteristic scarring (fibrosis) and cyst formation within the pancreas, first recognized in the 1930s.
mmunoreactive ypsinogen	Measurement of Immunoreactive trypsinogen in blood of newborn babies is an assay in rapidly increasing use as a screening test for cystic fibrosis.
inge eating	Binge eating is a pattern of disordered eating which consists of episodes of uncontrollable eating. It is sometimes as a symptom of binge eating disorder or compulsive overeating disorder. During such binges, a person rapidly consumes an excessive amount of food.
iotinidase deficiency	Biotinidase deficiency is an autosomal recessive metabolic disorder in which biotin is not released from proteins in the diet during digestion or from normal protein turnover in the cell. This situation results in biotin deficiency.
	Biotin, sometimes called vitamin B_7, is an important water-soluble nutrient that aids in the metabolism of fats, carbohydrates and proteins.

Chapter 13. COMMON AND UNCOMMON PROBLEMS OF THE TERM NEWBORN

Eating disorder	Eating disorders refer to a group of conditions defined by abnormal eating habits that may involve either insufficient or excessive food intake to the detriment of an individual's physical and mental health. Bulimia nervosa, anorexia nervosa, and binge eating disorder are the most common specific forms in the United Kingdom. Though primarily thought of as affecting females (an estimated 5-10 million being affected in the U.K)., eating disorders affect males as well Template:An estimated 10 - 15% of people with eating disorders are males (Gorgan, 1999).
Galactosemia	Galactosemia is a rare genetic metabolic disorder that affects an individual's ability to metabolize the sugar galactose properly. Although the sugar lactose can metabolize to galactose, galactosemia is not related to and should not be confused with lactose intolerance. Galactosemia follows an autosomal recessive mode of inheritance that confers a deficiency in an enzyme responsible for adequate galactose degradation.
Hypothyroidism	Hypothyroidism is a condition in which the thyroid gland does not make enough thyroid hormone.
	Iodine deficiency is often cited as the most common cause of hypothyroidism worldwide but it can be caused by many other factors. It can result from a lack of a thyroid gland or from iodine-131 treatment, and can also be associated with increased stress.
Mass spectrometry	Mass spectrometry is an analytical technique that measures the mass-to-charge ratio of charged particles. It is used for determining masses of particles, for determining the elemental composition of a sample or molecule, and for elucidating the chemical structures of molecules, such as peptides and other chemical compounds. MS works by ionizing chemical compounds to generate charged molecules or molecule fragments and measuring their mass-to-charge ratios.
Phenylketonuria	Phenylketonuria is an autosomal recessive metabolic genetic disorder characterized by a mutation in the gene for the hepatic enzyme phenylalanine hydroxylase (PAH), rendering it nonfunctional. This enzyme is necessary to metabolize the amino acid phenylalanine (Phe) to the amino acid tyrosine. When PAH activity is reduced, phenylalanine accumulates and is converted into phenylpyruvate (also known as phenylketone), which is detected in the urine.
Tandem mass spectrometry	Tandem mass spectrometry, also known as MS/MS, involves multiple steps of mass spectrometry selection, with some form of fragmentation occurring in between the stages.
	Multiple stages of mass analysis separation can be accomplished with individual mass spectrometer elements separated in space or in a single mass spectrometer with the MS steps separated in time.

Homocystinuria	Homocystinuria, is an inherited disorder of the metabolism of the amino acid methionine, often involving cystathionine beta synthase. It is an inherited autosomal recessive trait, which means a child needs to inherit a copy of the defective gene from each parent to be affected. This defect leads to a multisystemic disorder of the connective tissue, muscles, CNS, and cardiovascular system.
Maple syrup urine disease	Maple syrup urine disease also called branched-chain ketoaciduria, is an autosomal recessive metabolic disorder affecting branched-chain amino acids. It is one type of organic acidemia. The condition gets its name from the distinctive sweet odor of affected infants' urine.
Organic acid	An organic acid is an organic compound with acidic properties. The most common organic acid s are the carboxylic acids whose acidity is associated with their carboxyl group -COOH. Sulfonic acids, containing the group $-SO_2OH$, are relatively stronger acids. The relative stability of the conjugate base of the acid determines its acidity.
Tyrosinemia	Tyrosinemia is an error of metabolism, usually inborn, in which the body cannot effectively break down the amino acid tyrosine. Symptoms include liver and kidney disturbances and mental retardation. Untreated, tyrosinemia can be fatal.
Urea cycle disorder	An urea cycle disorder is responsible for removing ammonia from the blood stream. The urea cycle involves a series of biochemical steps in which nitrogen, a waste product of protein metabolism, is removed from the blood and converted to urea. Normally, the urea is transferred into the urine and removed from the body.
Propionic acidemia	Propionic acidemia, propionyl-CoA carboxylase deficiency and ketotic glycinemia, is an autosomal recessive metabolic disorder, classified as a branched-chain organic acidemia. The disorder presents in the early neonatal period with progressive encephalopathy. Death can occur quickly, due to secondary hyperammonemia, infection, cardiomyopathy, or basal ganglial stroke.
Continuous positive airway pressure	Continuous positive airway pressure is the use of continuous positive pressure to maintain a continuous level of positive airway pressure. It is functionally similar to P_{EEP}, except that PEEP is an applied pressure against exhalation and C_{PAP} is a pressure applied by a constant flow. The ventilator does not cycle during C_{PAP}, no additional pressure above the level of C_{PAP} is provided, and patients must initiate all of their breaths.
Mechanical ventilation	In medicine, mechanical ventilation is a method to mechanically assist or replace spontaneous breathing. This may involve a machine called a ventilator or the breathing may be assisted by a physician, respiratory therapist or other suitable person compressing a bag or set of bellows.

Chapter 13. COMMON AND UNCOMMON PROBLEMS OF THE TERM NEWBORN

Oxygen	Oxygen is the element with atomic number 8 and represented by the symbol O. Its name derives from the Greek roots ?ξ?ς (oxys) ('acid', literally 'sharp', referring to the sour taste of acids) and -γεν?ς (-genes) ('producer', literally 'begetter'), because at the time of naming, it was mistakenly thought that all acids required oxygen in their composition. At standard temperature and pressure, two atoms of the element bind to form dioxygen, a very pale blue, odorless, tasteless diatomic gas with the formula O_2.

Oxygen is a member of the chalcogen group on the periodic table and is a highly reactive nonmetallic element that readily forms compounds (notably oxides) with almost all other elements. |
| Respiratory failure | The term respiratory failure, in medicine, is used to describe inadequate gas exchange by the respiratory system, with the result that arterial oxygen and/or carbon dioxide levels cannot be maintained within their normal ranges. A drop in blood oxygenation is known as hypoxemia; a rise in arterial carbon dioxide levels is called hypercapnia. The normal reference values are: oxygen PaO_2 greater than 80 mmHg (11 kPa), and carbon dioxide $PaCO_2$ less than 45 mmHg (6.0 kPa). |
| Arnold-Chiari malformation | Arnold-Chiari malformation is a malformation of the brain. It consists of a downward displacement of the cerebellar tonsils through the foramen magnum, sometimes causing hydrocephalus as a result of obstruction of cerebrospinal fluid (CSF) outflow . The cerebrospinal fluid outflow is caused by phase difference in outflow and influx of blood in the vasculature of the brain. |
| Neural tube | In the developing vertebrate, the neural tube is the embryo's precursor to the central nervous system, which comprises the brain and spinal cord. The neural groove gradually deepens as the neural folds become elevated, and ultimately the folds meet and coalesce in the middle line and convert the groove into a closed tube, the neural tube or neural canal (which strictly speaking is the center of the neural tube), the ectodermal wall of which forms the rudiment of the nervous system.

There are 2 ways in which the neural tube develops: Primary neurulation and Secondary neurulation. |
| Neural tube defect | Neural tube defects (NTDs) are one of the most common birth defects, occurring in approximately one in 1,000 live births in the United States. An NTD is an opening in the spinal cord or brain that occurs very early in human development. |

1. In mammals, the _____s (also known as suprarenal glands) are endocrine glands that sit atop the kidneys; in humans, the right _____ is triangular shaped, while the left _____ is semilunar shaped. They are chiefly responsible for releasing hormones in response to stress through the synthesis of corticosteroids such as cortisol and catecholamines such as epinephrine (adrenaline) and norepinephrine. They also produce androgens.

   a. Adrenal gland
   b. Adrenalectomy
   c. Adrenarche
   d. Endocrine gland

2. _____ is an organic compound widely used as an automotive antifreeze and a precursor to polymers. In its pure form, it is an odorless, colorless, syrupy, liquid. _____ is toxic, and ingestion can result in death.

   a. Acrolein
   b. abdominal exam
   c. Acquired vision
   d. Ethylene glycol

3. The _____ of a disease is the mechanism by which the disease is caused. The term can also be used to describe the origin and development of the disease and whether it is acute, chronic or recurrent. The word comes from the Greek pathos, 'disease', and genesis, 'creation'.

   a. Pathogenesis
   b. KOH test
   c. Ballistocardiography
   d. BASDAI

4. _____ is a coagulation disturbance in newborns due to vitamin K deficiency. As a consequence of vitamin K deficiency there is an impaired production of coagulation factors II, VII, IX, X, C and S by the liver.

   Newborns are relatively vitamin K deficient for a variety of reasons.

   a. Bacteriophage
   b. Hemorrhagic disease of the newborn
   c. Behavioural genetics
   d. Diallel cross

5. . The _____, but also receives contributions from the 5th and 3rd cervical nerves (C3-C5) in humans.

   The _____s contain motor, sensory, and sympathetic nerve fibers. These nerves provide the only motor supply to the diaphragm as well as sensation to the central tendon.

   a. Transverse cervical nerve
   b. Great auricular nerve
   c. Phrenic nerve

1. a
2. d
3. a
4. b
5. c

You can take the complete Chapter Practice Test

for Chapter 13. COMMON AND UNCOMMON PROBLEMS OF THE TERM NEWBORN
on all key terms, persons, places, and concepts.

Online 99 Cents

http://www.epub219.49.13357.13.cram101.com/

Use www.Cram101.com for all your study needs

including Cram101's online interactive problem solving labs in

chemistry, statistics, mathematics, and more.

Chapter 14. SURGICAL

CHAPTER OUTLINE: KEY TERMS, PEOPLE, PLACES, CONCEPTS

Physical examination

Patient-controlled analgesia

Postoperative fever

Pathophysiology

Volvulus

Gastroesophageal reflux

Gastrointestinal series

Prognosis

Abdominal pain

Appendicitis

Differential diagnosis

Ovarian cyst

Computed tomography

Abdominal mass

Intubation

Acquired immune deficiency syndrome

Barium

Terminal sedation

Pyloric stenosis

	Rotavirus vaccine
	Rotavirus
	Inguinal hernia
	Infection
	Obstruction
	Gastrointestinal bleeding
	Asymptomatic
	Testicular torsion
	Appendix testis
	Epididymitis
	Seizure
	Abdominal trauma
	Concussion
	Epidural hematoma
	Skull fracture
	Subarachnoid hemorrhage
	Subdural hematoma
	Cardiopulmonary resuscitation
	Febrile seizure

CHAPTER OUTLINE: KEY TERMS, PEOPLE, PLACES, CONCEPTS

Status epilepticus

Chest radiograph

Heart failure

Trauma

Diagnostic peritoneal lavage

Child abuse

Imaging

Bites

Skeletal survey

Thoracic

Head injury

Chapter 14. SURGICAL

Physical examination	A physical examination, medical examination, or clinical examination (more popularly known as a check-up or medical) is the process by which a doctor investigates the body of a patient for signs of disease. It generally follows the taking of the medical history -- an account of the symptoms as experienced by the patient. Together with the medical history, the physical examination aids in determining the correct diagnosis and devising the treatment plan.
Patient-controlled analgesia	Patient-controlled analgesia is any method of allowing a person in pain to administer their own pain relief. The infusion is programmable by the prescriber. If it is programmed and functioning as intended, the machine is unlikely to deliver an overdose of medication.
Postoperative fever	Postoperative fever is a common condition challenging doctors to find the right diagnosis, because it can be a hallmark of serious underlying conditions. Between 40-50% of surgical patients develop postoperative fever depending on type of surgery but only a small percentage turn out to be due to infection. The most common causes have been summarized in a handy mnemonic: the five W's.
Pathophysiology	Pathophysiology sample values Pathophysiology is the study of the changes of normal mechanical, physical, and biochemical functions, either caused by a disease, or resulting from an abnormal syndrome. More formally, it is the branch of medicine which deals with any disturbances of body functions, caused by disease or prodromal symptoms. An alternative definition is 'the study of the biological and physical manifestations of disease as they correlate with the underlying abnormalities and physiological disturbances.' The study of pathology and the study of pathophysiology often involves substantial overlap in diseases and processes, but pathology emphasizes direct observations, while pathophysiology emphasizes quantifiable measurements.
Volvulus	A volvulus is a bowel obstruction with a loop of bowel that has abnormally twisted on itself. •volvulus neonatorum•volvulus of the small intestine•volvulus of the caecum (cecum), also cecal volvulus•sigmoid colon volvulus•gastric volvulusSigns and symptoms Regardless of cause, volvulus causes symptoms by two mechanisms:•One is bowel obstruction, manifested as abdominal distension and vomiting.•The other is ischemia (loss of blood flow) to the affected portion of intestine. Volvulus causes severe pain and progressive injury to the intestinal wall, with accumulation of gas and fluid in the portion of the bowel obstructed.

Gastroesophageal reflux	Gastroesophageal reflux disease (GERD), gastro-oesophageal reflux disease (GORD), gastric reflux disease, or acid reflux disease is defined as chronic symptoms or mucosal damage produced by the abnormal reflux in the oesophagus. This is commonly due to transient or permanent changes in the barrier between the oesophagus and the stomach. This can be due to incompetence of the lower esophageal sphincter, transient lower oesophageal sphincter relaxation, impaired expulsion of gastric reflux from the oesophagus, or a hiatal hernia.
Gastrointestinal series	A Gastrointestinal series is a radiologic examination of the upper and/or lower gastrointestinal tract. · Upper GI series · Lower GI series
Prognosis	Prognosis is a medical term to describe the likely outcome of an illness. When applied to large populations, prognostic estimates can be very accurate: for example the statement '45% of patients with severe septic shock will die within 28 days' can be made with some confidence, because previous research found that this proportion of patients died. However, it is much harder to translate this into a prognosis for an individual patient: additional information is needed to determine whether a patient belongs to the 45% who will succumb, or to the 55% who survive.
Abdominal pain	Abdominal pain can be one of the symptoms associated with transient disorders or serious disease. Making a definitive diagnosis of the cause of abdominal pain can be difficult, because many diseases can result in this symptom. Abdominal pain is a common problem.
Appendicitis	Appendicitis is a condition characterized by inflammation of the appendix. It is classified as a medical emergency and many cases require removal of the inflamed appendix, either by laparotomy or laparoscopy. Untreated, mortality is high, mainly because of the risk of rupture leading to peritonitis and shock.
Differential diagnosis	A differential diagnosis is a systematic diagnostic method used to identify the presence of an entity where multiple alternatives are possible (and the process may be termed differential diagnostic procedure), and may also refer to any of the included candidate alternatives (which may also be termed candidate condition). This method is essentially a process of elimination, or at least, rendering of the probabilities of candidate conditions to negligible levels. In this sense, probabilities are, in fact, imaginative parameters in the mind or hardware of the diagnostician or system, while in reality the target (such as a patient) either has a condition or not with an actual probability of either 0 or 100%.
Ovarian cyst	An ovarian cyst is any collection of fluid, surrounded by a very thin wall, within an ovary.

Chapter 14. SURGICAL

Any ovarian follicle that is larger than about two centimeters is termed an ovarian cyst. An ovarian cyst can be as small as a pea, or larger than an orange.

Computed tomography	Computed tomography is a medical imaging method employing tomography created by computer processing. Digital geometry processing is used to generate a three-dimensional image of the inside of an object from a large series of two-dimensional X-ray images taken around a single axis of rotation. Computed tomography produces a volume of data which can be manipulated, through a process known as 'windowing', in order to demonstrate various bodily structures based on their ability to block the X-ray/Röntgen beam.
Abdominal mass	An abdominal mass is any localized enlargement or swelling in the human abdomen. Depending on its location, the abdominal mass may be caused by an enlarged liver (hepatomegaly), enlarged spleen (splenomegaly), protruding kidney, a pancreatic mass, a retroperitoneal mass (a mass in the posterior of the peritoneum), an abdominal aortic aneurysm, or various tumours, such as those caused by abdominal carcinomatosis and omental metastasis. The treatments depend on the cause, and may range from watchful waiting to radical surgery.
Intubation	Intubation, is the insertion of a tube into an external or internal orifice of the body for the purpose of adding or removing fluids or air. It is sometimes considered synonymous with tracheal intubation, but it can also involve the gastrointestinal tract, as with balloon tamponade with a Sengstaken-Blakemore tube. Intubation into the trachea may be performed through the mouth (orotracheal intubation) or through the nose (nasotracheal intubation).
Acquired immune deficiency syndrome	Acquired immune deficiency syndrome or acquired immunodeficiency syndrome is a disease of the human immune system caused by the human immunodeficiency virus (HIV). This condition progressively reduces the effectiveness of the immune system and leaves individuals susceptible to opportunistic infections and tumors. HIV is transmitted through direct contact of a mucous membrane or the bloodstream with a bodily fluid containing HIV, such as blood, semen, vaginal fluid, preseminal fluid, and breast milk.
Barium	Barium is a chemical element with the symbol Ba and atomic number 56. It is the fifth element in Group 2, a soft silvery metallic alkaline earth metal.

Barium is never found in nature as a free element, due to its high chemical reactivity. Its oxide is historically known as baryta, but this oxide (in a similar way to calcium oxide, or quicklime) must be artificially produced since it reacts avidly with water and carbon dioxide, and is not found as a mineral.

Terminal sedation

In medicine, specifically in end-of-life care, terminal sedation is the palliative practice of relieving distress in a terminally ill person in the last hours or days of a dying patient's life, usually by means of a continuous intravenous or subcutaneous infusion of a sedative drug. This is a option of last resort for patients whose symptoms cannot be controlled by any other means. This should be differentiated from euthanasia as the goal of palliative sedation is to control symptoms through sedation but not shorten the patient's life, while in euthanasia the goal is to shorten life to relieve symptoms.

Pyloric stenosis

Pyloric stenosis is a condition that causes severe projectile non-bilious vomiting in the first few months of life. There is narrowing (stenosis) of the opening from the stomach to the first part of the small intestine known as the duodenum, due to enlargement (hypertrophy) of the muscle surrounding this opening (the pylorus, meaning 'gate'), which spasms when the stomach empties. This hypertrophy is felt classically as an olive-shaped mass in the middle upper part or right upper quadrant of the infant's abdomen.

Rotavirus vaccine

A rotavirus vaccine protects children from rotaviruses, which are the leading cause of severe diarrhea among infants and young children. Each year an estimated 453,000 children die from diarrhoeal disease caused by rotavirus, most of whom live in developing countries, and another two million are hospitalised. Rotavirus is highly contagious and resistant and, regardless of water quality and available sanitation nearly every child in the world is at risk of infection.

Rotavirus

Rotavirus is the most common cause of severe diarrhoea among infants and young children. It is a genus of double-stranded RNA virus in the family Reoviridae. By the age of five, nearly every child in the world has been infected with rotavirus at least once.

Inguinal hernia

An inguinal hernia is a protrusion of abdominal-cavity contents through the inguinal canal. They are very common (lifetime risk 27% for men, 3% for women), and their repair is one of the most frequently performed surgical operations.

There are two types of inguinal hernia, direct and indirect, which are defined by their relationship to the inferior epigastric vessels.

Infection

An infection is the invasion of body tissues by disease-causing microorganisms, their multiplication and the reaction of body tissues to these microorganisms and the toxins that they produce. Infections are caused by microorganisms such as viruses, prions, bacteria, and viroids, though larger organisms like macroparasites and fungi can also infect.

Chapter 14. SURGICAL

Obstruction	Obstruction is the act of blocking or impeding some performance · Obstruction theory, in mathematics · Obstruction of justice, the crime of interfering with law enforcement · Obstructing government administration · Propagation path Obstruction · Single Vegetative Obstruction Model · Obstructive jaundice · Obstructive sleep apnea · Airway Obstruction, a respiratory problem · Recurrent airway Obstruction · Bowel Obstruction, a blockage of the intestines. · Gastric outlet Obstruction · Distal intestinal Obstruction syndrome · Congenital lacrimal duct Obstruction · Obstruction, when a fielder illegally hinders a baserunner · Obstructing the field · The Five Obstructions, a 2003 film · Obstruction Island (Washington) · Emergency Workers (Obstruction) Act 2006
Gastrointestinal bleeding	Gastrointestinal bleeding, from the pharynx to the rectum. It has diverse causes, and a medical history, as well as physical examination, generally distinguishes between the main forms. The degree of bleeding can range from nearly undetectable to acute, massive, life-threatening bleeding.
Asymptomatic	In medicine, a disease is considered asymptomatic if a patient is a carrier for a disease or infection but experiences no symptoms. A condition might be asymptomatic if it fails to show the noticeable symptoms with which it is usually associated. Asymptomatic infections are also called subclinical infections.
Testicular torsion	Testicular torsion occurs when the spermatic cord to a testicle twists, cutting off the blood supply (a condition called ischemia). The most common symptom is the rapid onset of acute testicular pain; the most common underlying cause is a congenital malformation known as a 'bell-clapper deformity' wherein the testis is inadequately affixed of the spermatic cord allowing it to move too freely on its axis and become entangled. The diagnosis is often made clinically but if it is in doubt an ultrasound is helpful in evaluating the condition.
Appendix testis	The Appendix testis (or hydatid of Morgagni) is a vestigial remnant of the Müllerian duct, present on the upper pole of the testis and attached to the tunica vaginalis. It is present about 90% of the time. Although it has no physiological function, it can be medically significant in that it can, rarely, undergo torsion (i.e.

Epididymitis	Epididymitis is a medical condition characterized by discomfort or pain in of the epididymis, a curved structure at the back of the testicle in which sperm matures and is stored. Epididymitis is usually characterized as either acute or chronic: if acute, the onset of testicular pain is often accompanied by swelling, redness, and warmth in the scrotum; if chronic, pain may be the only symptom. In either form, testicular pain in one or both testes can vary from mild to severe.
Seizure	An epileptic Seizure, occasionally referred to as a fit, is defined as a transient symptom of 'abnormal excessive or synchronous neuronal activity in the brain'. The outward effect can be as dramatic as a wild thrashing movement (tonic-clonic Seizure) or as mild as a brief loss of awareness. It can manifest as an alteration in mental state, tonic or clonic movements, convulsions, and various other psychic symptoms (such as déjà vu or jamais vu).
Abdominal trauma	Abdominal trauma is an injury to the abdomen. It may be blunt or penetrating and may involve damage to the abdominal organs. Signs and symptoms include abdominal pain, tenderness, rigidity, and bruising of the external abdomen.
Concussion	Concussion is the most common type of traumatic brain injury. The terms mild brain injury, mild traumatic brain injury (MTBI), mild head injury (MHI), minor head trauma, and concussion may be used interchangeably, although the latter is often treated as a narrower category. The term 'concussion' has been used for centuries and is still commonly used in sports medicine, while 'MTBI' is a technical term used more commonly nowadays in general medical contexts.
Epidural hematoma	Epidural hematoma or extradural hematoma (haematoma) is a type of traumatic brain injury (TBI) in which a buildup of blood occurs between the dura mater (the tough outer membrane of the central nervous system) and the skull. The dura mater also covers the spine, so epidural bleeds may also occur in the spinal column. Often due to trauma, the condition is potentially deadly because the buildup of blood may increase pressure in the intracranial space and compress delicate brain tissue.
Skull fracture	Skull fracture is the term used to describe a break in one or more of the eight bones which form the cranial portion of the skull usually occurring as a result of blunt force trauma. If the force of the impact is excessive the bone may fracture at or near the site of the impact and may cause damage to the underlying physical structures contained within the skull such as the membranes, blood vessels, and brain, even in the absence of a fracture.
	While an uncomplicated skull fracture can occur without associated physical or neurological damage and is in itself usually not clinically significant, a fracture in healthy bone indicates that a substantial amount of force has been applied and increases the possibility of associated injury.

Chapter 14. SURGICAL

Subarachnoid hemorrhage	A subarachnoid hemorrhage or subarachnoid haemorrhage in British English, is bleeding into the subarachnoid space--the area between the arachnoid membrane and the pia mater surrounding the brain. This may occur spontaneously, usually from a ruptured cerebral aneurysm, or may result from head injury. Symptoms of SAH include a severe headache with a rapid onset ('thunderclap headache'), vomiting, confusion or a lowered level of consciousness, and sometimes seizures.
Subdural hematoma	A subdural hematoma or subdural haematoma (British spelling), also known as a subdural haemorrhage (SDH), is a type of hematoma, a form of traumatic brain injury. Blood gathers within the outermost meningeal layer, between the dura mater, which adheres to the skull, and the arachnoid mater, which envelops the brain. Usually resulting from tears in bridging veins which cross the subdural space, subdural hemorrhages may cause an increase in intracranial pressure (ICP), which can cause compression of and damage to delicate brain tissue.
Cardiopulmonary resuscitation	Cardiopulmonary resuscitation is an emergency procedure which is performed in an effort to manually preserve intact brain function until further measures are taken to restore spontaneous blood circulation and breathing in a person in cardiac arrest. It is indicated in those who are unresponsive with no breathing or abnormal breathing, for example agonal respirations. It may be performed both in and outside of a hospital.
Febrile seizure	A febrile seizure, is a convulsion associated with a significant rise in body temperature. They most commonly occur in children between the ages of 6 months to 6 years and are twice as common in boys as in girls. The direct cause of a febrile seizure is not known; however, it is normally precipitated by a recent upper respiratory infection or gastroenteritis.
Status epilepticus	Status epilepticus is a life-threatening condition in which the brain is in a state of persistent seizure. Definitions vary, but traditionally it is defined as one continuous unremitting seizure lasting longer than 30 minutes, or recurrent seizures without regaining consciousness between seizures for greater than 30 minutes. Treatment is, however, generally started after the seizure has lasted 5 minutes.
Chest radiograph	In medicine, a chest radiograph, commonly called a chest X-ray (CXR), is a projection radiograph of the chest used to diagnose conditions affecting the chest, its contents, and nearby structures. Chest radiographs are among the most common films taken, being diagnostic of many conditions.

Visit Cram101.com for full Practice Exams

eart failure	Heart failure often called congestive heart failure or congestive cardiac failure (CCF) is the inability of the heart to provide sufficient pump action to distribute blood flow to meet the needs of the body. Heart failure can cause a number of symptoms including shortness of breath, leg swelling, and exercise intolerance. The condition is diagnosed with echocardiography and blood tests.
rauma	Trauma refers to 'a body wound or shock produced by sudden physical injury, as from violence or accident.' It can also be described as 'a physical wound or injury, such as a fracture or blow.' Major trauma (defined by an Injury Severity Score of greater than 15) can result in secondary complications such as circulatory shock, respiratory failure and death. Resuscitation of a trauma patient often involves multiple management procedures. Trauma is the sixth leading cause of death worldwide, accounting for 10% of all mortality, and is a serious public health problem with significant social and economic costs.
iagnostic peritoneal vage	Diagnostic peritoneal lavage is a procedure where, after application of local anesthesia, a vertical skin incision is made one third of the distance from the umbilicus to the pubic symphysis. The linea alba is divided and the peritoneum entered after it has been picked up to prevent bowel perforation. A catheter is inserted towards the pelvis and aspiration of material attempted using a syringe.
hild abuse	Child abuse is the physical, sexual or emotional mistreatment or neglect of a child or children. In the United States, the Centers for Disease Control and Prevention (CDC) and the Department for Children And Families (DCF) define child maltreatment as any act or series of acts of commission or omission by a parent or other caregiver that results in harm, potential for harm, or threat of harm to a child. Child abuse can occur in a child's home, or in the organizations, schools or communities the child interacts with.
naging	Imaging is the representation or reproduction of an object's outward form; especially a visual representation (i.e., the formation of an image). · Chemical Imaging, the simultaneous measurement of spectra and pictures · Creation of a disk image, a file which contains the exact content of a non-volatile computer data storage medium.
ites	TT = Tetanus Toxoid; TIG: Tetanus Immune globulin Antihistamines are effective treatment for the symptoms from Bites. Many diseases such as malaria are transmitted by mosquitoes.

Chapter 14. SURGICAL

Skeletal survey	A skeletal survey is a series of X-rays of all the bones in the body, or at least the axial skeleton and the large cortical bones. A very common use is the diagnosis of multiple myeloma, where tumour deposits appear as 'punched-out' lesions. The standard set of X-rays for a skeletal survey includes X-rays of the skull, entire spine, pelvis, ribs, both humeri and femora (proximal long bones).
Thoracic	The thorax is a division of an animal's body that lies between the head and the abdomen.
	In mammals, the thorax is the region of the body formed by the sternum, the thoracic vertebrae and the ribs. It extends from the neck to the diaphragm, and does not include the upper limbs.
Head injury	Head injury refers to trauma of the head. This may or may not include injury to the brain. However, the terms traumatic brain injury and head injury are often used interchangeably in medical literature.

1.

_____ is a chemical element with the symbol Ba and atomic number 56. It is the fifth element in Group 2, a soft silvery metallic alkaline earth metal. _____ is never found in nature as a free element, due to its high chemical reactivity. Its oxide is historically known as baryta, but this oxide (in a similar way to calcium oxide, or quicklime) must be artificially produced since it reacts avidly with water and carbon dioxide, and is not found as a mineral.

a. Beryllium
b. Bioaccumulation
c. Barium
d. Bongkrek acid

2. _____ is the most common type of traumatic brain injury. The terms mild brain injury, mild traumatic brain injury (MTBI), mild head injury (MHI), minor head trauma, and _____ may be used interchangeably, although the latter is often treated as a narrower category. The term '_____' has been used for centuries and is still commonly used in sports medicine, while 'MTBI' is a technical term used more commonly nowadays in general medical contexts.

a. Decompressive craniectomy
b. Dementia pugilistica
c. Diffuse axonal injury
d. Concussion

3. . A _____, medical examination, or clinical examination (more popularly known as a check-up or medical) is the process by which a doctor investigates the body of a patient for signs of disease. It generally follows the taking of the medical history -- an account of the symptoms as experienced by the patient.

Chapter 14. SURGICAL

Together with the medical history, the _____ aids in determining the correct diagnosis and devising the treatment plan.

a. SOAP note
b. Taping
c. Physical examination
d. Bacteriophage

4. The thorax is a division of an animal's body that lies between the head and the abdomen.

In mammals, the thorax is the region of the body formed by the sternum, the _____ vertebrae and the ribs. It extends from the neck to the diaphragm, and does not include the upper limbs.

a. Thorax
b. Chest
c. Thoracic
d. Clavipectoral fascia

5. _____ is any method of allowing a person in pain to administer their own pain relief. The infusion is programmable by the prescriber. If it is programmed and functioning as intended, the machine is unlikely to deliver an overdose of medication.

a. Post-anesthesia care unit
b. Postanesthetic shivering
c. Patient-controlled analgesia
d. Preanesthetic agent

1. c
2. d
3. c
4. c
5. c

You can take the complete Chapter Practice Test

for Chapter 14. SURGICAL
on all key terms, persons, places, and concepts.

Online 99 Cents

http://www.epub219.49.13357.14.cram101.com/

Use www.Cram101.com for all your study needs

including Cram101's online interactive problem solving labs in

chemistry, statistics, mathematics, and more.

Health care

Home care

Primary care

Secondary care

Body mass

Body mass index

Diabetes mellitus

Insulin resistance

Obesity

Diabetes

Polycystic ovary syndrome

Apnea-hypopnea index

Atherosclerosis

Dyslipidemia

Hypertension

Sleep apnea

Mechanical ventilation

Airway management

Asthma

CHAPTER OUTLINE: KEY TERMS, PEOPLE, PLACES, CONCEPTS

Consequence

Respiratory failure

Down syndrome

Heart defect

Periodontal disease

Slipped capital femoral epiphysis

Fatty liver

Liver disease

Orthopedic

Idiopathic intracranial hypertension

Intracranial pressure

Nephrotic syndrome

Psychosocial

Renal failure

Cerebral palsy

Intraventricular hemorrhage

Differential diagnosis

Epidemiology

Etiological myth

Pathophysiology

Physical examination

Botulinum toxin

Nerve block

Abdominal mass

Imaging

Constraint-induced movement therapy

Carbon monoxide

Oxygen therapy

Gastroesophageal reflux

Prognosis

Cerebrospinal fluid

Hydrocephalus

Physiology

Hemolytic-uremic syndrome

Duchenne muscular dystrophy

Muscle biopsy

Muscular dystrophies

Motor neuron

CHAPTER OUTLINE: KEY TERMS, PEOPLE, PLACES, CONCEPTS

Heart failure

Arnold-Chiari malformation

Neural tube

Neural tube defect

Syringomyelia

Tethered spinal cord syndrome

Decubitus ulcer

Latex allergy

Bowel management

Autonomic dysreflexia

Precocious puberty

Independent living

Language development

Aspiration pneumonia

Central venous catheter

Air embolism

Breakage

Plasminogen activator

Tracheostomy

Timing

Respiratory distress

Advance directive

Granulation tissue

Feeding tube

Prevalence

Mortality rate

Pressure support

Phototherapy

Aplastic anemia

Infusion Therapy

Trace element

Health care	Health care is the diagnosis, treatment, and prevention of disease, illness, injury, and other physical and mental impairments in humans. Health care is delivered by practitioners in medicine, chiropractic, dentistry, nursing, pharmacy, allied health, and other care providers. It refers to the work done in providing primary care, secondary care and tertiary care, as well as in public health.
Home care	Home Care, (also referred to as domiciliary care or social care), is health care or supportive care provided in the patient's home by healthcare professionals (often referred to as home health care or formal care). Often, the term home care is used to distinguish non-medical care or custodial care, which is care that is provided by persons who are not nurses, doctors, or other licensed medical personnel, as opposed to home health care that is provided by licensed personnel. Professionals providing care Professionals providing home care include: Licensed practical nurses, Registered nurses, Home Care Aids, and Social workers.
Primary care	Primary care is the term for the health services by providers who act as the principal point of consultation for patients within a health care system. Such a professional can be a primary care physician, such as a general practitioner or family physician, or depending on the locality, health system organization, and patient's discretion, they may see a pharmacist, a physician assistant, a nurse practitioner, a nurse (such as in the United Kingdom), a clinical officer (such as in parts of Africa), or an Ayurvedic or other traditional medicine professional (such as in parts of Asia). Depending on the nature of the health condition, patients may then be referred for secondary or tertiary care.
Secondary care	Secondary care is the service provided by medical specialists who generally do not have first contact with patients, for example, cardiologists, urologists and dermatologists. In the United States, a physician might voluntarily limit his or her practice to secondary care by refusing patients who have not seen a primary care provider first, or a physician may be required, usually by various payment agreements, to limit the practice this way. However, specialists may take patients without a referral from another physician and it is up to the patient to determine whether self-referral is allowed by the insurance company.
Body mass	Although some people prefer the less-ambiguous term Body mass, the term body weight is overwhelmingly used in daily English speech as well as in the contexts of biological and medical sciences to describe the mass of an organism's body. Body weight is measured in kilograms throughout the world, although in some countries people more often measure and describe body weight in pounds or stones and pounds (e.g. among people in the Commonwealth of Nations) and thus may not be well acquainted with measurement in kilograms.

Body mass index	The body mass index or Quetelet index, is a heuristic proxy for human body fat based on an individual's weight and height. BMI does not actually measure the percentage of body fat. It was devised between 1830 and 1850 by the Belgian polymath Adolphe Quetelet during the course of developing 'social physics'.
Diabetes mellitus	Diabetes mellitus, often simply referred to as diabetes, is a group of metabolic diseases in which a person has high blood sugar, either because the body does not produce enough insulin, or because cells do not respond to the insulin that is produced. This high blood sugar produces the classical symptoms of polyuria (frequent urination), polydipsia (increased thirst) and polyphagia (increased hunger). The three main types of diabetes mellitus are:•Type 1 DM results from the body's failure to produce insulin, and presently requires the person to inject insulin.
Insulin resistance	Insulin resistance is the condition in which normal amounts of insulin are inadequate to produce a normal insulin response from fat, muscle and liver cells. Insulin resistance in fat cells reduces the effects of insulin and results in elevated hydrolysis of stored triglycerides in the absence of measures which either increase insulin sensitivity or which provide additional insulin. Increased mobilization of stored lipids in these cells elevates free fatty acids in the blood plasma.
Obesity	Obesity is a medical condition in which excess body fat has accumulated to the extent that it may have an adverse effect on health, leading to reduced life expectancy and/or increased health problems. Body mass index (BMI), a measurement which compares weight and height, defines people as overweight (pre-obese) if their BMI is between 25 and 30 kg/m^2, and obese when it is greater than 30 kg/m^2. Obesity increases the likelihood of various diseases, particularly heart disease, type 2 diabetes, obstructive sleep apnea, certain types of cancer, and osteoarthritis.
Diabetes	diabetes mellitus --often referred to as diabetes--is a condition in which the body either does not produce enough, or does not properly respond to, insulin, a hormone produced in the pancreas. Insulin enables cells to absorb glucose in order to turn it into energy. This causes glucose to accumulate in the blood , leading to various potential complications. Many types of diabetes are recognized: The principal three are: · Type 1: Results from the body's failure to produce insulin.
Polycystic ovary syndrome	Polycystic ovary syndrome is one of the most common female endocrine disorders.

	PCOS is a complex, heterogeneous disorder of uncertain etiology, but there is strong evidence that it can to a large degree be classified as a genetic disease.
	PCOS produces symptoms in approximately 5% to 10% of women of reproductive age (12-45 years old).
nea-hypopnea dex	The apnea-hypopnea index is an index of sleep apnea severity that combines apneas and hypopneas. The apneas (pauses in breathing) must last for at least 10 seconds and are associated with a decrease in blood oxygenation. Combining these gives an overall sleep apnea severity score that evaluates both number sleep disruptions and degree of oxygen desaturation (low blood level).
therosclerosis	Atherosclerosis is a condition in which an artery wall thickens as a result of the accumulation of fatty materials such as cholesterol. It is a syndrome affecting arterial blood vessels, a chronic inflammatory response in the walls of arteries, caused largely by the accumulation of macrophage white blood cells and promoted by low-density lipoproteins (plasma proteins that carry cholesterol and triglycerides) without adequate removal of fats and cholesterol from the macrophages by functional high density lipoproteins (HDL), . It is commonly referred to as a hardening or furring of the arteries.
yslipidemia	Dyslipidemia is a disruption in the amount of lipids in the blood. In societies of developed countries, most Dyslipidemias are hyperlipidemias; that is, an elevation of lipids in the blood, often due to diet and lifestyle. The prolonged elevation of insulin levels can lead to Dyslipidemia.
ypertension	Hypertension or high blood pressure, sometimes called arterial hypertension, is a chronic medical condition in which the blood pressure in the arteries is elevated. This requires the heart to work harder than normal to circulate blood through the blood vessels. Blood pressure involves two measurements, systolic and diastolic, which depend on whether the heart muscle is contracting (systole) or relaxed between beats (diastole).
eep apnea	Sleep apnea is a sleep disorder characterized by abnormal pauses in breathing or instances of abnormally low breathing, during sleep. Each pause in breathing, called an apnea, can last from a few seconds to minutes, and may occur 5 to 30 times or more an hour. Similarly, each abnormally low breathing event is called a hypopnea.
echanical ventilation	In medicine, mechanical ventilation is a method to mechanically assist or replace spontaneous breathing. This may involve a machine called a ventilator or the breathing may be assisted by a physician, respiratory therapist or other suitable person compressing a bag or set of bellows. Traditionally divided into negative-pressure ventilation, where air is essentially sucked into the lungs, or positive pressure ventilation, where air is pushed into the trachea.

Airway management	Airway management is the medical process of ensuring there is an open pathway between a patient's lungs and the outside world, as well as ensuring the lungs are safe from aspiration. Airway management is a primary consideration in cardiopulmonary resuscitation, anaesthesia, emergency medicine, intensive care medicine and first aid. Airway management is a high priority for clinical care.
Asthma	Asthma is the common chronic inflammatory disease of the airways characterized by variable and recurring symptoms, reversible airflow obstruction, and bronchospasm. Symptoms include wheezing, coughing, chest tightness, and shortness of breath. Asthma is clinically classified according to the frequency of symptoms, forced expiratory volume in 1 second (FEV1), and peak expiratory flow rate.
Consequence	Consequence, or a Consequence is the concept of a resulting effect Plural form · Consequences , a parlour game · Consequences (Buffy the Vampire Slayer), an episode of Buffy the Vampire Slayer · Consequences (New York Contemporary Five album), 1963 · Consequences (Dave Burrell album) · Consequences (Endwell album) · Consequences (Godley & Creme album) · Consequences (Kipling story), a short story by Rudyard Kipling · Consequences (Cather story), a short story by Willa Cather · Consequences (Torchwood), a novel based on the television series Torchwood · Consequences · Consequences (8 Simple Rules episode) · Consequences Creed, a professional wrestler
Respiratory failure	The term respiratory failure, in medicine, is used to describe inadequate gas exchange by the respiratory system, with the result that arterial oxygen and/or carbon dioxide levels cannot be maintained within their normal ranges. A drop in blood oxygenation is known as hypoxemia; a rise in arterial carbon dioxide levels is called hypercapnia. The normal reference values are: oxygen PaO_2 greater than 80 mmHg (11 kPa), and carbon dioxide $PaCO_2$ less than 45 mmHg (6.0 kPa).
Down syndrome	Down syndrome, also known as trisomy 21, is a chromosomal condition caused by the presence of all or part of a third copy of chromosome 21. It is named after John Langdon Down, the British physician who described the syndrome in 1866. The condition was clinically described earlier in the 19th century by Jean Etienne Dominique Esquirol in 1838 and Edouard Seguin in 1844. Down syndrome was identified as a chromosome 21 trisomy by Dr. Jérôme Lejeune in 1959. Down syndrome can be identified in a baby at birth, or by prenatal screening. The CDC estimates that about one of every 691 babies born in the United States each year is born with Down syndrome. Down syndrome occurs in all human populations, and analogous conditions have been found in other species such as chimpanzees.

Heart defect	A congenital Heart defect (C Heart defect) is a defect in the structure of the heart and great vessels of a newborn. Most Heart defect s either obstruct blood flow in the heart or vessels near it or cause blood to flow through the heart in an abnormal pattern, although other defects affecting heart rhythm (such as long QT syndrome) can also occur. Heart defect s are among the most common birth defects and are the leading cause of birth defect-related deaths.
Periodontal disease	Periodontal disease is a type of disease that affects one or more of the periodontal tissues:•alveolar bone•periodontal ligament•cementum•gingiva While many different diseases affect the tooth-supporting structures, plaque-induced inflammatory lesions make up the vast majority of periodontal diseases and have traditionally been divided into two categories:•gingivitis or•periodontitis. While in some sites or individuals, gingivitis never progresses to periodontitis, data indicates that gingivitis always precedes periodontitis.
Slipped capital femoral epiphysis	Slipped capital femoral epiphysis is a medical term referring to a fracture through the physis (the growth plate), which results in slippage of the overlying epiphysis. The capital (head of the femur) should sit squarely on the femoral neck. Abnormal movement along the growth plate results in the slip.
Fatty liver	Fatty liver, is a reversible condition where large vacuoles of triglyceride fat accumulate in liver cells via the process of steatosis (i.e. abnormal retention of lipids within a cell). Despite having multiple causes, fatty liver can be considered a single disease that occurs worldwide in those with excessive alcohol intake and those who are obese (with or without effects of insulin resistance). The condition is also associated with other diseases that influence fat metabolism.
Liver disease	Liver disease is an umbrella term referring to damage to or disease of the liver. The symptoms related to liver dysfunction include both physical signs and a variety of symptoms related to digestive problems, blood sugar problems, immune disorders, abnormal absorption of fats, and metabolism problems. The malabsorption of fats may lead to symptoms that include indigestion, reflux, deficit of fatsoluble vitamins, hemorrhoids, gall stones, intolerance to fatty foods, intolerance to alcohol, nausea and vomiting attacks, abdominal bloating, and constipation.
Orthopedic	Orthopedic surgery or Orthopedics (also spelled orthopaedics) is the branch of surgery concerned with conditions involving the musculoskeletal system.

	Orthopedic surgeons use both surgical and non-surgical means to treat musculoskeletal trauma, sports injuries, degenerative diseases, infections, tumors, and congenital conditions.
	Nicholas Andry coined the word 'orthopaedics', derived from Greek words for orthos and paideion ('child'), when he published Orthopaedia: or the Art of Correcting and Preventing Deformities in Children in 1741.
Idiopathic intracranial hypertension	Idiopathic intracranial hypertension sometimes called by the older names benign intracranial hypertension (BIH) or pseudotumor cerebri (PTC), is a neurological disorder that is characterized by increased intracranial pressure (pressure around the brain) in the absence of a tumor or other diseases. The main symptoms are headache, nausea and vomiting, as well as pulsatile tinnitus (buzzing in the ears synchronous with the pulse), double vision and other visual symptoms. If untreated, it may lead to swelling of the optic disc in the eye, which can progress to vision loss.
Intracranial pressure	Intracranial pressure is the pressure inside the skull and thus in the brain tissue and cerebrospinal fluid (CSF). The body has various mechanisms by which it keeps the ICP stable, with CSF pressures varying by about 1 mmHg in normal adults through shifts in production and absorption of CSF. CSF pressure has been shown to be influenced by abrupt changes in intrathoracic pressure during coughing (intraabdominal pressure), valsalva (Queckenstedt's maneuver), and communication with the vasculature (venous and arterial systems). ICP is measured in millimeters of mercury (mmHg) and, at rest, is normally 7-15 mmHg for a supine adult, and becomes negative (averaging −10 mmHg) in the vertical position.
Nephrotic syndrome	Nephrotic syndrome is a nonspecific disorder in which the kidneys are damaged, causing them to leak large amounts of protein (proteinuria at least 3.5 grams per day per $1.73m^2$ body surface area) from the blood into the urine. Kidneys affected by nephrotic syndrome have small pores in the podocytes, large enough to permit proteinuria (and subsequently hypoalbuminemia, because some of the protein albumin has gone from the blood to the urine) but not large enough to allow cells through (hence no hematuria). By contrast, in nephritic syndrome, RBCs pass through the pores, causing hematuria.
Psychosocial	For a concept to be psychosocial means it relates to one's psychological development in, and interaction with, a social environment. The individual needs not be fully aware of this relationship with his or her environment. It was first commonly used by psychologist Erik Erikson in his stages of social development.
Renal failure	Renal failure or kidney failure (formerly called renal insufficiency) describes a medical condition in which the kidneys fail to adequately filter toxins and waste products from the blood.

	The two forms are acute (acute kidney injury) and chronic (chronic kidney disease); a number of other diseases or health problems may cause either form of renal failure to occur.
	Renal failure is described as a decrease in glomerular filtration rate.
erebral palsy	Cerebral palsy is an umbrella term encompassing a group of non-progressive, non-contagious motor conditions that cause physical disability in human development, chiefly in the various areas of body movement.
	Cerebral refers to the cerebrum, which is the affected area of the brain (although the disorder most likely involves connections between the cortex and other parts of the brain such as the cerebellum), and palsy refers to disorder of movement. Furthermore, 'paralytic disorders' are not cerebral palsy - the condition of quadriplegia, therefore, should not be confused with spastic quadriplegia, nor tardive dyskinesia with dyskinetic cerebral palsy, nor diplegia with spastic diplegia, and so on.
traventricular emorrhage	An intraventricular hemorrhage, often abbreviated 'IVH,' is a bleeding into the brain's ventricular system, where the cerebrospinal fluid is produced and circulates through towards the subarachnoid space. It can result from physical trauma or from hemorrhaging in stroke.
	This type of hemorrhage is particularly common in infants, especially premature infants or those of very low birth weight.
ifferential diagnosis	A differential diagnosis is a systematic diagnostic method used to identify the presence of an entity where multiple alternatives are possible (and the process may be termed differential diagnostic procedure), and may also refer to any of the included candidate alternatives (which may also be termed candidate condition). This method is essentially a process of elimination, or at least, rendering of the probabilities of candidate conditions to negligible levels. In this sense, probabilities are, in fact, imaginative parameters in the mind or hardware of the diagnostician or system, while in reality the target (such as a patient) either has a condition or not with an actual probability of either 0 or 100%.
pidemiology	Epidemiology is the study of the distribution and patterns of health-events, health-characteristics and their causes or influences in well-defined populations. It is the cornerstone method of public health research and practice, and helps inform policy decisions and evidence-based medicine by identifying risk factors for disease and targets for preventive medicine and public policies. Epidemiologists are involved in the design of studies, collection and statistical analysis of data, and interpretation and dissemination of results (including peer review and occasional systematic review).
tiological myth	Etiology is the study of causation, or origination.

	The word is most commonly used in medical and philosophical theories, where it is used to refer to the study of why things occur, or even the reasons behind the way that things act, and is used in philosophy, physics, psychology, government, medicine, theology and biology in reference to the causes of various phenomena. An etiological myth is a myth intended to explain a name or create a mythic history for a place or family.
Pathophysiology	Pathophysiology sample values Pathophysiology is the study of the changes of normal mechanical, physical, and biochemical functions, either caused by a disease, or resulting from an abnormal syndrome. More formally, it is the branch of medicine which deals with any disturbances of body functions, caused by disease or prodromal symptoms. An alternative definition is 'the study of the biological and physical manifestations of disease as they correlate with the underlying abnormalities and physiological disturbances.' The study of pathology and the study of pathophysiology often involves substantial overlap in diseases and processes, but pathology emphasizes direct observations, while pathophysiology emphasizes quantifiable measurements.
Physical examination	A physical examination, medical examination, or clinical examination (more popularly known as a check-up or medical) is the process by which a doctor investigates the body of a patient for signs of disease. It generally follows the taking of the medical history -- an account of the symptoms as experienced by the patient. Together with the medical history, the physical examination aids in determining the correct diagnosis and devising the treatment plan.
Botulinum toxin	Botulinum toxin is a protein and neurotoxin produced by the bacterium Clostridium botulinum. Botulinum toxin can cause botulism, a serious and life-threatening illness in humans and animals. When introduced intravenously in monkeys, type A (Botox Cosmetic) of the toxin exhibits an LD_{50} of 40-56 ng, type C1 around 32 ng, type D 3200 ng, and type E 88 ng; these are some of the most potent neurotoxins known.
Nerve block	Regional nerve blockade, or more commonly nerve block, is a general term used to refer to the injection of local anesthetic onto or near nerves for temporary control of pain. It can also be used as a diagnostic tool to identify specific nerves as pain generators. Permanent nerve block can be produced by destruction of nerve tissue.
Abdominal mass	An abdominal mass is any localized enlargement or swelling in the human abdomen.

	Depending on its location, the abdominal mass may be caused by an enlarged liver (hepatomegaly), enlarged spleen (splenomegaly), protruding kidney, a pancreatic mass, a retroperitoneal mass (a mass in the posterior of the peritoneum), an abdominal aortic aneurysm, or various tumours, such as those caused by abdominal carcinomatosis and omental metastasis. The treatments depend on the cause, and may range from watchful waiting to radical surgery.
Imaging	Imaging is the representation or reproduction of an object's outward form; especially a visual representation (i.e., the formation of an image).
	· Chemical Imaging, the simultaneous measurement of spectra and pictures · Creation of a disk image, a file which contains the exact content of a non-volatile computer data storage medium.
Constraint-induced movement therapy	Constraint-induced movement therapy is a form of rehabilitation therapy that improves upper extremity function in stroke and other central nervous system damage victims by increasing the use of their affected upper limb.
	The focus of CIMT is to combine restraint of the unaffected limb and intensive use of the affected limb. Types of restraints include a sling or triangular bandage, a splint, a sling combined with a resting hand splint, a half glove, and a mitt.
Carbon monoxide	Carbon monoxide also called carbonous oxide, is a colorless, odorless, and tasteless gas that is slightly lighter than air. It can be toxic to humans and animals when encountered in higher concentrations, although it is also produced in normal animal metabolism in low quantities, and is thought to have some normal biological functions. In the atmosphere however, it is short lived and spatially variable, since it combines with oxygen to form carbon dioxide and ozone.
Oxygen therapy	Oxygen therapy is the administration of oxygen as a medical intervention, which can be for a variety of purposes in both chronic and acute patient care. Oxygen is essential for cell metabolism, and in turn, tissue oxygenation is essential for all normal physiological functions.
	Room air only contains 21% oxygen, and increasing the fraction of oxygen in the breathing gas increases the amount of oxygen in the blood.
Gastroesophageal reflux	Gastroesophageal reflux disease (GERD), gastro-oesophageal reflux disease (GORD), gastric reflux disease, or acid reflux disease is defined as chronic symptoms or mucosal damage produced by the abnormal reflux in the oesophagus.
	This is commonly due to transient or permanent changes in the barrier between the oesophagus and the stomach.

Prognosis	Prognosis is a medical term to describe the likely outcome of an illness. When applied to large populations, prognostic estimates can be very accurate: for example the statement '45% of patients with severe septic shock will die within 28 days' can be made with some confidence, because previous research found that this proportion of patients died. However, it is much harder to translate this into a prognosis for an individual patient: additional information is needed to determine whether a patient belongs to the 45% who will succumb, or to the 55% who survive.
Cerebrospinal fluid	Cerebrospinal fluid Liquor cerebrospinalis, is a clear, colorless, bodily fluid, that occupies the subarachnoid space and the ventricular system around and inside the brain and spinal cord. The CSF occupies the space between the arachnoid mater (the middle layer of the brain cover, meninges) and the pia mater (the layer of the meninges closest to the brain). It constitutes the content of all intra-cerebral (inside the brain, cerebrum) ventricles, cisterns, and sulci, as well as the central canal of the spinal cord.
Hydrocephalus	Hydrocephalus also known as 'water in the brain,' is a medical condition in which there is an abnormal accumulation of cerebrospinal fluid (CSF) in the ventricles, or cavities, of the brain. This may cause increased intracranial pressure inside the skull and progressive enlargement of the head, convulsion, tunnel vision, and mental disability. Hydrocephalus can also cause death.
Physiology	Physiology is the science of the function of living systems. This includes how organisms, organ systems, organs, cells, and bio-molecules carry out the chemical or physical functions that exist in a living system. The highest honor awarded in physiology is the Nobel Prize in Physiology or Medicine, awarded since 1901 by the Royal Swedish Academy of Sciences.
Hemolytic-uremic syndrome	Hemolytic-uremic syndrome , abbreviated HUS, is a disease characterized by hemolytic anemia (anemia caused by destruction of red blood cells), acute kidney failure (uremia) and a low platelet count (thrombocytopenia). It predominantly, but not exclusively, affects children. Most cases are preceded by an episode of infectious, sometimes bloody, diarrhea caused by E. coli O157:H7, which is acquired as a foodborne illness or from a contaminated water supply.
Duchenne muscular dystrophy	Duchenne muscular dystrophy is a recessive X-linked form of muscular dystrophy, which results in muscle degeneration, difficulty walking, breathing, and death. The incidence is 1 in 3,000. Females and males are affected, though females are rarely affected and are more often carriers. The disorder is caused by a mutation in the dystrophin gene, located in humans on the X chromosome (Xp21).
Muscle biopsy	In medicine, a muscle biopsy is a procedure in which a piece of muscle tissue is removed from an organism and examined microscopically.

A biopsy needle is usually inserted into a muscle, wherein a small amount of tissue remains. Alternatively, an 'open biopsy' can be performed by obtaining the muscle tissue through a small surgical incision.

Muscular dystrophies

Muscular dystrophy refers to a group of hereditary muscle diseases that weaken the muscles that move the human body. muscular dystrophies are characterized by progressive skeletal muscle weakness, defects in muscle proteins, and the death of muscle cells and tissue. Nine diseases including Duchenne, Becker, limb girdle, congenital, facioscapulohumeral, myotonic, oculopharyngeal, distal, and Emery-Dreifuss are always classified as muscular dystrophy but there are more than 100 diseases in total with similarities to muscular dystrophy.

Motor neuron

In vertebrates, the term motor neuron classically applies to neurons located in the central nervous system (or CNS) that project their axons outside the CNS and directly or indirectly control muscles. The motor neuron is often associated with efferent neuron, primary neuron, or alpha motor neurons.

Anatomy and physiology

According to their targets, motor neurons are classified into three broad categories:

Somatic motor neurons, which directly innervate skeletal muscles, involved in locomotion (such as the muscles of the limbs, abdominal, and intercostal muscles).

Heart failure

Heart failure often called congestive heart failure or congestive cardiac failure (CCF) is the inability of the heart to provide sufficient pump action to distribute blood flow to meet the needs of the body. Heart failure can cause a number of symptoms including shortness of breath, leg swelling, and exercise intolerance. The condition is diagnosed with echocardiography and blood tests.

Arnold-Chiari malformation

Arnold-Chiari malformation is a malformation of the brain. It consists of a downward displacement of the cerebellar tonsils through the foramen magnum, sometimes causing hydrocephalus as a result of obstruction of cerebrospinal fluid (CSF) outflow . The cerebrospinal fluid outflow is caused by phase difference in outflow and influx of blood in the vasculature of the brain.

Neural tube

In the developing vertebrate, the neural tube is the embryo's precursor to the central nervous system, which comprises the brain and spinal cord. The neural groove gradually deepens as the neural folds become elevated, and ultimately the folds meet and coalesce in the middle line and convert the groove into a closed tube, the neural tube or neural canal (which strictly speaking is the center of the neural tube), the ectodermal wall of which forms the rudiment of the nervous system.

Neural tube defect	Neural tube defects (NTDs) are one of the most common birth defects, occurring in approximately one in 1,000 live births in the United States. An NTD is an opening in the spinal cord or brain that occurs very early in human development. In the 3rd week of pregnancy called gastrulation, specialized cells on the dorsal side of the fetus begin to fuse and form the neural tube.
Syringomyelia	Syringomyelia is a generic term referring to a disorder in which a cyst or cavity forms within the spinal cord. This cyst, called a syrinx, can expand and elongate over time, destroying the spinal cord. The damage may result in pain, paralysis, weakness, and stiffness in the back, shoulders, and extremities.
Tethered spinal cord syndrome	Tethered spinal cord syndrome refers to a group of neurological disorders related to malformations of the spinal cord. The various forms include: tight filum terminale, lipomeningomyelocele, split cord malformations, dermal sinus tracts, dermoids, and cystoceles. All of the forms have in common the pulling of the spinal cord at the base of the spinal canal, literally a 'tethered cord'. The spinal cord normally hangs loose in the canal, free to move up and down with growth and bending and stretching, a tethered cord is held taut at the end. In children, a tethered can cause the spinal cord to stretch as they grow, in adults the spinal cord will stretch in the course of normal activity, usually leading to progressive spinal cord damage if left untreated. It is often associated with the closure of a spina bifida, although not always depending on the form it takes; for example it can be congenital such as in tight filum terminale, or the result of injury later in life.
Decubitus ulcer	Pressure ulcers, also known as decubitus ulcers or bedsores, are lesions caused by unrelieved pressure on soft tissues overlying a bony prominence which reduces or completely obstructs the blood flow to the superficial tissues. Most commonly this will be the sacrum or the hips, but other sites such as the elbows, knees, ankles or the back of the cranium can be affected. It is widely believed that other factors can influence the occurrence and development of pressure ulcers.
Latex allergy	Latex allergy is a medical term encompassing a range of allergic reactions to natural rubber latex. Latex is known to cause 2 of the 4 types of hypersensitivity. Type I The most serious and rare form, type I is an immediate and potentially life-threatening reaction, not unlike the severe reaction some people have to bee stings.
Bowel management	Bowel management is a medical approach to manage fecal incontinence or constipation. Bowel control is often a challenge for children who are born with anomalies in their anus or rectum, Hirschsprung's disease, and/or spina bifida.

Autonomic dysreflexia	Autonomic dysreflexia also known as autonomic hyperreflexia, is a potentially life threatening condition which can be considered a medical emergency requiring immediate attention. AD occurs most often in spinal cord-injured individuals with spinal lesions above the T6 spinal cord level; although, it has been known to occur in patients with a lesion as low as T10. Acute AD is a reaction of the autonomic (involuntary) nervous system to overstimulation. It is characterised by severe paroxysmal hypertension (episodic high blood pressure) associated with throbbing headaches, profuse sweating, nasal stuffiness, flushing of the skin above the level of the lesion, bradycardia, apprehension and anxiety, which is sometimes accompanied by cognitive impairment.
Precocious puberty	As a medical term, precocious puberty describes puberty occurring at an unusually early age. In most of these children, the process is normal in every respect except the unusually early age, and simply represents a variation of normal development. In a minority of children, the early development is triggered by a disease such as a tumor or injury of the brain.
Independent living	Independent living, as seen by its advocates, is a philosophy, a way of looking at disability and society, and a worldwide movement of people with disabilities working for self-determination, self-respect and equal opportunities. In the context of eldercare, independent living is seen as a step in the continuum of care, with assisted living being the next step.

In most countries, proponents of the IL Movement claim preconceived notions and a predominantly medical view of disability contribute to negative attitudes towards people with disabilities, portraying them as sick, defective and deviant persons, as objects of professional intervention, as a burden for themselves and their families, dependent on other people's charity. |
| Language development | Language development is a process starting early in human life, when a person begins to acquire language by learning it as it is spoken and by mimicry. Children's language development moves from simple to complex. Infants start without language. |
| Aspiration pneumonia | Aspiration pneumonia is bronchopneumonia that develops due to the entrance of foreign materials that enter the bronchial tree, usually oral or gastric contents (including food, saliva, or nasal secretions). Depending on the acidity of the aspirate, a chemical pneumonitis can develop, and bacterial pathogens (particularly anaerobic bacteria) may add to the inflammation.

Aspiration pneumonia is often caused by an incompetent swallowing mechanism, such as occurs in some forms of neurological disease (a common cause being strokes) or while a person is intoxicated. |
| Central venous catheter | In medicine, a central venous catheter is a catheter placed into a large vein in the neck (internal jugular vein), chest (subclavian vein or axillary vein) or groin (femoral vein). |

It is used to administer medication or fluids, obtain blood tests (specifically the 'mixed venous oxygen saturation'), and directly obtain cardiovascular measurements such as the central venous pressure.

There are several types of central venous catheters:Non-tunneled vs. tunneled catheters

Non-tunneled catheters are fixed in place at the site of insertion, with the catheter and attachments protruding directly.

Air embolism	An air embolism, is a pathological condition caused by gas bubbles in a vascular system. The most common context is a human body, in which case it refers to gas bubbles in the bloodstream (embolism in a medical context refers to any large moving mass or defect in the blood stream). However air embolisms may also occur in the xylem of vascular plants, especially when suffering from water stress.
Breakage	Breakage is a term used in accounting to indicate gift cards that have been sold but never redeemed. Revenue from breakage is almost entirely profit, since companies need not provide any goods or services for unredeemed gift cards. Breakage is a term used in sales, distribution, and multi-level marketing organizations to indicate commissions that are lost for the failure to meet certain conditions or requirements.
Plasminogen activator	A plasminogen activator is a serine protease which converts plasminogen to plasmin, thus promoting fibrinolysis. Types include:•Tissue plasminogen activator•Urokinase It is inhibited by plasminogen activator inhibitor-1 and plasminogen activator inhibitor-2. .
Tracheostomy	Tracheotomy and Tracheostomy are surgical procedures on the neck to open a direct airway through an incision in the trachea (the windpipe). They are performed by paramedics, veterinarians, emergency physicians and surgeons. Both surgical and percutaneous techniques are now widely used.
Timing	Timing is the spacing of events in time. Some typical uses are: · The act of measuring the elapsed time of something or someone, often at athletic events such as swimming or running, where participants are timed with a device such as a stopwatch. · Engine Timing, for various functions such as ignition, cam Timing to control poppet valve Timing and overlap, and fuel injection Timing.

	· see ignition Timing · Timing light, · Timing mark · Comic Timing by a comedian or actor, an element of humor. · In phonology, the rhythm of a spoken language.
espiratory distress	Respiratory distress is a medical term that refers to both difficulty in breathing, and to the psychological experience associated with such difficulty, even if there is no physiological basis for experiencing such distress. The physical presentation of respiratory distress is generally referred to as labored breathing,s while the sensation of respiratory distress is called shortness of breath or dyspnea. Respiratory distress occurs in connection with various physical ailments, such as acute respiratory distress syndrome, a serious reaction to various forms of injuries to the lung, and infant respiratory distress syndrome, a syndrome in premature infants caused by developmental insufficiency of surfactant production and structural immaturity in the lungs.
dvance directive	Advance health care directives, also known as living wills, Advance directives, are instructions given by individuals specifying what actions should be taken for their health in the event that they are no longer able to make decisions due to illness or incapacity. A living will is one form of Advance directive, leaving instructions for treatment. Another form authorizes a specific type of power of attorney or health care proxy, where someone is appointed by the individual to make decisions on their behalf when they are incapacitated.
ranulation tissue	Granulation tissue is the perfused, fibrous connective tissue that replaces a fibrin clot in healing wounds. Granulation tissue typically grows from the base of a wound and is able to fill wounds of almost any size it heals. In addition, it is also found in ulcers like esophageal ulcer.
eding tube	A feeding tube is a medical device used to provide nutrition to patients who cannot obtain nutrition by swallowing. The state of being fed by a feeding tube is called gavage, enteral feeding or tube feeding. Placement may be temporary for the treatment of acute conditions or lifelong in the case of chronic disabilities.
revalence	In epidemiology, the prevalence of a health-related state (typically disease, but also other things like smoking or seatbelt use) in a statistical population is defined as the total number of cases of the risk factor in the population at a given time, or the total number of cases in the population, divided by the number of individuals in the population. It is used as an estimate of how common a disease is within a population over a certain period of time. It helps physicians or other health professionals understand the probability of certain diagnoses and is routinely used by epidemiologists, health care providers, government agencies and insurers.
ortality rate	Mortality rate is a measure of the number of deaths (in general, or due to a specific cause) in a population, scaled to the size of that population, per unit of time. Mortality rate is typically expressed in units of deaths per 1000 individuals per year; thus, a mortality rate of 9.5 (out of 1000) in a population of 100,000 would mean 950 deaths per year in that entire population, or 0.95% out of the total.

Pressure support	Pressure Support (PS) is a spontaneous mode of ventilation also named Pressure Support Ventilation. The patient initiates the breath and the ventilator delivers support with the preset pressure value. With support from the ventilator, the patient also regulates the respiratory rate and the tidal volume.
Phototherapy	Light therapy or Phototherapy consists of exposure to daylight or to specific wavelengths of light using lasers, light-emitting diodes, fluorescent lamps, dichroic lamps or very bright, full-spectrum light, for a prescribed amount of time and, in some cases, at a specific time of day. Light therapy is used to treat Acne vulgaris, seasonal affective disorder, neonatal jaundice, and is part of the standard treatment regimen for delayed sleep phase syndrome with some support for its use with non-seasonal psychiatric disorders.
	Sunlight was long known to improve acne, and this was thought to be due to antibacterial and other effects of the ultraviolet spectrum; which cannot be used as a treatment due to the likelihood of skin damage in the long term.
Aplastic anemia	Aplastic anemia is a condition where bone marrow does not produce sufficient new cells to replenish blood cells. The condition, as the name indicates, involves both aplasia and anemia. Typically, anemia refers to low red blood cell counts, but aplastic anemia patients have lower counts of all three blood cell types: red blood cells, white blood cells, and platelets, termed pancytopenia.
Infusion Therapy	In medicine, infusion therapy deals with all aspects of fluid and medication infusion, usually via the intravenous route. A special infusion pump can be used for this purpose.
	Infusion therapy involves the administration of medication through a needle or catheter.
Trace element	In analytical chemistry, a trace element is an element in a sample that has an average concentration of less than 100 parts per million measured in atomic count, or less than 100 micrograms per gram.
	In biochemistry, a trace element is a dietary mineral that is needed in very minute quantities for the proper growth, development, and physiology of the organism.
	In geochemistry, a trace element is a chemical element whose concentration is less than 1000 ppm or 0.1% of a rock's composition.

1. Regional nerve blockade, or more commonly _____, is a general term used to refer to the injection of local anesthetic onto or near nerves for temporary control of pain. It can also be used as a diagnostic tool to identify specific nerves as pain generators. Permanent _____ can be produced by destruction of nerve tissue.

   a. Paracervical block
   b. Retrobulbar block
   c. Spinal anaesthesia
   d. Nerve block

2. The _____ is an index of sleep apnea severity that combines apneas and hypopneas. The apneas (pauses in breathing) must last for at least 10 seconds and are associated with a decrease in blood oxygenation. Combining these gives an overall sleep apnea severity score that evaluates both number sleep disruptions and degree of oxygen desaturation (low blood level).

   a. Apnea-hypopnea index
   b. Intrapleural pressure
   c. Open lung ventilation
   d. Oxygenation

3. _____ is a medical approach to manage fecal incontinence or constipation. Bowel control is often a challenge for children who are born with anomalies in their anus or rectum, Hirschsprung's disease, and/or spina bifida. Some patients have a poor prognosis and will never be able to control their bowel, and so benefit from _____ techniques.

   a. Bowel management
   b. BUN-to-creatinine ratio
   c. Canadian Association of Gastroenterology
   d. Cecal bascule

4. A congenital _____ (C _____) is a defect in the structure of the heart and great vessels of a newborn. Most _____ s either obstruct blood flow in the heart or vessels near it or cause blood to flow through the heart in an abnormal pattern, although other defects affecting heart rhythm (such as long QT syndrome) can also occur. _____ s are among the most common birth defects and are the leading cause of birth defect-related deaths.

   a. Double aortic arch
   b. Baffle
   c. Heart defect
   d. Congenital heart defect

5. . _____ is the pressure inside the skull and thus in the brain tissue and cerebrospinal fluid (CSF). The body has various mechanisms by which it keeps the ICP stable, with CSF pressures varying by about 1 mmHg in normal adults through shifts in production and absorption of CSF. CSF pressure has been shown to be influenced by abrupt changes in intrathoracic pressure during coughing (intraabdominal pressure), valsalva (Queckenstedt's maneuver), and communication with the vasculature (venous and arterial systems). ICP is measured in millimeters of mercury (mmHg) and, at rest, is normally 7-15 mmHg for a supine adult, and becomes negative (averaging −10 mmHg) in the vertical position.

Chapter 15. HOSPITAL CARE OF CHILDREN WITH COMPLEX AND CHRONIC CONDITIC

a. Oligoclonal band

b. Orbital apex syndrome

c. Intracranial hypertension syndrome

d. Intracranial pressure

1. d
2. a
3. a
4. c
5. d

You can take the complete Chapter Practice Test

for Chapter 15. HOSPITAL CARE OF CHILDREN WITH COMPLEX AND CHRONIC CONDITIONS
on all key terms, persons, places, and concepts.

Online 99 Cents

http://www.epub219.49.13357.15.cram101.com/

Use www.Cram101.com for all your study needs

including Cram101's online interactive problem solving labs in

chemistry, statistics, mathematics, and more.

CHAPTER OUTLINE: KEY TERMS, PEOPLE, PLACES, CONCEPTS

| | FLACC scale |

| | Pain assessment |

| | ACE inhibitor |

| | Dosing |

| | Pharmacokinetics |

| | Side effect |

| | Tolerance |

| | Infusion |

| | Pain management |

| | Palliative care |

| | Patient-controlled analgesia |

| | Cochrane Library |

| | Regional analgesia |

| | Tramadol |

| | Diabetes insipidus |

| | Heart failure |

| | Hypertensive crisis |

| | Local anesthetic |

| | Transdermal |

Bupivacaine

Ropivacaine

Nausea

Sedation

Urinary retention

Asthma

Respiratory system

Respiratory tract

Upper respiratory tract infection

Oxygen

Capnography

Pulse oximetry

Chloral hydrate

Intravenous

Midazolam

Procedural sedation

Dexmedetomidine

Pentobarbital

Propofol

	Nitrous oxide
	Ketamine
	Flumazenil
	Naloxone

CHAPTER HIGHLIGHTS & NOTES: KEY TERMS, PEOPLE, PLACES, CONCEPTS

LACC scale	The Face, Legs, Activity, Cry, Consolability scale or FLACC scale is a measurement used to assess pain for children between the ages of 2 months-7years or individuals that are unable to communicate their pain. The scale is scored between a range of 0-10 with 0 representing no pain. The scale has 5 criteria which are each assigned a score of 0, 1 or 2.
ain assessment	Pain is often regarded as the fifth vital sign in regard to healthcare because it is accepted now in healthcare that pain, like other vital signs, is an objective sensation rather than subjective. As a result nurses are trained and expected to assess pain. Pain assessment and re-assessment after administration of analgesics or pain management is regulated in healthcare facilities by accreditation bodies, like the Joint Commission.
CE inhibitor	ACE inhibitors are a group of drugs used primarily for the treatment of hypertension (high blood pressure) and congestive heart failure. Originally synthesized from compounds found in pit viper venom, they inhibit angiotensin-converting enzyme (ACE), a component of the blood pressure-regulating renin-angiotensin system.
osing	Dosing generally applies to feeding chemicals or medicines in small quantities into a process fluid or to a living being at intervals or to atmosphere at intervals to give sufficient time for the chemical or medicine to react or show the results. In the case of human beings or animals the word dose is generally used but in the case of inanimate objects the word dosing is used. In engineering

Chapter 16. SEDATION AND PAIN MANAGEMENT

Pharmacokinetics	Pharmacokinetics, is a branch of pharmacology dedicated to the determination of the fate of substances administered externally to a living organism. The substances of interest include pharmaceutical agents, hormones, nutrients, and toxins.
	Pharmacokinetics is often studied in conjunction with pharmacodynamics.
Side effect	In medicine, a side effect is an effect, whether therapeutic or adverse, that is secondary to the one intended; although the term is predominantly employed to describe adverse effects, it can also apply to beneficial, but unintended, consequences of the use of a drug.
	Occasionally, drugs are prescribed or procedures performed specifically for their side effects; in that case, said side effect ceases to be a side effect, and is now an intended effect. For instance, X-rays were historically (and are currently) used as an imaging technique; the discovery of their oncolytic capability led to their employ in radiotherapy (ablation of malignant tumors).
Tolerance	Toleration and tolerance are terms used in social, cultural and religious contexts to describe attitudes which are 'tolerant' (or moderately respectful) of practices or group memberships that may be disapproved of by those in the majority. In practice, tolerance indicates support for practices that prohibit ethnic and religious discrimination. Conversely, 'in tolerance ' may be used to refer to the discriminatory practices sought to be prohibited.
Infusion	An infusion is the outcome of steeping plants that have desired chemical compounds or flavors in a solvent such as water or oil or alcohol.
	The first recorded use of essential oils was in the 10th or 11th century by the Persian polymath Avicenna, possibly in The Canon of Medicine. Preparation techniques
	An infusion is a very simple chemical process used with botanicals that are volatile and dissolve readily, or release their active ingredients easily, in water, oil or alcohol.
Pain management	Pain management is a branch of medicine employing an interdisciplinary approach for easing the suffering and improving the quality of life of those living with pain. The typical pain management team includes medical practitioners, clinical psychologists, physiotherapists, occupational therapists, and nurse practitioners. Pain sometimes resolves promptly once the underlying trauma or pathology has healed, and is treated by one practitioner, with drugs such as analgesics and (occasionally) anxiolytics.
Palliative care	Palliative care is an area of healthcare that focuses on relieving and preventing the suffering of patients. Unlike hospice care, palliative medicine is appropriate for patients in all disease stages, including those undergoing treatment for curable illnesses and those living with chronic diseases, as well as patients who are nearing the end of life.

Patient-controlled analgesia	Patient-controlled analgesia is any method of allowing a person in pain to administer their own pain relief. The infusion is programmable by the prescriber. If it is programmed and functioning as intended, the machine is unlikely to deliver an overdose of medication.
Cochrane Library	The Cochrane Library is a collection of databases in medicine and other healthcare specialties provided by the Cochrane Collaboration and other organisations. At its core is the collection of Cochrane Reviews, a database of systematic reviews and meta-analyses which summarize and interpret the results of medical research. The Cochrane Library aims to make the results of well-conducted controlled trials readily available and is a key resource in evidence-based medicine.
Regional analgesia	Regional analgesia blocks passage of pain impulses through a nerve by depositing an analgesic drug close to the nerve trunk, cutting off sensory innervation to the region it supplies. The drug is normally injected at a site where the nerve is unprotected by bone.
Tramadol	Tramadol hydrochloride (trademarked as Conzip, Ryzolt, Ultracet, Ultram in the USA,Ralivia in Canada) is a centrally acting synthetic analgesic used to treat moderate to moderately-severe pain. The drug has a wide range of applications, including treatment of rheumatoid arthritis, restless legs syndrome and fibromyalgia. It was launched and marketed as Tramal by the German pharmaceutical company Grünenthal GmbH in 1977.
Diabetes insipidus	Diabetes insipidus is a condition characterized by excessive thirst and excretion of large amounts of severely diluted urine, with reduction of fluid intake having no effect on the concentration of the urine. There are several different types of DI, each with a different cause. The most common type in humans is central DI, caused by a deficiency of arginine vasopressin (AVP), also known as antidiuretic hormone (ADH).
Heart failure	Heart failure often called congestive heart failure or congestive cardiac failure (CCF) is the inability of the heart to provide sufficient pump action to distribute blood flow to meet the needs of the body. Heart failure can cause a number of symptoms including shortness of breath, leg swelling, and exercise intolerance. The condition is diagnosed with echocardiography and blood tests.
Hypertensive crisis	A hypertensive emergency is severe hypertension (high blood pressure) with acute impairment of an organ system (especially the central nervous system, cardiovascular system and/or the renal system) and the possibility of irreversible organ-damage. In case of a hypertensive emergency, the blood pressure should be lowered aggressively over minutes to hours with an antihypertensive agent.

Chapter 16. SEDATION AND PAIN MANAGEMENT

Local anesthetic	A local anesthetic is a drug that causes reversible local anesthesia, generally for the aim of having local analgesic effect, that is, inducing absence of pain sensation, although other local senses are often affected as well. Also, when it is used on specific nerve pathways (nerve block), paralysis (loss of muscle power) can be achieved as well. Clinical local anesthetics belong to one of two classes: aminoamide and aminoester local anesthetics.
Transdermal	Transdermal is a route of administration wherein active ingredients are delivered across the skin for systemic distribution. Examples include transdermal patches used for medicine delivery, and transdermal implants used for medical or aesthetic purposes. Obstacles Although the skin is a large and logical target for drug delivery, its basic functions limit its utility for this purpose.
Bupivacaine	Bupivacaine ( ) is a local anaesthetic drug belonging to the amino amide group. It is commonly marketed under various trade names, including Marcain, Marcaine (CareStream Dental), Sensorcaine (Astra Zeneca) and Vivacaine (Septodont). Bupivacaine is indicated for local anesthesia including infiltration, nerve block, epidural, and intrathecal anesthesia.
Ropivacaine	Ropivacaine ( ) is a local anaesthetic drug belonging to the amino amide group. The name ropivacaine refers to both the racemate and the marketed S-enantiomer. Ropivacaine hydrochloride is commonly marketed by AstraZeneca under the trade name Naropin.
Nausea	Nausea, is a sensation of unease and discomfort in the upper stomach with an involuntary urge to vomit. It often, but not always, precedes vomiting. A person can suffer nausea without vomiting.
Sedation	Sedation is the reduction of irritability or agitation by administration of sedative drugs, generally to facilitate a medical procedure or diagnostic procedure. Drugs which can be used for sedation include propofol, etomidate, ketamine, fentanyl, and midazolam. Sedation is now typically used in procedures such as endoscopy, vasectomy, RSI (Rapid Sequence Intubation), or minor surgery and in dentistry for reconstructive surgery, some cosmetic surgeries, removal of wisdom teeth, or for high-anxiety patients.
Urinary retention	Urinary retention, is a lack of ability to urinate.

It is a common complication of benign prostatic hyperplasia (BPH), although it can also be caused by nerve dysfunction, constipation, infection, or medications (including anticholinergics, antidepressants, COX-2 inhibitors, amphetamines and opiates). Diagnosis and/or treatment may require use of a catheter or prostatic stent.

sthma	Asthma is the common chronic inflammatory disease of the airways characterized by variable and recurring symptoms, reversible airflow obstruction, and bronchospasm. Symptoms include wheezing, coughing, chest tightness, and shortness of breath. Asthma is clinically classified according to the frequency of symptoms, forced expiratory volume in 1 second (FEV1), and peak expiratory flow rate.
espiratory system	The respiratory system is the biological system of an organism that introduces respiratory gases to the interior and performs gas exchange. In humans and other mammals, the anatomical features of the respiratory system include airways, lungs, and the respiratory muscles. Molecules of oxygen and carbon dioxide are passively exchanged, by diffusion, between the gaseous external environment and the blood.
espiratory tract	In humans the respiratory tract is the part of the anatomy involved with the process of respiration.
	The respiratory tract is divided into 3 segments:•Upper respiratory tract: nose and nasal passages, paranasal sinuses, and throat or pharynx•Respiratory airways: voice box or larynx, trachea, bronchi, and bronchioles•Lungs: respiratory bronchioles, alveolar ducts, alveolar sacs, and alveoli
	The respiratory tract is a common site for infections. Upper respiratory tract infections are probably the most common infections in the world.
oper respiratory ict infection	Upper respiratory tract infections (URI or URTI) are the illnesses caused by an acute infection which involves the upper respiratory tract: nose, sinuses, pharynx or larynx. This commonly includes: tonsillitis, pharyngitis, laryngitis, sinusitis, otitis media, and the common cold.
	Common URI terms are defined as follows:•Rhinitis - Inflammation of the nasal mucosa•Rhinosinusitis or sinusitis - Inflammation of the nares and paranasal sinuses, including frontal, ethmoid, maxillary, and sphenoid•Nasopharyngitis (rhinopharyngitis or the common cold) - Inflammation of the nares, pharynx,hypopharynx, uvula, and tonsils•Pharyngitis - Inflammation of the pharynx, hypopharynx, uvula, and tonsils•Epiglottitis (supraglottitis) - Inflammation of the superior portion of the larynx and supraglottic area•Laryngitis - Inflammation of the larynx•Laryngotracheitis - Inflammation of the larynx, trachea, and subglottic area•Tracheitis - Inflammation of the trachea and subglottic areaSigns and symptoms

Chapter 16. SEDATION AND PAIN MANAGEMENT

Oxygen

Oxygen is the element with atomic number 8 and represented by the symbol O. Its name derives from the Greek roots ?ξ?ς (oxys) ('acid', literally 'sharp', referring to the sour taste of acids) and -γεν?ς (-genes) ('producer', literally 'begetter'), because at the time of naming, it was mistakenly thought that all acids required oxygen in their composition. At standard temperature and pressure, two atoms of the element bind to form dioxygen, a very pale blue, odorless, tasteless diatomic gas with the formula O_2.

Oxygen is a member of the chalcogen group on the periodic table and is a highly reactive nonmetallic element that readily forms compounds (notably oxides) with almost all other elements.

Capnography

Capnography is the monitoring of the concentration or partial pressure of carbon dioxide (CO_2) in the respiratory gases. Its main development has been as a monitoring tool for use during anaesthesia and intensive care. It is usually presented as a graph of expiratory CO_2 plotted against time, or, less commonly, but more usefully, expired volume.

Pulse oximetry

Pulse oximetry is a non-invasive method allowing the monitoring of the oxygenation of a patient's hemoglobin.

A sensor is placed on a thin part of the patient's body, usually a fingertip or earlobe, or in the case of an infant, across a foot. Light of two different wavelengths is passed through the patient to a photodetector.

Chloral hydrate

Chloral hydrate is a sedative and hypnotic drug as well as a chemical reagent and precursor. The name chloral hydrate indicates that it is formed from chloral (trichloroacetaldehyde) by the addition of one molecule of water. Its chemical formula is $C_2H_3Cl_3O_2$.

Intravenous

Intravenous therapy or IV therapy is the giving of liquid substances directly into a vein. The word intravenous simply means 'within a vein'. Therapies administered intravenously are often called specialty pharmaceuticals.

Midazolam

Midazolam is a short-acting drug in the benzodiazepine class that is used for treatment of acute seizures, moderate to severe insomnia, and for inducing sedation and amnesia before medical procedures. It possesses profoundly potent anxiolytic, amnestic, hypnotic, anticonvulsant, skeletal muscle relaxant, and sedative properties. Midazolam has a fast recovery time and is the most commonly used benzodiazepine as a premedication for sedation; less commonly it is used for induction and maintenance of anesthesia.

rocedural sedation	Procedural sedation is defined as 'a technique of administering sedatives or dissociative agents with or without analgesics to induce a state that allows the patient to tolerate unpleasant procedures while maintaining cardiorespiratory function.' It was previously referred to as conscious sedation. This technique is often used in the emergency department for the performance of painful or uncomfortable procedures. It has been used for setting fractures, draining abscesses, reducing dislocations, performing endoscopy, imaging procedures in patients unable to hold still, cardioversion and during dental procedures.
exmedetomidine	Dexmedetomidine is a sedative medication used by intensive care units and anesthetists. It is relatively unique in its ability to provide sedation without causing respiratory depression. Like clonidine, it is an agonist of α_2-adrenergic receptors in certain parts of the brain.
entobarbital	Pentobarbital is a short-acting barbiturate that was first synthesized in 1928. Pentobarbital is available as both a free acid and a sodium salt, the former of which is only slightly soluble in water and ethanol. One brand name for this drug is Nembutal, coined by Dr. John S. Lundy, who started using it in 1930, from the structural formula of the sodium salt--Na (sodium) + ethyl + methyl + butyl + al (common suffix for barbiturates). Approved Pentobarbital's FDA-approved human uses include treatment of seizures and preoperative (and other) sedation; it is also approved as a short-term hypnotic.
ropofol	Propofol is a short-acting, intravenously administered hypnotic agent. Its uses include the induction and maintenance of general anesthesia, sedation for mechanically ventilated adults, and procedural sedation. Propofol is also commonly used in veterinary medicine.
itrous oxide	Nitrous oxide, commonly known as laughing gas or sweet air, is a chemical compound with the formula N_2O. It is an oxide of nitrogen. At room temperature, it is a colorless, non-flammable gas, with a slightly sweet odor and taste.
etamine	Ketamine is a drug used in human and veterinary medicine. Its hydrochloride salt is sold as Ketanest, Ketaset, and Ketalar. Pharmacologically, ketamine is classified as an NMDA receptor antagonist.
lumazenil	Flumazenil is a benzodiazepine antagonist available for injection only, and the only benzodiazepine receptor antagonist on the market today. It was first introduced in 1987 by Hoffmann-La Roche under the trade name Anexate, but only approved by the FDA on December 20, 1991. Some years ago an oral preparation was under development, though it had low bio-availability and was thus abandoned.

Chapter 16. SEDATION AND PAIN MANAGEMENT

Naloxone	Naloxone is an opioid antagonist drug developed by Sankyo in the 1960s. Naloxone is a drug used to counter the effects of opiate overdose, for example heroin or morphine overdose. Naloxone is specifically used to counteract life-threatening depression of the central nervous system and respiratory system.

1. An _____ is the outcome of steeping plants that have desired chemical compounds or flavors in a solvent such as water or oil or alcohol.

   The first recorded use of essential oils was in the 10th or 11th century by the Persian polymath Avicenna, possibly in The Canon of Medicine. Preparation techniques

   An _____ is a very simple chemical process used with botanicals that are volatile and dissolve readily, or release their active ingredients easily, in water, oil or alcohol.

   a. abdominal exam
   b. Receptor antagonist
   c. Infusion
   d. combination therapy

2. _____ hydrochloride (trademarked as Conzip, Ryzolt, Ultracet, Ultram in the USA,Ralivia in Canada) is a centrally acting synthetic analgesic used to treat moderate to moderately-severe pain. The drug has a wide range of applications, including treatment of rheumatoid arthritis, restless legs syndrome and fibromyalgia. It was launched and marketed as Tramal by the German pharmaceutical company Grünenthal GmbH in 1977.

   a. Tybamate
   b. Valaciclovir
   c. Valganciclovir
   d. Tramadol

3. . _____ is an area of healthcare that focuses on relieving and preventing the suffering of patients. Unlike hospice care, palliative medicine is appropriate for patients in all disease stages, including those undergoing treatment for curable illnesses and those living with chronic diseases, as well as patients who are nearing the end of life. Palliative medicine utilizes a multidisciplinary approach to patient care, relying on input from physicians, pharmacists, nurses, chaplains, social workers, psychologists, and other allied health professionals in formulating a plan of care to relieve suffering in all areas of a patient's life.

   a. Palliative sedation
   b. Palliative care

c. Russell and Fern de Greeff Hospice House

d. Symptomatic treatment

4. _____ is a non-invasive method allowing the monitoring of the oxygenation of a patient's hemoglobin.

A sensor is placed on a thin part of the patient's body, usually a fingertip or earlobe, or in the case of an infant, across a foot. Light of two different wavelengths is passed through the patient to a photodetector.

a. Reflex bradycardia

b. Pulse oximetry

c. Regurgitant fraction

d. Regurgitation

5. _____ blocks passage of pain impulses through a nerve by depositing an analgesic drug close to the nerve trunk, cutting off sensory innervation to the region it supplies. The drug is normally injected at a site where the nerve is unprotected by bone.

a. Resiniferatoxin

b. Regional analgesia

c. RUB A535

d. Salicylamide

1. c
2. d
3. b
4. b
5. b

You can take the complete Chapter Practice Test

for Chapter 16. SEDATION AND PAIN MANAGEMENT
on all key terms, persons, places, and concepts.

Online 99 Cents

http://www.epub219.49.13357.16.cram101.com/

Use www.Cram101.com for all your study needs

including Cram101's online interactive problem solving labs in

chemistry, statistics, mathematics, and more.

Chapter 17. CHILD ABUSE AND NEGLECT

CHAPTER OUTLINE: KEY TERMS, PEOPLE, PLACES, CONCEPTS

Child abuse

Risk factor

Differential diagnosis

Physical examination

Imaging

Sexual abuse

Documentation

Abdominal pain

Chlamydia trachomatis

Neisseria gonorrhoeae

Sexually transmitted

Multiple sclerosis

Epidemiology

Medical history

Medical record

Delays

Literature review

Child abuse	Child abuse is the physical, sexual or emotional mistreatment or neglect of a child or children. In the United States, the Centers for Disease Control and Prevention (CDC) and the Department for Children And Families (DCF) define child maltreatment as any act or series of acts of commission or omission by a parent or other caregiver that results in harm, potential for harm, or threat of harm to a child. Child abuse can occur in a child's home, or in the organizations, schools or communities the child interacts with.
Risk factor	In epidemiology, a risk factor is a variable associated with an increased risk of disease or infection. Sometimes, determinant is also used, being a variable associated with either increased or decreased risk.
	Risk factors or determinants are correlational and not necessarily causal, because correlation does not prove causation.
Differential diagnosis	A differential diagnosis is a systematic diagnostic method used to identify the presence of an entity where multiple alternatives are possible (and the process may be termed differential diagnostic procedure), and may also refer to any of the included candidate alternatives (which may also be termed candidate condition). This method is essentially a process of elimination, or at least, rendering of the probabilities of candidate conditions to negligible levels. In this sense, probabilities are, in fact, imaginative parameters in the mind or hardware of the diagnostician or system, while in reality the target (such as a patient) either has a condition or not with an actual probability of either 0 or 100%.
Physical examination	A physical examination, medical examination, or clinical examination (more popularly known as a check-up or medical) is the process by which a doctor investigates the body of a patient for signs of disease. It generally follows the taking of the medical history -- an account of the symptoms as experienced by the patient. Together with the medical history, the physical examination aids in determining the correct diagnosis and devising the treatment plan.
Imaging	Imaging is the representation or reproduction of an object's outward form; especially a visual representation (i.e., the formation of an image).
	· Chemical Imaging, the simultaneous measurement of spectra and pictures · Creation of a disk image, a file which contains the exact content of a non-volatile computer data storage medium.
Sexual abuse	Sexual abuse is the forcing of undesired sexual behavior by one person upon another. When that force is immediate, of short duration, or infrequent, it is called sexual assault. The offender is referred to as a sexual abuser or (often pejoratively) molester. The term also covers any behavior by any adult towards a child to stimulate either the adult or child sexually. When the victim is younger than the age of consent, it is referred to as child sexual abuse.

Chapter 17. CHILD ABUSE AND NEGLECT

Documentation	Documentation is a term with many meanings, the most common of which are:•A set of documents provided on paper, or online, or on digital or analog media, such as audio tape or CDs.•The process of documenting knowledge, as in scientific articles.•The process of providing evidence.•The writing of product documentation, such as software documentation.•A synonym for the term document.•A synonym for the term bibliography.•A field of study and a profession founded by Paul Otlet (1868-1944) and Henri La Fontaine (1854-1943), which is also termed documentation science. Professionals educated in this field are termed documentalists. This field changed its name to information science in 1968, but some uses of the term documentation still exists and there have been efforts to reintroduce the term documentation as a field of study.Documentation composure

Documentation may include•written information for any read, projection or technical performing,•data media of any format and for any reproduction,•other content.

Common types of documentation include user guides, white papers, on-line help, quick-reference guides. |
| Abdominal pain | Abdominal pain can be one of the symptoms associated with transient disorders or serious disease. Making a definitive diagnosis of the cause of abdominal pain can be difficult, because many diseases can result in this symptom. Abdominal pain is a common problem. |
| Chlamydia trachomatis | Chlamydia trachomatis, an obligate intracellular human pathogen, is one of three bacterial species in the genus Chlamydia. C. trachomatis is a Gram-negative bacteria, therefore its cell wall components retain the counter-stain safranin and appear pink under a light microscope.

The inclusion bodies of Chlamydia trachomatis were first described in 1907, the Chlamydia trachomatis agent was first cultured in the yolk sacs of eggs by Feifan Tang et al in 1957. |
| Neisseria gonorrhoeae | Neisseria gonorrhoeae, or gonococcus, is a species of Gram-negative coffee bean-shaped diplococci bacteria responsible for the sexually transmitted infection gonorrhea.

N. gonorrhoea was first described by Albert Neisser in 1879. Microbiology

Neisseria are fastidious Gram-negative cocci that require nutrient supplementation to grow in laboratory cultures. |
| Sexually transmitted | A sexually transmitted disease is an illness that has a significant probability of transmission between humans or animals by means of sexual contact, including vaginal intercourse, oral sex, and anal sex. |

	While in the past, these illnesses have mostly been referred to as sexually transmitted Ds or VD, in recent years the term sexually transmitted infection has been preferred, as it has a broader range of meaning; a person may be infected, and may potentially infect others, without showing signs of disease. Some sexually transmitted Is can also be transmitted via use of an IV drug needle after its use by an infected person, as well as through childbirth or breastfeeding.
Multiple sclerosis	Multiple sclerosis is a disease in which the fatty myelin sheaths around the axons of the brain and spinal cord are damaged, leading to demyelination and scarring as well as a broad spectrum of signs and symptoms. Disease onset usually occurs in young adults, and it is more common in females. It has a prevalence that ranges between 2 and 150 per 100,000. Multiple sclerosis was first described in 1868 by Jean-Martin Charcot.
Epidemiology	Epidemiology is the study of the distribution and patterns of health-events, health-characteristics and their causes or influences in well-defined populations. It is the cornerstone method of public health research and practice, and helps inform policy decisions and evidence-based medicine by identifying risk factors for disease and targets for preventive medicine and public policies. Epidemiologists are involved in the design of studies, collection and statistical analysis of data, and interpretation and dissemination of results (including peer review and occasional systematic review).
Medical history	The medical history or anamnesis (abbr. Hx) of a patient is information gained by a physician by asking specific questions, either of the patient or of other people who know the person and can give suitable information (in this case, it is sometimes called heteroanamnesis), with the aim of obtaining information useful in formulating a diagnosis and providing medical care to the patient. The medically relevant complaints reported by the patient or others familiar with the patient are referred to as symptoms, in contrast with clinical signs, which are ascertained by direct examination on the part of medical personnel.
Medical record	The terms medical record, health record, and medical chart are used somewhat interchangeably to describe the systematic documentation of a single patient's medical history and care across time within one particular health care provider's jurisdiction.. The medical record includes a variety of types of 'notes' entered over time by health care professionals, recording observations and administration of drugs and therapies, orders for the administration of drugs and therapies, test results, x-rays, reports, etc. The maintenance of complete and accurate medical records is a requirement of health care providers and is generally enforced as a licensing or certification prerequisite.
Delays	Delays are an English indie band formed in Southampton, consisting of brothers Greg and Aaron Gilbert, Colin Fox and Rowly. The band's sound combines guitar and synths and features Greg Gilbert's distinctive falsetto lead vocals. They have released three critically acclaimed albums to date, all of which have charted high in the UK.

Literature review	A literature review is a body of text that aims to review the critical points of current knowledge including substantive findings as well as theoretical and methodological contributions to a particular topic. Literature reviews are secondary sources, and as such, do not report any new or original experimental work. Most often associated with academic-oriented literature, such as a thesis, a literature review usually precedes a research proposal and results section.

1. _____, an obligate intracellular human pathogen, is one of three bacterial species in the genus Chlamydia. C. trachomatis is a Gram-negative bacteria, therefore its cell wall components retain the counter-stain safranin and appear pink under a light microscope.

   The inclusion bodies of _____ were first described in 1907, the _____ agent was first cultured in the yolk sacs of eggs by Feifan Tang et al in 1957.

   a. Aeromonas veronii
   b. Ischemia
   c. Chlamydia trachomatis
   d. General formal ontology

2. In epidemiology, a _____ is a variable associated with an increased risk of disease or infection. Sometimes, determinant is also used, being a variable associated with either increased or decreased risk.

   _____s or determinants are correlational and not necessarily causal, because correlation does not prove causation.

   a. Rule of three
   b. Risk factor
   c. Standardized mortality ratio
   d. Surrogate endpoint

3. . _____ is the physical, sexual or emotional mistreatment or neglect of a child or children. In the United States, the Centers for Disease Control and Prevention (CDC) and the Department for Children And Families (DCF) define child maltreatment as any act or series of acts of commission or omission by a parent or other caregiver that results in harm, potential for harm, or threat of harm to a child. _____ can occur in a child's home, or in the organizations, schools or communities the child interacts with.

   a. Baby farming
   b. Child abuse

Chapter 17. CHILD ABUSE AND NEGLECT

c. Chernokozovo

d. Child Exploitation Tracking System

4. A _____ is a systematic diagnostic method used to identify the presence of an entity where multiple alternatives are possible (and the process may be termed differential diagnostic procedure), and may also refer to any of the included candidate alternatives (which may also be termed candidate condition). This method is essentially a process of elimination, or at least, rendering of the probabilities of candidate conditions to negligible levels. In this sense, probabilities are, in fact, imaginative parameters in the mind or hardware of the diagnostician or system, while in reality the target (such as a patient) either has a condition or not with an actual probability of either 0 or 100%.

a. Hospital emergency codes

b. Differential diagnosis

c. Gliosis

d. Health Sciences Descriptors

5. _____ can be one of the symptoms associated with transient disorders or serious disease. Making a definitive diagnosis of the cause of _____ can be difficult, because many diseases can result in this symptom. _____ is a common problem.

a. Abdominal pain

b. Ischemia

c. Findability

d. General formal ontology

1. c
2. b
3. b
4. b
5. a

You can take the complete Chapter Practice Test

for Chapter 17. CHILD ABUSE AND NEGLECT
on all key terms, persons, places, and concepts.

Online 99 Cents

http://www.epub219.49.13357.17.cram101.com/

Use www.Cram101.com for all your study needs

including Cram101's online interactive problem solving labs in

chemistry, statistics, mathematics, and more.

Chapter 18. NUTRITION

_____	Body mass
_____	Body mass index
_____	Body weight
_____	Physical examination
_____	Basal metabolic rate
_____	C-reactive protein
_____	Nitrogen balance
_____	Transferrin
_____	Transthyretin
_____	Basal animal metabolic rate
_____	Neonatal sepsis
_____	Renal failure
_____	Health care
_____	Social history
_____	Miliary tuberculosis
_____	Parenteral nutrition
_____	Amino acid
_____	Protease inhibitor
_____	Protein

Chapter 18. NUTRITION

CHAPTER OUTLINE: KEY TERMS, PEOPLE, PLACES, CONCEPTS

	Fanconi anemia
	Monitoring
	Trace element

CHAPTER HIGHLIGHTS & NOTES: KEY TERMS, PEOPLE, PLACES, CONCEPTS

Body mass	Although some people prefer the less-ambiguous term Body mass, the term body weight is overwhelmingly used in daily English speech as well as in the contexts of biological and medical sciences to describe the mass of an organism's body. Body weight is measured in kilograms throughout the world, although in some countries people more often measure and describe body weight in pounds or stones and pounds (e.g. among people in the Commonwealth of Nations) and thus may not be well acquainted with measurement in kilograms. Most hospitals, even in the United States, now use kilograms for calculations, but use kilograms and pounds together for other purposes.
Body mass index	The body mass index or Quetelet index, is a heuristic proxy for human body fat based on an individual's weight and height. BMI does not actually measure the percentage of body fat. It was devised between 1830 and 1850 by the Belgian polymath Adolphe Quetelet during the course of developing 'social physics'.
Body weight	The term body weight is used in daily English speech as well as in the contexts of biological and medical sciences to describe the Earth's gravitational pull on an organism's body. Body weight is measured in kilograms throughout the world, although in some countries it is still measured in pounds (e.g. United States) or stones and pounds (e.g. among people in the United Kingdom) and thus some people may not be well acquainted with measurement in kilograms. Most hospitals, even in the United States, now use kilograms for calculations, but use kilograms and pounds together for other purposes.
Physical examination	A physical examination, medical examination, or clinical examination (more popularly known as a check-up or medical) is the process by which a doctor investigates the body of a patient for signs of disease. It generally follows the taking of the medical history -- an account of the symptoms as experienced by the patient.

Chapter 18. NUTRITION

Basal metabolic rate	Basal Metabolic Rate and the closely related resting metabolic rate (RMR), is the amount of energy expended daily by humans and other animals at rest. Rest is defined as existing in a neutrally temperate environment while in the post-absorptive state. In plants, different considerations apply.
C-reactive protein	C-reactive protein is a protein found in the blood, the levels of which rise in response to inflammation (i.e. C-reactive protein is an acute-phase protein). Its physiological role is to bind to phosphocholine expressed on the surface of dead or dying cells (and some types of bacteria) in order to activate the complement system via the C1Q complex. CRP is synthesized by the liver in response to factors released by fat cells (adipocytes).
Nitrogen balance	nitrogen balance is the measure of nitrogen output subtracted from nitrogen input. Blood urea nitrogen can be used in estimating nitrogen balance, as can the urea concentration in urine. A positive value is often found during periods of growth, tissue repair or pregnancy.
Transferrin	Transferrin Transferrins are iron-binding blood plasma glycoproteins that control the level of free iron in biological fluids. Human transferrin is encoded by the TF gene. Transferrin glycoproteins bind iron very tightly, but reversibly.
Transthyretin	Transthyretin is a serum and cerebrospinal fluid carrier of the thyroid hormone thyroxine (T4) and retinol binding protein bound to retinol. This is how transthyretin gained its name, transports thyroxine and retinol. The liver secretes transthyretin into the blood, and the choroid plexus secretes TTR into the cerebrospinal fluid.
Basal animal metabolic rate	Basal animal metabolic rate is the amount of daily energy expended by animals while at rest in a neutrally temperate environment, in the post-absorptive state (meaning that the digestive system is inactive, which requires about twelve hours of fasting in humans). In plants, different considerations apply. The release of energy in this state is sufficient only for the functioning of the vital organs, the heart, lungs, nervous system, kidneys, liver, intestine, sex organs, muscles, and skin.

Neonatal sepsis	In common clinical usage, neonatal sepsis specifically refers to the presence of a bacterial blood stream infection (BSI) (such as meningitis, pneumonia, pyelonephritis, or gastroenteritis) in the setting of fever. Criteria with regards to hemodynamic compromise or respiratory failure are not useful clinically because these symptoms often do not arise in neonates until death is imminent and unpreventable. It is difficult to clinically exclude sepsis in newborns less than 90 days old that have fever (defined as a temperature > 38°C (100.4°F).
Renal failure	Renal failure or kidney failure (formerly called renal insufficiency) describes a medical condition in which the kidneys fail to adequately filter toxins and waste products from the blood. The two forms are acute (acute kidney injury) and chronic (chronic kidney disease); a number of other diseases or health problems may cause either form of renal failure to occur. Renal failure is described as a decrease in glomerular filtration rate.
Health care	Health care is the diagnosis, treatment, and prevention of disease, illness, injury, and other physical and mental impairments in humans. Health care is delivered by practitioners in medicine, chiropractic, dentistry, nursing, pharmacy, allied health, and other care providers. It refers to the work done in providing primary care, secondary care and tertiary care, as well as in public health.
Social history	Social history, often called the new social history, is a branch of History that includes history of ordinary people and their strategies of coping with life. In its 'golden age' it was a major growth field in the 1960s and 1970s among scholars, and still is well represented in history departments. In two decades from 1975 to 1995, the proportion of professors of history in American universities identifying with social history rose from 31% to 41%, while the proportion of political historians fell from 40% to 30%. In the history departments of British universities in 2007, of the 5723 faculty members, 1644 (29%) identified themselves with social history while political history came next with 1425 (25%).
Miliary tuberculosis	Miliary tuberculosis is a form of tuberculosis that is characterized by a wide dissemination into the human body and by the tiny size of the lesions (1-5 mm). Its name comes from a distinctive pattern seen on a chest X-ray of many tiny spots distributed throughout the lung fields with the appearance similar to millet seeds--thus the term 'miliary' tuberculosis. Miliary TB may infect any number of organs, including the lungs, liver, and spleen.
Parenteral nutrition	Parenteral nutrition is feeding a person intravenously, bypassing the usual process of eating and digestion. The person receives nutritional formulae that contain nutrients such as glucose, amino acids, lipids and added vitamins and dietary minerals.

Chapter 18. NUTRITION

Amino acid	In chemistry, an Amino acid is a molecule containing both amine and carboxyl functional groups. These molecules are particularly important in biochemistry, where this term refers to alpha- Amino acid s with the general formula $H_2NCHRCOOH$, where R is an organic substituent. In the alpha Amino acid s, the amino and carboxylate groups are attached to the same carbon atom, which is called the α-carbon.
Protease inhibitor	Protease inhibitors are a class of drugs used to treat or prevent infection by viruses, including HIV and Hepatitis C. Protease inhibitors prevent viral replication by inhibiting the activity of proteases, e.g.HIV-1 protease, enzymes used by the viruses to cleave nascent proteins for final assembly of new virons.
	Protease inhibitors have been developed or are presently undergoing testing for treating various viruses:•HIV/AIDS: antiretroviral protease inhibitors (saquinavir, ritonavir, indinavir, nelfinavir, amprenavir etc).•Hepatitis C: experimental agents: BILN 2061 (All clinical trials of BILN 2061 have been suspended due to cardiac issues), VX 950 (trade name Telaprevir), or SCH 503034
	Given the specificity of the target of these drugs there is the risk, as in antibiotics, of the development of drug-resistant mutated viruses. To reduce this risk it is common to use several different drugs together that are each aimed at different targets.
Protein	Proteins are biochemical compounds consisting of one or more polypeptides typically folded into a globular or fibrous form, facilitating a biological function.
	A polypeptide is a single linear polymer chain of amino acids bonded together by peptide bonds between the carboxyl and amino groups of adjacent amino acid residues. The sequence of amino acids in a protein is defined by the sequence of a gene, which is encoded in the genetic code.
Fanconi anemia	Fanconi anemia is a genetic disease with an incidence of 1 per 350,000 births, with a higher frequency in Ashkenazi Jews and Afrikaners in South Africa.
	FA is the result of a genetic defect in a cluster of proteins responsible for DNA repair. As a result, the majority of FA patients develop cancer, most often acute myelogenous leukemia, and 90% develop bone marrow failure (the inability to produce blood cells) by age 40. About 60-75% of FA patients have congenital defects, commonly short stature, abnormalities of the skin, arms, head, eyes, kidneys, and ears, and developmental disabilities. Around 75% of FA patients have some form of endocrine problem, with varying degrees of severity.
Monitoring	In medicine, monitoring is the evaluation of a disease or condition over time.

Chapter 18. NUTRITION

It can be performed by continuously measuring certain parameters (for example, by continuously measuring vital signs by a bedside monitor), and/or by repeatedly performing medical tests (such as blood glucose monitoring in people with diabetes mellitus).

Transmitting data from a monitor to a distant monitoring station is known as telemetry or biotelemetry.

ace element

In analytical chemistry, a trace element is an element in a sample that has an average concentration of less than 100 parts per million measured in atomic count, or less than 100 micrograms per gram.

In biochemistry, a trace element is a dietary mineral that is needed in very minute quantities for the proper growth, development, and physiology of the organism.

In geochemistry, a trace element is a chemical element whose concentration is less than 1000 ppm or 0.1% of a rock's composition.

1. The term _____ is used in daily English speech as well as in the contexts of biological and medical sciences to describe the Earth's gravitational pull on an organism's body. _____ is measured in kilograms throughout the world, although in some countries it is still measured in pounds (e.g. United States) or stones and pounds (e.g. among people in the United Kingdom) and thus some people may not be well acquainted with measurement in kilograms. Most hospitals, even in the United States, now use kilograms for calculations, but use kilograms and pounds together for other purposes.

    a. Body weight
    b. Fat Head
    c. Ghrelin
    d. Hogging

2. _____ is feeding a person intravenously, bypassing the usual process of eating and digestion. The person receives nutritional formulae that contain nutrients such as glucose, amino acids, lipids and added vitamins and dietary minerals. It is called total _____ or total nutrient admixture (TNA) when no food is given by other routes.

    a. Passive leg raising test
    b. PIM2
    c. Positive airway pressure
    d. Parenteral nutrition

. In medicine, monitoring is the evaluation of a disease or condition over time.

Chapter 18. NUTRITION

CHAPTER QUIZ: KEY TERMS, PEOPLE, PLACES, CONCEPTS

It can be performed by continuously measuring certain parameters (for example, by continuously measuring vital signs by a bedside monitor), and/or by repeatedly performing medical tests (such as blood glucose monitoring in people with diabetes mellitus).

Transmitting data from a monitor to a distant _____ station is known as telemetry or biotelemetry.

a. Pediatric ependymoma
b. Receptor editing
c. Monitoring
d. Visceral pain

4. Although some people prefer the less-ambiguous term _____, the term body weight is overwhelmingly used in daily English speech as well as in the contexts of biological and medical sciences to describe the mass of an organism's body. Body weight is measured in kilograms throughout the world, although in some countries people more often measure and describe body weight in pounds or stones and pounds (e.g. among people in the Commonwealth of Nations) and thus may not be well acquainted with measurement in kilograms. Most hospitals, even in the United States, now use kilograms for calculations, but use kilograms and pounds together for other purposes.

a. abdominal exam
b. Aeromonas veronii
c. Body mass
d. Ametropia

5. _____ is the measure of nitrogen output subtracted from nitrogen input.

Blood urea nitrogen can be used in estimating _____, as can the urea concentration in urine.

A positive value is often found during periods of growth, tissue repair or pregnancy.

a. Barr body
b. Body surface area
c. brainstem
d. Nitrogen balance

ANSWER KEY
Chapter 18. NUTRITION

1. a
2. d
3. c
4. c
5. d

You can take the complete Chapter Practice Test

for Chapter 18. NUTRITION
on all key terms, persons, places, and concepts.

Online 99 Cents

http://www.epub219.49.13357.18.cram101.com/

Use www.Cram101.com for all your study needs

including Cram101's online interactive problem solving labs in

chemistry, statistics, mathematics, and more.

CHAPTER OUTLINE: KEY TERMS, PEOPLE, PLACES, CONCEPTS

Anaphylaxis

Opioid

Pathogenesis

Latex allergy

Exercise-induced anaphylaxis

Latex

Risk factor

Airway management

Differential diagnosis

Prognosis

Anaphylactic shock

Patient education

Erythema multiforme

Herpes simplex

Mycoplasma pneumoniae

Toxic epidermal necrolysis

Etiological myth

Koebner phenomenon

Serotonin syndrome

Chapter 19. Emergency MEDICINE
CHAPTER OUTLINE: KEY TERMS, PEOPLE, PLACES, CONCEPTS

_____ Kawasaki disease

_____ Physical examination

_____ ACE inhibitor

_____ Metabolic acidosis

_____ Basic metabolic panel

_____ Osmol gap

_____ Anorexia nervosa

_____ Drug overdose

_____ Arterial blood

_____ Arterial blood gas

_____ Blood gas

_____ Gastric lavage

_____ Blood cell

_____ Opioid overdose

_____ Palliative care

_____ Arginine vasopressin

_____ Liver failure

_____ Extracellular fluid

_____ Renal failure

Chapter 19. Emergency MEDICINE

Carbon monoxide

Chemical burn

Hydrocarbon

Chelation therapy

Lead poisoning

Carbon monoxide poisoning

EDTA

Oxygen therapy

Epidemiology

Cardiopulmonary resuscitation

Hypotension

Respiratory failure

Pathophysiology

Bacterial vaginosis

Chest compressions

Life support

Sexual abuse

Ventricular tachycardia

Medication

Ventricular fibrillation

Bradycardia

Foreign body

Supraventricular tachycardia

Tachycardia

Abdominal trauma

Endotracheal tube

Volume expander

Naloxone

Umbilical vein

Amniotic fluid

Bicarbonate

Bronchopulmonary dysplasia

Anaphylaxis	Anaphylaxis is defined as 'a serious allergic reaction that is rapid in onset and may cause death'. It typically results in a number of symptoms including an itchy rash, throat swelling, and low blood pressure. Common causes include insect bites, foods, and medications.
Opioid	An opioid is a psychoactive chemical that works by binding to opioid receptors, which are found principally in the central and peripheral nervous system and the gastrointestinal tract. The receptors in these organ systems mediate both the beneficial effects and the side effects of opioids. Opioids are among the world's oldest known drugs; the use of the opium poppy for its therapeutic benefits predates recorded history.
Pathogenesis	The pathogenesis of a disease is the mechanism by which the disease is caused. The term can also be used to describe the origin and development of the disease and whether it is acute, chronic or recurrent. The word comes from the Greek pathos, 'disease', and genesis, 'creation'.
Latex allergy	Latex allergy is a medical term encompassing a range of allergic reactions to natural rubber latex. Latex is known to cause 2 of the 4 types of hypersensitivity. Type I The most serious and rare form, type I is an immediate and potentially life-threatening reaction, not unlike the severe reaction some people have to bee stings.
Exercise-induced anaphylaxis	Exercise-induced anaphylaxis (EIA) is a syndrome in which the symptoms of anaphylaxis occur related to exercise. In some incidents, individuals experienced anaphylaxis only after combination exposure to a triggering agent and increased physical activity shortly after the ingestion of the triggering agent. In these individuals, either the exercise or ingestion of the triggering agent alone does not cause anaphylaxis.
Latex	Latex is the stable dispersion (emulsion) of polymer microparticles in an aqueous medium. Latexes may be natural or synthetic. Latex as found in nature is a milky sap-like fluid found in 10% of all flowering plants (angiosperms).
Risk factor	In epidemiology, a risk factor is a variable associated with an increased risk of disease or infection. Sometimes, determinant is also used, being a variable associated with either increased or decreased risk.

Chapter 19. Emergency MEDICINE

irway management	Airway management is the medical process of ensuring there is an open pathway between a patient's lungs and the outside world, as well as ensuring the lungs are safe from aspiration. Airway management is a primary consideration in cardiopulmonary resuscitation, anaesthesia, emergency medicine, intensive care medicine and first aid. Airway management is a high priority for clinical care.
ifferential diagnosis	A differential diagnosis is a systematic diagnostic method used to identify the presence of an entity where multiple alternatives are possible (and the process may be termed differential diagnostic procedure), and may also refer to any of the included candidate alternatives (which may also be termed candidate condition). This method is essentially a process of elimination, or at least, rendering of the probabilities of candidate conditions to negligible levels. In this sense, probabilities are, in fact, imaginative parameters in the mind or hardware of the diagnostician or system, while in reality the target (such as a patient) either has a condition or not with an actual probability of either 0 or 100%.
rognosis	Prognosis is a medical term to describe the likely outcome of an illness. When applied to large populations, prognostic estimates can be very accurate: for example the statement '45% of patients with severe septic shock will die within 28 days' can be made with some confidence, because previous research found that this proportion of patients died. However, it is much harder to translate this into a prognosis for an individual patient: additional information is needed to determine whether a patient belongs to the 45% who will succumb, or to the 55% who survive.
naphylactic shock	Anaphylactic shock, the most severe type of anaphylaxis, occurs when an allergic response triggers a quick release of large quantities of immunological mediators (histamines, prostaglandins, and leukotrienes) from mast cells, leading to systemic vasodilation (associated with a sudden drop in blood pressure) and edema of bronchial mucosa (resulting in bronchoconstriction and difficulty breathing.) Anaphylactic shock can lead to death in a matter of minutes if left untreated. Due in part to the variety of definitions, an estimated 1.24% to 16.8% of the population of the United States is considered 'at risk' for having an anaphylactic reaction if they are exposed to one or more allergens, especially penicillin and insect stings.
atient education	Patient education is the process by which health professionals and others impart information to patients that will alter their health behaviors or improve their health status. Education providers may include: physicians, pharmacists, registered dietitians, nurses, hospital discharge planners, medical social workers, psychologists, disease or disability advocacy groups, special interest groups, and pharmaceutical companies.

| Erythema multiforme | Erythema multiforme is a skin condition of unknown cause, possibly mediated by deposition of immune complex (mostly IgM) in the superficial microvasculature of the skin and oral mucous membrane that usually follows an infection or drug exposure. It is a common disorder, with peak incidence in the second and third decades of life.

The condition varies from a mild, self-limited rash (E. multiforme minor) to a severe, life-threatening form known as erythema multiforme major (or erythema multiforme majus) that also involves mucous membranes. |
| --- | --- |
| Herpes simplex | Herpes simplex is a viral disease from the herpesviridae family caused by both Herpes simplex virus type 1 (HSV-1) and type 2 (HSV-2). Infection with the herpes virus is categorized into one of several distinct disorders based on the site of infection. Oral herpes, the visible symptoms of which are colloquially called cold sores or fever blisters, is an infection of the face or mouth. |
| Mycoplasma pneumoniae | Mycoplasma pneumoniae is a very small bacterium in the class Mollicutes. It causes the disease Mycoplasma pneumonia, a form of bacterial pneumonia.

This species lacks a peptidoglycan cell wall, like all other Molicutes. |
| Toxic epidermal necrolysis | Toxic epidermal necrolysis is a rare, life-threatening dermatological condition that is usually induced by a reaction to medications. It is characterized by the detachment of the top layer of skin (the epidermis) from the lower layers of the skin (the dermis) all over the body.

There is broad agreement in medical literature that TEN can be considered a more severe form of Stevens-Johnson syndrome, and debate whether it falls on a spectrum of disease that includes erythema multiforme. |
| Etiological myth | Etiology is the study of causation, or origination.

The word is most commonly used in medical and philosophical theories, where it is used to refer to the study of why things occur, or even the reasons behind the way that things act, and is used in philosophy, physics, psychology, government, medicine, theology and biology in reference to the causes of various phenomena. An etiological myth is a myth intended to explain a name or create a mythic history for a place or family. |
| Koebner phenomenon | The Koebner phenomenon, refers to skin lesions appearing on lines of trauma. The Koebner phenomenon may result from either a linear exposure or irritation. Conditions demonstrating linear lesions after a linear exposure to a causative agent include: molluscum contagiosum, warts and toxicodendron dermatitis (a dermatitis caused by a genus of plants including poison ivy). |

Chapter 19. Emergency MEDICINE

rotonin syndrome	Serotonin syndrome is a potentially life-threatening adverse drug reaction that may occur following therapeutic drug use, inadvertent interactions between drugs, overdose of particular drugs, or the recreational use of certain drugs. Serotonin syndrome is not an idiosyncratic drug reaction; it is a predictable consequence of excess serotonergic activity at central nervous system (CNS) and peripheral serotonin receptors. For this reason, some experts strongly prefer the terms serotonin toxicity or serotonin toxidrome because these more accurately reflect the fact that it is a form of poisoning.
wasaki disease	Kawasaki disease also known as Kawasaki syndrome, lymph node syndrome and mucocutaneous lymph node syndrome, is an autoimmune disease in which the medium-sized blood vessels throughout the body become inflamed. It is largely seen in children under five years of age. It affects many organ systems, mainly those including the blood vessels, skin, mucous membranes and lymph nodes; however its rare but most serious effect is on the heart where it can cause fatal coronary artery aneurysms in untreated children.
ysical examination	A physical examination, medical examination, or clinical examination (more popularly known as a check-up or medical) is the process by which a doctor investigates the body of a patient for signs of disease. It generally follows the taking of the medical history -- an account of the symptoms as experienced by the patient. Together with the medical history, the physical examination aids in determining the correct diagnosis and devising the treatment plan.
CE inhibitor	ACE inhibitors are a group of drugs used primarily for the treatment of hypertension (high blood pressure) and congestive heart failure. Originally synthesized from compounds found in pit viper venom, they inhibit angiotensin-converting enzyme (ACE), a component of the blood pressure-regulating renin-angiotensin system.
etabolic acidosis	In medicine, metabolic acidosis is a condition that occurs when the body produces too much acid or when the kidneys are not removing enough acid from the body. If unchecked, metabolic acidosis leads to acidemia, i.e., blood pH is low (less than 7.35) due to increased production of hydrogen by the body or the inability of the body to form bicarbonate (HCO_3^-) in the kidney. Its causes are diverse, and its consequences can be serious, including coma and death.
sic metabolic panel	A basic metabolic panel is a set of seven or eight blood chemical tests. It is one of the most common lab tests ordered by health care providers. It provides key information that has a variety of applications in guiding the medical management of a patient.
smol gap	Osmol gap in medical science is the difference between measured serum osmolality and calculated serum osmolarity. There are a variety of ions and molecules dissolved in the serum.

Anorexia nervosa	The differential diagnoses of anorexia nervosa (AN) include various medical and psychological conditions which may be misdiagnosed as (AN), in some cases these conditions may be comorbid with anorexia nervosa (AN). The misdiagnosis of AN is not uncommon. In one instance a case of achalasia was misdiagnosed as AN and the patient spent two months confined to a psychiatric hospital.
Drug overdose	The term drug overdose describes the ingestion or application of a drug or other substance in quantities greater than are recommended or generally practiced. An overdose may result in a toxic state or death. The word 'overdose' implies that there is a common safe dosage and usage for the drug; therefore, the term is commonly only applied to drugs, not poisons, though even certain poisons are harmless at a low enough dosage.
Arterial blood	Arterial blood is the oxygenated blood in the circulatory system found in the lungs, the left chambers of the heart, and in the arteries. It is bright red in color, while venous blood is dark red in color (but looks purple through the opaque skin). It is the contralateral term to venous blood.
Arterial blood gas	An arterial blood gas is a blood test that is performed using blood from an artery. It involves puncturing an artery with a thin needle and syringe and drawing a small volume of blood. The most common puncture site is the radial artery at the wrist, but sometimes the femoral artery in the groin or other sites are used.
Blood gas	Blood gas is a term used to describe a laboratory test of blood where the purpose is primarily to measure ventilation and oxygenation. The source is generally noted by an added word to the beginning; arterial blood gases come from arteries, venous blood gases come from veins and capillary blood gases come from capillaries. •pH -- The acidity or basicity of the blood.•PaCO2 -- The partial pressure of carbon dioxide in the blood.•PaO2 -- The partial pressure of oxygen in the blood.•HCO3 -- The level of bicarbonate in the blood.•BE -- The base-excess of bicarbonate in the blood.Purposes for testing •Acidosis•Diabetic ketoacidosis•Lactic acidosis•Metabolic acidosis•Respiratory acidosis•Respiratory alkalosisAbnormal results Abnormal results may be due to lung, kidney, or metabolic diseases.
Gastric lavage	Gastric lavage, also commonly called stomach pumping or gastric irrigation, is the process of cleaning out the contents of the stomach. It has been used for over 200 years as a means of eliminating poisons from the stomach. Such devices are normally used on a person who has ingested a poison or overdosed on a drug or consumed too much alcohol.
Blood cell	A blood cell, is a cell produced by haematopoiesis and normally found in blood.

	In mammals, these fall into three general categories:•Red blood cells -- Erythrocytes•White blood cells -- Leukocytes•Platelets -- Thrombocytes. Together, these three kinds of blood cells add up to a total 45% of the blood tissue by volume, with the remaining 55% of the volume composed of plasma, the liquid component of blood. This volume percentage (e.g., 45%) of cells to total volume is called hematocrit, determined by centrifuge or flow cytometry.
pioid overdose	An opioid overdose is an acute condition due to excessive use of narcotics. It should not be confused with opioid dependency. Opiate overdose symptoms and signs include: decreased level of consciousness and pinpoint pupil except with meperidine (Demerol) where one sees dilated pupils, known as pinpoint pupils.
alliative care	Palliative care is an area of healthcare that focuses on relieving and preventing the suffering of patients. Unlike hospice care, palliative medicine is appropriate for patients in all disease stages, including those undergoing treatment for curable illnesses and those living with chronic diseases, as well as patients who are nearing the end of life. Palliative medicine utilizes a multidisciplinary approach to patient care, relying on input from physicians, pharmacists, nurses, chaplains, social workers, psychologists, and other allied health professionals in formulating a plan of care to relieve suffering in all areas of a patient's life.
rginine vasopressin	Arginine vasopressin, also known as vasopressin, argipressin or antidiuretic hormone (ADH), is a hormone found in most mammals, including humans. Vasopressin is a peptide hormone. It is derived from a preprohormone precursor that is synthesized in the hypothalamus and stored in vesicles at the posterior pituitary. Most of it is stored in the posterior pituitary to be released into the blood stream; however, some of it is also released directly into the brain.
iver failure	Liver failure is the inability of the liver to perform its normal synthetic and metabolic function as part of normal physiology. Two forms are recognised, acute and chronic. Acute liver failure is defined as 'the rapid development of hepatocellular dysfunction, specifically coagulopathy and mental status changes (encephalopathy) in a patient without known prior liver disease'.
xtracellular fluid	Extracellular fluid or extracellular fluid volume (ECFV) usually denotes all body fluid outside of cells. The remainder is called intracellular fluid.

Renal failure	Renal failure or kidney failure (formerly called renal insufficiency) describes a medical condition in which the kidneys fail to adequately filter toxins and waste products from the blood. The two forms are acute (acute kidney injury) and chronic (chronic kidney disease); a number of other diseases or health problems may cause either form of renal failure to occur.
	Renal failure is described as a decrease in glomerular filtration rate.
Carbon monoxide	Carbon monoxide also called carbonous oxide, is a colorless, odorless, and tasteless gas that is slightly lighter than air. It can be toxic to humans and animals when encountered in higher concentrations, although it is also produced in normal animal metabolism in low quantities, and is thought to have some normal biological functions. In the atmosphere however, it is short lived and spatially variable, since it combines with oxygen to form carbon dioxide and ozone.
Chemical burn	A chemical burn occurs when living tissue is exposed to a corrosive substance such as a strong acid or base. Chemical burns follow standard burn classification and may cause extensive tissue damage. The main types of irritant and/or corrosive products are: acids, bases, oxidizers, solvents, reducing agents and alkylants.
Hydrocarbon	In organic chemistry, a Hydrocarbon is an organic compound consisting entirely of hydrogen and carbon. Hydrocarbons from which one hydrogen atom has been removed are functional groups, called hydrocarbyls. Aromatic Hydrocarbons (arenes), alkanes, alkenes, cycloalkanes and alkyne-based compounds are different types of Hydrocarbons.
Chelation therapy	Chelation therapy is the administration of chelating agents to remove heavy metals from the body. Chelation therapy has a long history of use in clinical toxicology. Poison centers around the world are using this form of metal detoxification.
Lead poisoning	Lead poisoning is a medical condition caused by increased levels of the heavy metal lead in the body. Lead interferes with a variety of body processes and is toxic to many organs and tissues including the heart, bones, intestines, kidneys, and reproductive and nervous systems. It interferes with the development of the nervous system and is therefore particularly toxic to children, causing potentially permanent learning and behavior disorders.
Carbon monoxide poisoning	Carbon monoxide poisoning occurs after enough inhalation of carbon monoxide (CO). Carbon monoxide is a toxic gas, but, being colorless, odorless, tasteless, and initially non-irritating, it is very difficult for people to detect. Carbon monoxide is a product of incomplete combustion of organic matter due to insufficient oxygen supply to enable complete oxidation to carbon dioxide (CO_2).
EDTA	EDTA is a widely used initialism for the organic compound ethylenediaminetetraacetic acid . The conjugate base is named ethylenediaminetetraacetate.

Chapter 19. Emergency MEDICINE

Oxygen therapy	Oxygen therapy is the administration of oxygen as a medical intervention, which can be for a variety of purposes in both chronic and acute patient care. Oxygen is essential for cell metabolism, and in turn, tissue oxygenation is essential for all normal physiological functions. Room air only contains 21% oxygen, and increasing the fraction of oxygen in the breathing gas increases the amount of oxygen in the blood.
Epidemiology	Epidemiology is the study of the distribution and patterns of health-events, health-characteristics and their causes or influences in well-defined populations. It is the cornerstone method of public health research and practice, and helps inform policy decisions and evidence-based medicine by identifying risk factors for disease and targets for preventive medicine and public policies. Epidemiologists are involved in the design of studies, collection and statistical analysis of data, and interpretation and dissemination of results (including peer review and occasional systematic review).
Cardiopulmonary resuscitation	Cardiopulmonary resuscitation is an emergency procedure which is performed in an effort to manually preserve intact brain function until further measures are taken to restore spontaneous blood circulation and breathing in a person in cardiac arrest. It is indicated in those who are unresponsive with no breathing or abnormal breathing, for example agonal respirations. It may be performed both in and outside of a hospital.
Hypotension	In physiology and medicine, hypotension is abnormally low blood pressure, especially in the arteries of the systemic circulation. It is best understood as a physiological state, rather than a disease. It is often associated with shock, though not necessarily indicative of it.
Respiratory failure	The term respiratory failure, in medicine, is used to describe inadequate gas exchange by the respiratory system, with the result that arterial oxygen and/or carbon dioxide levels cannot be maintained within their normal ranges. A drop in blood oxygenation is known as hypoxemia; a rise in arterial carbon dioxide levels is called hypercapnia. The normal reference values are: oxygen PaO_2 greater than 80 mmHg (11 kPa), and carbon dioxide $PaCO_2$ less than 45 mmHg (6.0 kPa).
Pathophysiology	Pathophysiology sample values Pathophysiology is the study of the changes of normal mechanical, physical, and biochemical functions, either caused by a disease, or resulting from an abnormal syndrome. More formally, it is the branch of medicine which deals with any disturbances of body functions, caused by disease or prodromal symptoms. An alternative definition is 'the study of the biological and physical manifestations of disease as they correlate with the underlying abnormalities and physiological disturbances.'

Bacterial vaginosis	Bacterial vaginosis is the most common cause of vaginal infection. It is less commonly referred to as vaginal bacteriosis. It is not considered to be a sexually transmitted infection by the CDC. Bacterial vaginosis is not transmitted through sexual intercourse but is more common in women who are sexually active.
Chest compressions	Cardiopulmonary resuscitation (CPR) is an emergency procedure for people in cardiac arrest or, in some circumstances, respiratory arrest. CPR is performed in hospitals and in the community. CPR involves physical interventions to create artificial circulation through rhythmic pressing on the patient's chest to manually pump blood through the heart, called chest compressions, and usually also involves the rescuer exhaling into the patient (or using a device to simulate this) to inflate the lungs and pass oxygen in to the blood, called artificial respiration.
Life support	Life support in medicine is a broad term that applies to any therapy used to sustain a patient's life while they are critically ill or injured, as part of intensive-care medicine. There are many therapies and techniques that may be used by clinicians to achieve the goal of sustaining life. Some examples include:•Feeding tube•Total parenteral nutrition•Mechanical ventilation•Heart/Lung bypass•Urinary catheterization•Dialysis•Cardiopulmonary resuscitation•Defibrillation•Artificial pacemaker These techniques are applied most commonly in the Emergency Department, Intensive Care Unit and, Operating Rooms.
Sexual abuse	Sexual abuse is the forcing of undesired sexual behavior by one person upon another. When that force is immediate, of short duration, or infrequent, it is called sexual assault. The offender is referred to as a sexual abuser or (often pejoratively) molester. The term also covers any behavior by any adult towards a child to stimulate either the adult or child sexually. When the victim is younger than the age of consent, it is referred to as child sexual abuse.
Ventricular tachycardia	Ventricular tachycardia is a tachycardia, or fast heart rhythm, that originates in one of the ventricles of the heart. This is a potentially life-threatening arrhythmia because it may lead to ventricular fibrillation, asystole, and sudden death. Ventricular tachycardia can be classified based on its morphology:•Monomorphic ventricular tachycardia means that the appearance of all the beats match each other in each lead of a surface electrocardiogram (ECG).
Medication	A pharmaceutical drug, also referred to as medicine, medication or medicament, can be loosely defined as any chemical substance intended for use in the medical diagnosis, cure, treatment, or prevention of disease.

medications can be classified in various ways, such as by chemical properties, mode or route of administration, biological system affected, or therapeutic effects. An elaborate and widely used classification system is the Anatomical Therapeutic Chemical Classification System (ATC system).

ventricular fibrillation	Ventricular fibrillation is a condition in which there is uncoordinated contraction of the cardiac muscle of the ventricles in the heart, making them quiver rather than contract properly. Ventricular fibrillation is the most commonly identified arrythmia in cardiac arrest patients. While there is some activity, the lay person is usually unable to detect it by palpating (feeling) the major pulse points of the carotid and femoral arteries.
Bradycardia	Bradycardia, in the context of adult medicine, is the resting heart rate of under 60 beats per minute, though it is seldom symptomatic until the rate drops below 50 beats/min. It may cause cardiac arrest in some patients, because those with bradycardia may not be pumping enough oxygen to their hearts. It sometimes results in fainting, shortness of breath, and if severe enough, death.
Foreign body	A foreign body is any object originating outside the body. In machinery, it can mean any unwanted intruding object.
	Most references to foreign bodies involve propulsion through natural orifices into hollow organs.
Supraventricular tachycardia	Supraventricular tachycardia is a general term that refers to any rapid heart rhythm originating above the ventricular tissue. Supraventricular tachycardias can be contrasted to the potentially more dangerous ventricular tachycardias - rapid rhythms that originate within the ventricular tissue.
	Although technically an SVT can be due to any supraventricular cause, the term is often used by clinicians to refer to one specific cause of SVT, namely Paroxysmal supraventricular tachycardia.
Tachycardia	Tachycardia comes from the Greek words tachys (rapid or accelerated) and kardia (of the heart). Tachycardia typically refers to a heart rate that exceeds the normal range. A heart rate over 100 beats per minute is generally accepted as tachycardia.
Abdominal trauma	Abdominal trauma is an injury to the abdomen. It may be blunt or penetrating and may involve damage to the abdominal organs. Signs and symptoms include abdominal pain, tenderness, rigidity, and bruising of the external abdomen.
Endotracheal tube	An Endotracheal tube is used in general anaesthesia, intensive care and emergency medicine for airway management and mechanical ventilation.

The tube is inserted into a patient's trachea in order to ensure that the airway is not closed off and that air is able to reach the lungs. The Endotracheal tube is regarded as the most reliable available method for protecting a patient's airway.

Volume expander	A volume expander is a type of intravenous therapy that has the function of providing volume for the circulatory system. It may be used for fluid replacement.
	When blood is lost, the greatest immediate need is to stop further blood loss.

| Naloxone | Naloxone is an opioid antagonist drug developed by Sankyo in the 1960s. Naloxone is a drug used to counter the effects of opiate overdose, for example heroin or morphine overdose. Naloxone is specifically used to counteract life-threatening depression of the central nervous system and respiratory system. |

Umbilical vein	The umbilical vein is a vein present during fetal development that carries oxygenated blood from the placenta to the growing fetus.
	The blood pressure inside the umbilical vein is approximately 20 mmHg. Closure
	Within a week of birth, the infant's umbilical vein is completely obliterated and is replaced by a fibrous cord called the round ligament of the liver (also called ligamentum teres hepatis).

Amniotic fluid	Amniotic fluid is the nourishing and protecting liquid contained by the amniotic sac of a pregnant woman.
	From the very beginning of the formation of the extracoelomal cavity, amniotic fluid [AF] can be detected. This firstly water-like fluid originates from the maternal plasma, and passes through the fetal membranes by osmotic and hydrostatic forces.

Bicarbonate	
	In inorganic chemistry, Bicarbonate is an intermediate form in the deprotonation of carbonic acid. Its chemical formula is HCO_3^-.
	Bicarbonate serves a crucial biochemical role in the physiological pH buffering system.

| Bronchopulmonary dysplasia | Bronchopulmonary dysplasia is a chronic lung disorder that is most common among children who were born prematurely, with low birthweights and who received prolonged mechanical ventilation to treat respiratory distress syndrome. |

Chapter 19. Emergency MEDICINE

. _____ is a medical condition caused by increased levels of the heavy metal lead in the body. Lead interferes with a variety of body processes and is toxic to many organs and tissues including the heart, bones, intestines, kidneys, and reproductive and nervous systems. It interferes with the development of the nervous system and is therefore particularly toxic to children, causing potentially permanent learning and behavior disorders.

a. Mesothelioma
b. Metal fume fever
c. Nosocomial infection
d. Lead poisoning

. _____ is an opioid antagonist drug developed by Sankyo in the 1960s. _____ is a drug used to counter the effects of opiate overdose, for example heroin or morphine overdose. _____ is specifically used to counteract life-threatening depression of the central nervous system and respiratory system.

a. Nevirapine
b. Niclosamide
c. Naloxone
d. Nitrous oxide

. _____ also called carbonous oxide, is a colorless, odorless, and tasteless gas that is slightly lighter than air. It can be toxic to humans and animals when encountered in higher concentrations, although it is also produced in normal animal metabolism in low quantities, and is thought to have some normal biological functions. In the atmosphere however, it is short lived and spatially variable, since it combines with oxygen to form carbon dioxide and ozone.

a. Carbon monoxide
b. Certain safety factor
c. Chemical safety assessment
d. Chloracne

. _____, also commonly called stomach pumping or gastric irrigation, is the process of cleaning out the contents of the stomach. It has been used for over 200 years as a means of eliminating poisons from the stomach. Such devices are normally used on a person who has ingested a poison or overdosed on a drug or consumed too much alcohol.

a. Hemoperfusion
b. Mithridatism
c. Snake antivenom
d. Gastric lavage

. _____ is an area of healthcare that focuses on relieving and preventing the suffering of patients. Unlike hospice care, palliative medicine is appropriate for patients in all disease stages, including those undergoing treatment for curable illnesses and those living with chronic diseases, as well as patients who are nearing the end of life. Palliative medicine utilizes a multidisciplinary approach to patient care, relying on input from physicians, pharmacists, nurses, chaplains, social workers, psychologists, and other allied health professionals in formulating a plan of care to relieve suffering in all areas of a patient's life.

a. Palliative sedation

b. Patient safety

c. Russell and Fern de Greeff Hospice House

d. Palliative care

1. d
2. c
3. a
4. d
5. d

You can take the complete Chapter Practice Test

for Chapter 19. Emergency MEDICINE
on all key terms, persons, places, and concepts.

Online 99 Cents

http://www.epub219.49.13357.19.cram101.com/

Use www.Cram101.com for all your study needs

including Cram101's online interactive problem solving labs in

chemistry, statistics, mathematics, and more.

CHAPTER OUTLINE: KEY TERMS, PEOPLE, PLACES, CONCEPTS

	Psychosis
	Risk factor
	Protective factor
	Risk assessment
	Aggression
	Chemical restraint
	Atypical antipsychotic
	Delirium
	Side effect
	Terminal sedation
	Hallucination
	Thought disorder
	Bipolar disorder
	Mood disorder
	Schizophrenia
	Case study
	Dysthymic disorder
	Differential diagnosis
	Posttraumatic stress disorder

Trichomonas vaginalis

Bulimia nervosa

Reuptake inhibitor

Acute stress over reaction

Palliative care

Conversion disorder

Somatoform disorder

Prognosis

Anorexia nervosa

Eating disorder

Antipsychotic

Pharmacology

Stimulant

Bupropion

Maprotiline

Monoamine oxidase

Monoamine oxidase inhibitor

Lithium

Dosing

CHAPTER OUTLINE: KEY TERMS, PEOPLE, PLACES, CONCEPTS

Akathisia

Beta-adrenergic agonist

Extrapyramidal symptoms

Parkinsonism

Tardive dyskinesia

Malignant hyperthermia

Neuroleptic malignant syndrome

Serotonin syndrome

Dantrolene

Cystic fibrosis

Hemolytic-uremic syndrome

Ventricular tachycardia

Ventricular septal defect

Parenteral nutrition

Cardiovascular physiology

Pathophysiology

Kawasaki disease

Lupus erythematosus

Systemic lupus erythematosus

	Dermatomyositis
	Rocky Mountains
	High-mobility group
	Adrenal hyperplasia
	Turner syndrome
	Congenital adrenal hyperplasia
	Inguinal hernia
	Cardiopulmonary resuscitation
	Tachycardia

CHAPTER HIGHLIGHTS & NOTES: KEY TERMS, PEOPLE, PLACES, CONCEPTS

sychosis

Psychosis means abnormal condition of the mind, and is a generic psychiatric term for a mental state often described as involving a 'loss of contact with reality'. People suffering from psychosis are described as psychotic. Psychosis is given to the more severe forms of psychiatric disorder, during which hallucinations and delusions and impaired insight may occur.

isk factor

In epidemiology, a risk factor is a variable associated with an increased risk of disease or infection. Sometimes, determinant is also used, being a variable associated with either increased or decreased risk.

Risk factors or determinants are correlational and not necessarily causal, because correlation does not prove causation.

Protective factor	Protective factors are conditions or attributes (skills, strengths, resources, supports or coping strategies) in individuals, families, communities or the larger society that help people deal more effectively with stressful events and mitigate or eliminate risk in families and communities.
	Protective factors include:•Adoptive parents having an accurate understanding of their adopted children's pre-adoption medical and behavioral problems •Assistance of adoption professionals in the home of adopted children
	Some risks that adopted children are prone to :•Self-mutilation•Delinquency•Trouble with the law•Substance abuse•Thievery.
Risk assessment	Risk assessment is a step in a risk management procedure. Risk assessment is the determination of quantitative or qualitative value of risk related to a concrete situation and a recognized threat (also called hazard). Quantitative risk assessment requires calculations of two components of risk (R):, the magnitude of the potential loss (L), and the probability (p) that the loss will occur.
Aggression	Aggression, in its broadest sense, is behavior, or a disposition, that is forceful, hostile or attacking. It may occur either in retaliation or without provocation. In narrower definitions that are used in social sciences and behavioral sciences, aggression is an intention to cause harm or an act intended to increase relative social dominance.
Chemical restraint	A Chemical restraint is a form of medical restraint in which a drug is used to restrict the freedom or movement of a patient or in some cases to sedate a patient. These are used in emergency, acute, and psychiatric settings to control unruly patients who are interfering with their care or who are otherwise harmful to themselves or others in their vicinity.
	Drugs that are often used as Chemical restraints include benzodiazepine, lorazepam, and haloperidol.
Atypical antipsychotic	The atypical antipsychotics (AAP) (also known as second generation antipsychotics) are a group of antipsychotic tranquilizing drugs used to treat psychiatric conditions. Some atypical antipsychotics are FDA approved for use in the treatment of schizophrenia. Some carry FDA approved indications for acute mania, bipolar depression, psychotic agitation, bipolar maintenance, and other indications.
Delirium	Delirium is a common and severe neuropsychiatric syndrome with core features of acute onset and fluctuating course, attentional deficits and generalized severe disorganization of behavior. It typically involves other cognitive deficits, changes in arousal (hyperactive, hypoactive, or mixed), perceptual deficits, altered sleep-wake cycle, and psychotic features such as hallucinations and delusions.

Chapter 20. PSYCHIATRIC HOSPITALIZATION

e effect	In medicine, a side effect is an effect, whether therapeutic or adverse, that is secondary to the one intended; although the term is predominantly employed to describe adverse effects, it can also apply to beneficial, but unintended, consequences of the use of a drug. Occasionally, drugs are prescribed or procedures performed specifically for their side effects; in that case, said side effect ceases to be a side effect, and is now an intended effect. For instance, X-rays were historically (and are currently) used as an imaging technique; the discovery of their oncolytic capability led to their employ in radiotherapy (ablation of malignant tumors).
rminal sedation	In medicine, specifically in end-of-life care, terminal sedation is the palliative practice of relieving distress in a terminally ill person in the last hours or days of a dying patient's life, usually by means of a continuous intravenous or subcutaneous infusion of a sedative drug. This is a option of last resort for patients whose symptoms cannot be controlled by any other means. This should be differentiated from euthanasia as the goal of palliative sedation is to control symptoms through sedation but not shorten the patient's life, while in euthanasia the goal is to shorten life to relieve symptoms.
llucination	A hallucination, in the broadest sense of the word, is a perception in the absence of a stimulus. In a stricter sense, hallucinations are defined as perceptions in a conscious and awake state in the absence of external stimuli which have qualities of real perception, in that they are vivid, substantial, and located in external objective space. The latter definition distinguishes hallucinations from the related phenomena of dreaming, which does not involve wakefulness; illusion, which involves distorted or misinterpreted real perception; imagery, which does not mimic real perception and is under voluntary control; and pseudohallucination, which does not mimic real perception, but is not under voluntary control.
ought disorder	In psychiatry, thought disorder or formal thought disorder is a term used to describe incomprehensible language, either speech or writing, that is presumed to reflect thinking. There are different types. For example, language may be difficult to understand if it switches quickly from one unrelated idea to another (flight of ideas) or if it is long-winded and very delayed at reaching its goal (circumstantiality) or if words are inappropriately strung together resulting in gibberish (word salad).
polar disorder	Bipolar disorder, historically known as manic-depressive disorder, is a psychiatric diagnosis that describes a category of mood disorders defined by the presence of one or more episodes of abnormally elevated energy levels, cognition, and mood with or without one or more depressive episodes. The elevated moods are clinically referred to as mania or, if milder, hypomania. Individuals who experience manic episodes also commonly experience depressive episodes, or symptoms, or a mixed state in which features of both mania and depression are present at the same time.

Mood disorder	Mood disorder is the term designating a group of diagnoses in the Diagnostic and Statistical Manual of Mental Disorders (DSM IV TR) classification system where a disturbance in the person's mood is hypothesized to be the main underlying feature. The classification is known as mood (affective) disorders in ICD 10. English psychiatrist Henry Maudsley proposed an overarching category of affective disorder.
Schizophrenia	Schizophrenia is a mental disorder characterized by a breakdown of thought processes and by poor emotional responsiveness. It most commonly manifests itself as auditory hallucinations, paranoid or bizarre delusions, or disorganized speech and thinking, and it is accompanied by significant social or occupational dysfunction. The onset of symptoms typically occurs in young adulthood, with a global lifetime prevalence of about 0.3-0.7%.
Case study	A case study is an intensive analysis of an individual unit (e.g., a person, group, or event) stressing developmental factors in relation to context. The case study is common in social sciences and life sciences. Case studies may be descriptive or explanatory.
Dysthymic disorder	Dysthymic disorder is a chronic mood disorder that falls within the depression spectrum, the opposite of hyperthymia. It is considered a chronic depression, but with less severity than major depressive disorder. This disorder tends to be a chronic, long-lasting illness.
Differential diagnosis	A differential diagnosis is a systematic diagnostic method used to identify the presence of an entity where multiple alternatives are possible (and the process may be termed differential diagnostic procedure), and may also refer to any of the included candidate alternatives (which may also be termed candidate condition). This method is essentially a process of elimination, or at least, rendering of the probabilities of candidate conditions to negligible levels. In this sense, probabilities are, in fact, imaginative parameters in the mind or hardware of the diagnostician or system, while in reality the target (such as a patient) either has a condition or not with an actual probability of either 0 or 100%.
Posttraumatic stress disorder	Posttraumatic stress disorder is a severe anxiety disorder that can develop after exposure to any event that results in psychological trauma. This event may involve the threat of death to oneself or to someone else, or to one's own or someone else's physical, sexual, or psychological integrity, overwhelming the individual's ability to cope. As an effect of psychological trauma, PTSD is less frequent and more enduring than the more commonly seen acute stress response.
Trichomonas vaginalis	Trichomonas vaginalis is an anaerobic, flagellated protozoan, a form of microorganism. The parasitic microorganism is the causative agent of trichomoniasis, and is the most common pathogenic protozoan infection of humans in industrialized countries.

Chapter 20. PSYCHIATRIC HOSPITALIZATION

Bulimia nervosa	Bulimia nervosa is an eating disorder characterized by binge eating and purging or consuming a large amount of food in a short amount of time, followed by an attempt to rid oneself of the food consumed, usually by purging (vomiting) and/or by laxative, diuretics or excessive exercise. Bulimia nervosa is considered to be less life threatening than anorexia, however the occurrence of bulimia nervosa is higher. Bulimia nervosa is nine times more likely to occur in women than men (Barker 2003).
reuptake inhibitor	A reuptake inhibitor also known as a transporter blocker, is a drug that inhibits the plasmalemmal transporter-mediated reuptake of a neurotransmitter from the synapse into the pre-synaptic neuron, leading to an increase in the extracellular concentrations of the neurotransmitter and therefore an increase in neurotransmission. Various drugs utilize reuptake inhibition to exert their psychological and physiological effects, including many antidepressants and psychostimulants. Most known reuptake inhibitors affect the monoamine neurotransmitters serotonin, norepinephrine (and epinephrine), and dopamine.
Acute stress over reaction	Acute stress over reaction is a psychological condition arising in response to a terrifying event. It should not be confused with the unrelated circulatory condition of shock. 'Acute stress response' was first described by Walter Cannon in the 1920s as a theory that animals react to threats with a general discharge of the sympathetic nervous system.
Palliative care	Palliative care is an area of healthcare that focuses on relieving and preventing the suffering of patients. Unlike hospice care, palliative medicine is appropriate for patients in all disease stages, including those undergoing treatment for curable illnesses and those living with chronic diseases, as well as patients who are nearing the end of life. Palliative medicine utilizes a multidisciplinary approach to patient care, relying on input from physicians, pharmacists, nurses, chaplains, social workers, psychologists, and other allied health professionals in formulating a plan of care to relieve suffering in all areas of a patient's life.
Conversion disorder	Conversion disorder is where patients suffer apparently neurological symptoms, such as numbness, blindness, paralysis, or fits, but without a neurological cause. It is thought that these problems arise in response to difficulties in the patient's life, and conversion is considered a psychiatric disorder in the Diagnostic and Statistical Manual of Mental Disorders fourth edition (DSM-IV). Formerly known as 'hysteria', the disorder has arguably been known for millennia, though it came to greatest prominence at the end of the 19th century, when the neurologists Jean-Martin Charcot and Sigmund Freud and psychiatrist Pierre Janet focused their studies on the subject.

Somatoform disorder	In psychology, a somatoform disorder is a mental disorder characterized by physical symptoms that suggest physical illness or injury - symptoms that cannot be explained fully by a general medical condition, direct effect of a substance, or attributable to another mental disorder (e.g. panic disorder). The symptoms that result from a somatoform disorder are due to mental factors. In people who have a somatoform disorder, medical test results are either normal or do not explain the person's symptoms.
Prognosis	Prognosis is a medical term to describe the likely outcome of an illness. When applied to large populations, prognostic estimates can be very accurate: for example the statement '45% of patients with severe septic shock will die within 28 days' can be made with some confidence, because previous research found that this proportion of patients died. However, it is much harder to translate this into a prognosis for an individual patient: additional information is needed to determine whether a patient belongs to the 45% who will succumb, or to the 55% who survive.
Anorexia nervosa	The differential diagnoses of anorexia nervosa (AN) include various medical and psychological conditions which may be misdiagnosed as (AN), in some cases these conditions may be comorbid with anorexia nervosa (AN). The misdiagnosis of AN is not uncommon. In one instance a case of achalasia was misdiagnosed as AN and the patient spent two months confined to a psychiatric hospital.
Eating disorder	Eating disorders refer to a group of conditions defined by abnormal eating habits that may involve either insufficient or excessive food intake to the detriment of an individual's physical and mental health. Bulimia nervosa, anorexia nervosa, and binge eating disorder are the most common specific forms in the United Kingdom. Though primarily thought of as affecting females (an estimated 5-10 million being affected in the U.K)., eating disorders affect males as well Template:An estimated 10 - 15% of people with eating disorders are males (Gorgan, 1999).
Antipsychotic	An antipsychotic is a tranquilizing psychiatric medication primarily used to manage psychosis (including delusions or hallucinations, as well as disordered thought), particularly in schizophrenia and bipolar disorder, and is increasingly being used in the management of non-psychotic disorders. A first generation of antipsychotics, known as typical antipsychotics, was discovered in the 1950s. Most of the drugs in the second generation, known as atypical antipsychotics, have been developed more recently, although the first atypical antipsychotic, clozapine, was discovered in the 1950s and introduced clinically in the 1970s.
Pharmacology	Pharmacology is the branch of medicine and biology concerned with the study of drug action, where a drug can be broadly defined as any man-made, natural, or endogenous (within the cell) molecule which exerts a biochemical and/or physiological effect on the cell, tissue, organ, or organism. More specifically, it is the study of the interactions that occur between a living organism and chemicals that affect normal or abnormal biochemical function.

mulant	Stimulants are psychoactive drugs which induce temporary improvements in either mental or physical function or both. Examples of these kinds of effects may include enhanced alertness, wakefulness, and locomotion, among others. Due to their effects typically having an 'up' quality to them, stimulants are also occasionally referred to as 'uppers'.
propion	Bupropion is an atypical antidepressant and smoking cessation aid. The drug is a non-tricyclic antidepressant and differs from most commonly prescribed antidepressants such as SSRIs, as its primary pharmacological action is thought to be norepinephrine-dopamine reuptake inhibition. It binds selectively to the dopamine transporter, but its behavioural effects have often been attributed to its inhibition of norepinephrine reuptake.
protiline	Maprotiline is a tetracyclic antidepressant (TeCA). It is a strong norepinephrine reuptake inhibitor with only weak effects on serotonin and dopamine reuptake. It exerts blocking effects at the following postsynaptic receptors:•Strong : H_1•Moderate : $5\text{-}HT_2$, $alpha_1$•Weak : D_2, mACh The pharmacologic profile of Maprotiline explains its antidepressant, sedative, anxiolytic, and sympathomimetic activities.
noamine oxidase	L-Monoamine oxidases (MAO) (EC 1.4.3.4) are a family of enzymes that catalyze the oxidation of monoamines. They are found bound to the outer membrane of mitochondria in most cell types in the body. The enzyme was originally discovered by Mary Bernheim (née Hare) in the liver and was named tyramine oxidase.
noamine oxidase ibitor	Monoamine oxidase inhibitors (MAOIs) are a class of antidepressant drugs prescribed for the treatment of depression. They are particularly effective in treating atypical depression. Because of potentially lethal dietary and drug interactions, monoamine oxidase inhibitors have historically been reserved as a last line of treatment, used only when other classes of antidepressant drugs (for example selective serotonin reuptake inhibitors and tricyclic antidepressants) have failed.
hium	Lithium is a soft, silver-white metal that belongs to the alkali metal group of chemical elements. It is represented by the symbol Li, and it has the atomic number three. Under standard conditions it is the lightest metal and the least dense solid element.
sing	Dosing generally applies to feeding chemicals or medicines in small quantities into a process fluid or to a living being at intervals or to atmosphere at intervals to give sufficient time for the chemical or medicine to react or show the results.

In the case of human beings or animals the word dose is generally used but in the case of inanimate objects the word dosing is used. In engineering

The word dosing is very commonly used by engineers in thermal power stations, in water treatment or in any industry where steam is being generated.

Akathisia	Akathisia, is a syndrome characterized by unpleasant sensations of inner restlessness that manifests itself with an inability to sit still or remain motionless . It can be a side effect of medications, mainly neuroleptic antipsychotics especially the phenothiazines (such as perphenazine and chlorpromazine), thioxanthenes (such as flupenthixol and zuclopenthixol) and butyrophenones (such as haloperidol (Haldol)), piperazines (such as ziprasidone), antiemetics (such as metoclopramide and promethazine), and stimulants (such as antidepressants and amphetamines). Akathisia can also, to a lesser extent, be caused by Parkinson's disease and related syndromes, and likely other neurological diseases.
Beta-adrenergic agonist	Beta-adrenergic agonists are adrenergic agonists which act upon the beta receptors. β_1 agonists β_1 agonists: stimulates adenylyl cyclase activity; opening of calcium channel. (cardiac stimulants; used to treat cardiogenic shock, acute heart failure, bradyarrhythmias).
Extrapyramidal symptoms	The extrapyramidal system can be affected in a number of ways, which are revealed in a range of extrapyramidal symptoms also known as extrapyramidal side-effects (EPSE), such as akinesia (inability to initiate movement) and akathisia (inability to remain motionless). Extrapyramidal symptoms are various movement disorders such as acute dystonic reactions, pseudoparkinsonism, or akathisia suffered as a result of taking dopamine antagonists, usually antipsychotic (neuroleptic) drugs, which are often used to control psychosis. The Simpson-Angus Scale (SAS) and the Barnes Akathisia Rating Scale (BARS) are used to measure extrapyramidal symptoms.
Parkinsonism	Parkinsonism is a neurological syndrome characterized by tremor, hypokinesia, rigidity, and postural instability. The underlying causes of parkinsonism are numerous, and diagnosis can be complex. While the neurodegenerative condition Parkinson's disease (PD) is the most common cause of parkinsonism, a wide-range of other etiologies may lead to a similar set of symptoms, including some toxins, a few metabolic diseases, and a handful of non-PD neurological conditions.

Chapter 20. PSYCHIATRIC HOSPITALIZATION

Tardive dyskinesia	Tardive dyskinesia is a difficult-to-treat form of dyskinesia, a disorder resulting in involuntary, repetitive body movements. In this form of dyskinesia, the involuntary movements are tardive, meaning they have a slow or belated onset. This neurological disorder frequently appears after long-term or high-dose use of antipsychotic drugs, or in children and infants as a side effect from usage of drugs for gastrointestinal disorders.
Malignant hyperthermia	Malignant hyperthermia or malignant hyperpyrexia is a rare life-threatening condition that is usually triggered by exposure to certain drugs used for general anesthesia; specifically, the volatile anesthetic agents and the neuromuscular blocking agent, succinylcholine. In susceptible individuals, these drugs can induce a drastic and uncontrolled increase in skeletal muscle oxidative metabolism, which overwhelms the body's capacity to supply oxygen, remove carbon dioxide, and regulate body temperature, eventually leading to circulatory collapse and death if not treated quickly. Susceptibility to MH is often inherited as an autosomal dominant disorder, for which there are at least 6 genetic loci of interest, most prominently the ryanodine receptor gene (RYR1).
Neuroleptic malignant syndrome	Neuroleptic malignant syndrome is a life-threatening neurological disorder most often caused by an adverse reaction to neuroleptic or antipsychotic drugs. NMS typically consists of muscle rigidity, fever, autonomic instability, and cognitive changes such as delirium, and is associated with elevated plasma creatine phosphokinase. The incidence of neuroleptic malignant syndrome has decreased since it was first described, due to changes in prescribing habits, but NMS is still a potential danger to patients being treated with antipsychotic medication.
Serotonin syndrome	Serotonin syndrome is a potentially life-threatening adverse drug reaction that may occur following therapeutic drug use, inadvertent interactions between drugs, overdose of particular drugs, or the recreational use of certain drugs. Serotonin syndrome is not an idiosyncratic drug reaction; it is a predictable consequence of excess serotonergic activity at central nervous system (CNS) and peripheral serotonin receptors. For this reason, some experts strongly prefer the terms serotonin toxicity or serotonin toxidrome because these more accurately reflect the fact that it is a form of poisoning.
Dantrolene	Dantrolene sodium is a muscle relaxant that acts by abolishing excitation-contraction coupling in muscle cells, probably by action on the ryanodine receptor. It is the only specific and effective treatment for malignant hyperthermia, a rare, life-threatening disorder triggered by general anesthesia. It is also used in the management of neuroleptic malignant syndrome, muscle spasticity (e.g. after strokes, in paraplegia, cerebral palsy, or patients with multiple sclerosis), 3,4-methylenedioxy methylamphetamine ('ecstasy') intoxication, serotonin syndrome, and 2,4-dinitrophenol poisoning.

Cystic fibrosis	Cystic fibrosis is an autosomal recessive genetic disorder affecting most critically the lungs, and also the pancreas, liver, and intestine. It is characterized by abnormal transport of chloride and sodium across an epithelium, leading to thick, viscous secretions.

The name cystic fibrosis refers to the characteristic scarring (fibrosis) and cyst formation within the pancreas, first recognized in the 1930s. |
| Hemolytic-uremic syndrome | Hemolytic-uremic syndrome , abbreviated HUS, is a disease characterized by hemolytic anemia (anemia caused by destruction of red blood cells), acute kidney failure (uremia) and a low platelet count (thrombocytopenia). It predominantly, but not exclusively, affects children. Most cases are preceded by an episode of infectious, sometimes bloody, diarrhea caused by E. coli O157:H7, which is acquired as a foodborne illness or from a contaminated water supply. |
| Ventricular tachycardia | Ventricular tachycardia is a tachycardia, or fast heart rhythm, that originates in one of the ventricles of the heart. This is a potentially life-threatening arrhythmia because it may lead to ventricular fibrillation, asystole, and sudden death.

Ventricular tachycardia can be classified based on its morphology:•Monomorphic ventricular tachycardia means that the appearance of all the beats match each other in each lead of a surface electrocardiogram (ECG). |
| Ventricular septal defect | A ventricular septal defect is a defect in the ventricular septum, the wall dividing the left and right ventricles of the heart.

The ventricular septum consists of an inferior muscular and superior membranous portion and is extensively innervated with conducting cardiomyocytes.

The membranous portion, which is close to the atrioventricular node, is most commonly affected in adults and older children in the United States. |
| Parenteral nutrition | Parenteral nutrition is feeding a person intravenously, bypassing the usual process of eating and digestion. The person receives nutritional formulae that contain nutrients such as glucose, amino acids, lipids and added vitamins and dietary minerals. It is called total parenteral nutrition or total nutrient admixture (TNA) when no food is given by other routes. |
| Cardiovascular physiology | Cardiovascular physiology is the study of the circulatory system. More specifically, it addresses the physiology of the heart ('cardio') and blood vessels ('vascular').

These subjects are sometimes addressed separately, under the names cardiac physiology and circulatory physiology. |

Chapter 20. PSYCHIATRIC HOSPITALIZATION

thophysiology	Pathophysiology sample values
	Pathophysiology is the study of the changes of normal mechanical, physical, and biochemical functions, either caused by a disease, or resulting from an abnormal syndrome. More formally, it is the branch of medicine which deals with any disturbances of body functions, caused by disease or prodromal symptoms.
	An alternative definition is 'the study of the biological and physical manifestations of disease as they correlate with the underlying abnormalities and physiological disturbances.'
	The study of pathology and the study of pathophysiology often involves substantial overlap in diseases and processes, but pathology emphasizes direct observations, while pathophysiology emphasizes quantifiable measurements.
wasaki disease	Kawasaki disease also known as Kawasaki syndrome, lymph node syndrome and mucocutaneous lymph node syndrome, is an autoimmune disease in which the medium-sized blood vessels throughout the body become inflamed. It is largely seen in children under five years of age. It affects many organ systems, mainly those including the blood vessels, skin, mucous membranes and lymph nodes; however its rare but most serious effect is on the heart where it can cause fatal coronary artery aneurysms in untreated children.
pus erythematosus	Lupus erythematosus is a category for a collection of diseases with similar underlying problems with immunity (autoimmune disease). Symptoms of these diseases can affect many different body systems, including joints, skin, kidneys, blood cells, heart, and lungs. Four main types of lupus exist: systemic lupus erythematosus, discoid lupus erythematosus, drug-induced lupus erythematosus, and neonatal lupus erythematosus.
stemic lupus rthematosus	Systemic lupus erythematosus often abbreviated to SLE or lupus, is a systemic autoimmune disease that can affect any part of the body. As occurs in other autoimmune diseases, the immune system attacks the body's cells and tissue, resulting in inflammation and tissue damage. It is a Type III hypersensitivity reaction caused by antibody-immune complex formation.
rmatomyositis	Dermatomyositis is a connective-tissue disease related to polymyositis (PM) that is characterized by inflammation of the muscles and the skin. While DM most frequently affects the skin and muscles, it is a systemic disorder that may also affect the joints, the esophagus, the lungs, and, less commonly, the heart.
	The cause is unknown, but it may result from either a viral infection or an autoimmune reaction.
cky Mountains	The Rocky Mountains are a major mountain range in western North America.

	The North American Rocky Mountains stretch more than 4,800 kilometres (2,980 mi) from the northernmost part of British Columbia, in western Canada, to New Mexico, in the southwestern United States. The range's highest peak is Mount Elbert located in Colorado at 14,440 feet (4,401 m) above sea level. Though part of North America's Pacific Cordillera, the Rockies are distinct from the Pacific Coast Ranges or the Pacific Mountain System (as it is known in the United States), which are located directly adjacent to the Pacific coast.
High-mobility group	High-Mobility Group is a group of chromosomal proteins that help with transcription, replication, recombination, and DNA repair. The proteins are subdivided into 3 superfamilies each containing a characteristic functional domain:•A - contains an AT-hook domain •A1•A2•B - contains a -box domain •B1•B2•B3•B4•N - contains a nucleosomal binding domain domain •N1•N2•N3•N4•Sex-Determining Region Y Protein•TCF Transcription Factors •Lymphoid enhancer-binding factor 1•T Cell Transcription Factor 1 Proteins containing any of these embedded in their sequence are known as motif proteins. -box proteins are found in a variety of eukaryotic organisms.
Adrenal hyperplasia	Congenital adrenal hyperplasia refers to any of several autosomal recessive diseases resulting from mutations of genes for enzymes mediating the biochemical steps of production of cortisol from cholesterol by the adrenal glands (steroidogenesis). Most of these conditions involve excessive or deficient production of sex steroids and can alter development of primary or secondary sex characteristics in some affected infants, children, or adults. Associated conditions The symptoms of CAH vary depending upon the form of CAH and the gender of the patient.
Turner syndrome	Turner syndrome, of which monosomy X (absence of an entire sex chromosome, the Barr body) is most common. It is a chromosomal abnormality in which all or part of one of the sex chromosomes is absent (unaffected humans have 46 chromosomes, of which two are sex chromosomes). Typical females have two X chromosomes, but in Turner syndrome, one of those sex chromosomes is missing or has other abnormalities.
Congenital adrenal hyperplasia	Congenital adrenal hyperplasia refers to any of several autosomal recessive diseases resulting from mutations of genes for enzymes mediating the biochemical steps of production of cortisol from cholesterol by the adrenal glands (steroidogenesis).

Most of these conditions involve excessive or deficient production of sex steroids and can alter development of primary or secondary sex characteristics in some affected infants, children, or adults. Associated conditions

The symptoms of CAH vary depending upon the form of CAH and the gender of the patient.

guinal hernia

An inguinal hernia is a protrusion of abdominal-cavity contents through the inguinal canal. They are very common (lifetime risk 27% for men, 3% for women), and their repair is one of the most frequently performed surgical operations.

There are two types of inguinal hernia, direct and indirect, which are defined by their relationship to the inferior epigastric vessels.

ardiopulmonary suscitation

Cardiopulmonary resuscitation is an emergency procedure which is performed in an effort to manually preserve intact brain function until further measures are taken to restore spontaneous blood circulation and breathing in a person in cardiac arrest. It is indicated in those who are unresponsive with no breathing or abnormal breathing, for example agonal respirations. It may be performed both in and outside of a hospital.

chycardia

Tachycardia comes from the Greek words tachys (rapid or accelerated) and kardia (of the heart). Tachycardia typically refers to a heart rate that exceeds the normal range. A heart rate over 100 beats per minute is generally accepted as tachycardia.

1. _____s are psychoactive drugs which induce temporary improvements in either mental or physical function or both. Examples of these kinds of effects may include enhanced alertness, wakefulness, and locomotion, among others. Due to their effects typically having an 'up' quality to them, _____s are also occasionally referred to as 'uppers'.

   a. Stimulant
   b. Benzodiazepine
   c. Benzodiazepine dependence
   d. Benzodiazepine withdrawal syndrome

2. _____ is a medical term to describe the likely outcome of an illness. When applied to large populations, prognostic estimates can be very accurate: for example the statement '45% of patients with severe septic shock will die within 28 days' can be made with some confidence, because previous research found that this proportion of patients died. However, it is much harder to translate this into a _____ for an individual patient: additional information is needed to determine whether a patient belongs to the 45% who will succumb, or to the 55% who survive.

   a. differential diagnosis
   b. Prognosis
   c. History of the present illness
   d. Gliosis

3. _____ sodium is a muscle relaxant that acts by abolishing excitation-contraction coupling in muscle cells, probably by action on the ryanodine receptor. It is the only specific and effective treatment for malignant hyperthermia, a rare, life-threatening disorder triggered by general anesthesia. It is also used in the management of neuroleptic malignant syndrome, muscle spasticity (e.g. after strokes, in paraplegia, cerebral palsy, or patients with multiple sclerosis), 3,4-methylenedioxy methylamphetamine ('ecstasy') intoxication, serotonin syndrome, and 2,4-dinitrophenol poisoning.

   a. Bacteriophage
   b. Course
   c. Dantrolene
   d. Degeneration

4. _____ is an eating disorder characterized by binge eating and purging or consuming a large amount of food in a short amount of time, followed by an attempt to rid oneself of the food consumed, usually by purging (vomiting) and/or by laxative, diuretics or excessive exercise. _____ is considered to be less life threatening than anorexia, however the occurrence of _____ is higher. _____ is nine times more likely to occur in women than men (Barker 2003).

   a. Bulimia nervosa
   b. Childhood disintegrative disorder
   c. Clinical formulation
   d. Cluttering

5. . In medicine, a _____ is an effect, whether therapeutic or adverse, that is secondary to the one intended; although the term is predominantly employed to describe adverse effects, it can also apply to beneficial, but unintended,

consequences of the use of a drug.

Chapter 20. PSYCHIATRIC HOSPITALIZATION

Occasionally, drugs are prescribed or procedures performed specifically for their _____s; in that case, said _____ ceases to be a _____, and is now an intended effect. For instance, X-rays were historically (and are currently) used as an imaging technique; the discovery of their oncolytic capability led to their employ in radiotherapy (ablation of malignant tumors).

a. Mechanism of action
b. Side effect
c. clinical pharmacology
d. combination therapy

1. a
2. b
3. c
4. a
5. b

You can take the complete Chapter Practice Test

for Chapter 20. PSYCHIATRIC HOSPITALIZATION
on all key terms, persons, places, and concepts.

Online 99 Cents

http://www.epub219.49.13357.20.cram101.com/

Use www.Cram101.com for all your study needs

including Cram101's online interactive problem solving labs in

chemistry, statistics, mathematics, and more.

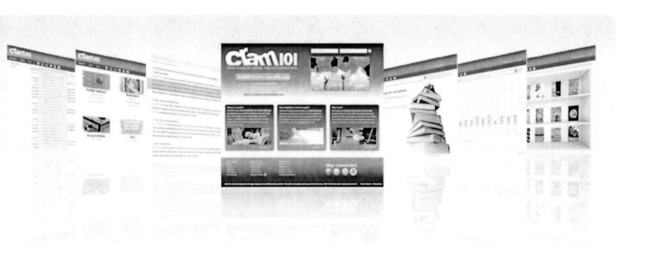